SOFT TISSUE PAIN AND DISABILITY

SOFT TISSUE PAIN AND DISABILITY
EDITION 3

RENE CAILLIET, MD

Professor Emeritus and Chairman
Department of Physical Medicine and Rehabilitation
University of Southern California
School of Medicine
Los Angeles, California

 F. A. DAVIS COMPANY • Philadelphia

F. A. Davis Company
1915 Arch Street
Philadelphia, PA 19103

Printed in the United States of America

Last digit indicates print number: 10 9 8 7 6 5 4 3 2

Publisher, Nursing: Robert G. Martone
Production Editor: Glenn L. Fechner
Cover Designer: Louis J. Forgione

As new scientific information becomes available through basic and clinical research, recommended treatments and drug therapies undergo changes. The author and publisher have done everything possible to make this book accurate, up to date, and in accord with accepted standards at the time of publication. The authors, editors, and publisher are not responsible for errors or omissions or for consequences from application of the book, and make no warranty, expressed or implied, in regard to the contents of the book. Any practice described in this book should be applied by the reader in accordance with professional standards of care used in regard to the unique circumstances that may apply in each situation. The reader is advised always to check product information (package inserts) for changes and new information regarding dose and contraindications before administering any drug. Caution is especially urged when using new or infrequently ordered drugs.

Library of Congress Cataloging-in-Publication Data

Cailliet, Rene.
 Soft tissue pain and disability / Rene Cailliet; illustrations by
R. Cailliet.—Ed. 3.
  p. cm.
 Includes bibliographical references and index.
 ISBN 0-8036-0110-7
 1. Myalgia. 2. Musculoskeletal system—Wounds and injuries.
3. Overuse injuries. 4. Pain. I. Title.
 [DNLM: 1. Soft Tissue Injuries. 2. Collagen Diseases.
3. Connective Tissue—injuries. 4. Musculoskeletal System—
injuries. 5. Pain.   WD 375 C134s 1996]
RC925.5.C24 1996
616'.0472—dc20
DNLM/DLC
for Library of Congress   95-39159
                                                                CIP

Preface

This third edition has been totally rewritten to reflect the latest thinking in assessment, diagnosis, and treatment of painful and disabling conditions. Because the first two editions were so well received it became apparent that the practitioner, chiropractor, physical therapist, occupational therapist, athletic trainer, occupational physician, attorney, and worker's compensation adviser have recognized that *soft tissue injuries* play a major role in daily practice.

Pain is an important consideration in treating disabilities and impairment today. The focus of daily care has addressed pain as the predominant concern with regard to function. This is, however, changing with the advent of athletic injuries where quicker return to play has become the goal. Return to work has also been become the primary goal of care for those injured industrially.

The tremendous cost of injury to society has been detailed in the press. In the halls of congress, debate has focused the attention of ordinary people in the country as well as that of medical professionals.

In considering the scope of the national problem, the U.S. Department of Health and Human Services in 1992[1] emphasized the role of musculoskeletal injuries. In 1993, the National Institute for Occupational Safety and Health (NIOSH) developed and published a *Suggested List of Ten Leading Work Related Diseases and Injuries* with most, if not all, related to the soft tissue.

The following statistics were offered:

(1) Musculoskeletal injuries were the leading cause of disability during a person's working years, afflicting 19 million persons, (see no. 5) with nearly half the work force affected at some time during their working lives.

(2) Musculoskeletal injuries were ranked first among health problems affecting the quality of life.

(3) The cost of musculoskeletal injuries based on earnings and worker's compensation payments exceeded that of any single health disorder.

(4) Musculoskeletal injuries accounted for a third of annual worker's compensation claims paid out.

(5) Musculoskeletal injuries are expected to increase, with larger numbers of older workers performing manual labor in certain industries.

Though cost estimates vary greatly, most authorities believe the medical workers' compensation costs are believed to range from **$20** to **$40 BILLION** annually in the United States. The value of the lost quality of life cannot be estimated.

Repetitive stress injuries, especially involving soft tissues, are rapidly increasing in frequency and severity, at exhorbitant cost to society in terms of discomfort, disability, and medical and compensation expense. *The Wall Street Journal* (July 14, 1994) wrote a lead article entitled "Out of Hand: Is It an Epidemic or Largely a Fad? The Debate Over Repetitive Stress Injury Heats Up." The article claimed it was ". . . a multibillion dollar question."

The article stated that repetitive stress disorders (RSD) or cumulative trauma disorders (CTD) largely afflicted office workers who used personal computers but others also suffer: 1396 out of 10,000 workers in a meat packing plant and 44 out of 10,000 employees of a newspaper. The author proceeded with the statement ". . . preventing RSD is largely a matter of simple ergonomics, the adjustment of job tasks and work stations. The jury is out on how much certain ergonomic measures help . . . common remedies such as splints and wrist rests may actually make matters worse."

When these medical conditions cause the Wall Street Journal to ponder the severity of soft tissue problems initiated or aggravated by RSD, professional clinical studies are justified.

Soft tissue pain and impairment are very justifiably being researched and the study results are implemented. This text attempts a complete update of recent etiologies, mechanisms, and management of these injuries. Pain has been analyzed by me in other places[2] but impairment and resultant disability are the focus of this book.

RENE CAILLIET, MD

REFERENCES

1. US Department of Health and Human Services, Public Health Service NIOSH 1991 Conference Summary, November 1992.
2. Cailliet, R: Pain: Mechanisms and Management, ed 1. FA Davis, Philadelphia, 1993.

Contents

Illustrations .... **xv**

Chapter 1   Concepts of Pain and Impairment **1**

Connective Tissue 1
    Dense Connective Tissue 3
    Collagen 3
    Tendons 6
    Muscle 6
Metabolic Effects of Inactivity and Injury 9

**Chapter 2   Pain: Mechanisms, Assessment,
              and Management** **14**

Neuroanatomic Basis 14
Modulation 27
Role of the Cerebral Cortex in Pain Perception 32
Chronic Pain Mechanisms 34
Pain Mediated Through the Sympathetic
    Nervous System 37
Hyperalgesia in Reflex Sympathetic Dystrophy 46
Chronic Fatigue Syndrome 52

**Chapter 3   The Muscle Component of Soft Tissue
              Function and Pain** **60**

Spindle Cell: Gamma System 60
Fibromyalgia Syndromes 72
    Pathophysiology 74
    Management of Fibromyalgia Syndromes 77

Chapter 4   Treatment Modalities **84**

Pharmacology   84
Physical Intervention   87
    Modalities   88
    Modalities for Elongation   91
Exercise   91
Manual Therapy   94
Analgesic Nerve Blocks   95

Chapter 5   Low Back Pain **101**

Functional Anatomy   103
    Functional Unit   103
    Zygapophyseal Joints   105
    Neural Tissues Within the Functional Unit   109
Normal Body Mechanics   113
History   116
Examination of the Low Back Pain Patient   122
    Techniques of Examination   123
Tissue Sites of Pain and Their Manifestations   124
    Tissue Sources of Pain   124
    Examination of Muscles and Tendons   125
    Facet Pathology and Examination   125
Lumbar Disk Pain: Its Examination   126
Standard Physical Examination Tests   127
    Lordosis   127
    Lumbar Flexion   128
    Lateral and Rotational Flexibility   129
    Hamstring Flexibility   130
Strength Testing   133
    Lumbar Extension   135
Objective Neurologic Examination   136
    Neurologic Determination of
        Nerve Root Involvement   140
    Tests to Increase Intrathecal Pressure   143
    Confirmatory Tests for Sciatic Radiculitis   147
    Test for Malingering   148
Treatment Protocol for Low Back Pain   149
Analgesic Nerve Block In Treating Pain   150
Exercise Treatment of Acute Low Back Pain   150
Manipulation   156
Spinal Stenosis   158

Spondylolysis and Spondylolisthesis 161
   Symptoms 162
   Treatment 162
Piriformis Syndrome 162

Chapter 6   Neck and Upper Back Pain **171**

Upper Cervical Complex 171
   Occipital Neuralgia 173
   Muscular Component of Cervical Pathology 179
   Neck Muscle Proprioception and Motor Control 179
   Examination of the Upper Cervical Complex 181
Lower Cervical Segment Examination 185
Examination of the Cervical Spine 187
   Objectives of Examination 188
   Bony and Soft Tissue Palpation 188
   Nerve Function Testing 189
   Range of Motion Testing 189
Clinical Entities 194
   Upper Cervical Segment (Occiput–Atlas–Axis) 194
   Lower Cervical Segment Pain and Impairment 195
   Cervical Zygapophyseal Joint Pain 196
Neurologic Examination (Nerves Emanating From
   Cervical Spine) 198
   Cervicogenic Headache 199
   Hyperextension-Hyperflexion Cervical Injuries:
     Whiplash Syndrome 201
Lesions of the Cervical Cord 206
   Treatment Protocols for Cervical Pain 209
Facet Joint Injections 214
Temporomandibular Joint Pain 216
Upper Thoracic Pain 232

Chapter 7   Neurovascular Compression Syndromes **239**

Thoracic Outlet Syndrome 239
   Symptoms and Signs 240
Anterior Scalene Syndrome 246
   Symptoms and Signs 247
   Treatment 247
Costoclavicular Syndrome 248
   Symptoms and Signs 249

Treatment 249
Hyperabduction Syndrome 250
    Treatment 250
Brachial Plexus Injuries 251
Lesions of the Trunk 254
    Upper Plexus (Trunk) Lesions 254
    Middle Plexus (Trunk) Lesions 254
    Lower Plexus (Trunk) Lesions 254
Lesions of the Cords 254
    Signs and Symptoms 254
    Therapy 255
Brachial Plexus Compression 255

Chapter 8   Shoulder Pain and Impairment **259**

Glenohumeral Joint 259
    Muscular Action 261
    Pathogenic Factors 267
    History and Examination 270
    Diagnostic Procedures 271
    Treatment 279
Shoulder Dislocation 289
Acromioclavicular Joint 289
Sternoclavicular Joint 293

Chapter 9   Elbow Pain **295**

Trauma 295
Nerve Damage 297
    Ulnar Nerve 297
    Radial Nerve 298
    Baseball Elbow 300
    Epicondylalgia 302

Chapter 10   Wrist and Hand Pain **310**

Carpal Tunnel Syndrome 310
    Pathophysiology of Nerve Compression 315
    Treatment 317
Pronator Teres Median Nerve Compression 329
    Symptoms and Signs 331

Treatment of the PTS 332
Anterior Interosseous Syndrome 332
Ulnar Nerve Compression 332
Cubital Tunnel Syndrome 335
    Symptoms of Cubital Tunnel
        Ulnar Nerve Compression 338
    Treatment 339
    Surgical Intervention 339
Tendon Problems 339
    Common Tendinitis 339
    Tendon Rupture 343
    Flexor Tendon Injury 344
    Specific Tendinitis Problems of the Hand 346
Fractures and Dislocations 354
    Principles of Treatment 355

Chapter 11   Hip Pain and Impairment **362**

Functional Anatomy 362
Hip Joint Motions 368
    Walking 369
    Standing 371
Pain Mechanisms of the Hip 375
    Degenerative Arthritis 377
Pelvic Trauma 383

Chapter 12   Knee Pain **388**

Ligaments 388
Menisci 397
Nerve Supply to the Knee 398
Muscles 398
Functional Anatomy 399
Patellofemoral Articulation 401
Clinical Evaluation of Knee Pain and Disability 404
    Collateral Ligament Injury 407
    Medial Collateral Ligament 407
    Lateral Collateral Ligament Injuries 409
    Cruciate Ligament Injuries 410
    Treatment of Anterior Cruciate Ligament Injuries 413
    Meniscus Injuries 415
    Anterior Knee Pain 420

Chapter 13   Foot and Ankle Pain **428**

The Foot 428
Ankle Joint 428
Ankle Injuries 433
    Injury Evaluation 435
    Radiologic Evaluation 436
    Treatment—Acute Injury 436
    Stress Fractures 439
Subtalar Joint 439
The Painful Foot 441
    Evaluation of the Painful Foot 442
    Acute Foot Strain 443
    Chronic Foot Pain 443
    Heel Pain 446
Transverse Tarsal Joint 449
    Metatarsalgia 452
    Morton's Syndrome 454
    Interdigital Neuritis 456
    March Fracture 458
    Hallux Valgus 459
    Hallux Rigidus 461
    Hammertoe 462
Rupture of the Achilles Tendon 464
The Diabetic Foot 465
Orthotic Devices 467

Chapter 14   Causalgia and Other Reflex
Sympathetic Dystrophies **470**

Reflex Sympathetic Dystrophy 470
Reflex Sympathetic Dystrophy in Lower Extremity 479
Leg-Ankle-Foot RSD Syndrome 479
    Mechanism of LAF Syndrome 481
    Diagnosis 482
    Treatment 484

Chapter 15   Psychologic Concepts of Soft Tissue Pain **489**

Panic and Anxiety Disorders 492
Pain Behavior 495
    Facial Expression of Pain 495
    The "Undesirable Patient" 496

Psychologic Testing in Patients With Chronic Pain   497
Secondary Gain Concept   501

Chapter 16   Workers' Compensation **507**

Problems With the System   507
Proposed Remedies   508
Disability and Impairment   511
Medical Report   512
Ergonomic Approaches for the Clinical Assessment of
   Occupational Musculoskeletal Disorders   513

**Chapter 17   Neuromusculoskeletal Basis of Soft Tissue
                 Pain and Impairment**   517

Stretch Reflex   523
Supraspinal Motor Centers   524

Index **529**

Illustrations

1–1.	Formation of connective tissue	2
1–2.	Tropocollagen trihelix fiber (schematic)	4
1–3.	Collagen fibers	5
1–4.	The role of type IX collagen in cartilage	5
1–5.	Muscle microscopic structure	7
1–6.	Cross section of a peripheral nerve	8
1–7.	Degrees of nerve injury	9
1–8.	A node of Ranvier	10
1–9.	Tourniquet-induced nerve degeneration	10
1–10.	Nerve regeneration	11
2–1.	Nociceptive substances liberated from trauma	17
2–2.	Schematic concept of vasochemical sequelae of trauma	17
2–3.	Neural patterns causing muscle spasm in response to pain	18
2–4.	Neural patterns emanating from skin blood vessels and muscles causing spasm	19
2–5.	Sensory fibers entering the dorsal horn	20
2–6.	Major ascending sensory pathways of the spinal cord carrying pain mediating fibers	21
2–7.	Ascending and descending tracts of the spinal cord	22
2–8.	Thalamic pathways	23
2–9.	Thalamocortical projections	24
2–10.	The reticular system	25
2–11.	Sensory and motor tracts on the spinal cord	26
2–12.	Nociceptive transmission and inhibition at the dorsal horn level	27
2–13.	The synapse	29
2–14.	Neurotransmission: wiring transmission versus volume transmission (schematic)	30
2–15.	Wire transmission versus volume transmission	30

2–16.	"Mismatched" transmitters and receptors: a concept . . .	31
2–17.	Kneeling man perceiving pain (Descartes)	33
2–18.	Sequence of neurohormonal aspects of stress	34
2–19.	Modifiers of sensory (pain) transmission	35
2–20.	Pharmacologic sites of action of pain pattern interruption	36
2–21.	Autonomic nervous system: anatomic	38
2–22.	Autonomic compared with somatic	39
2–23.	Transmission sequence of the peripheral autonomic nervous system	39
2–24.	Axoplasmic neural transport	40
2–25.	Components of a spinal nerve	41
2–26.	The ventricular system of the brain	42
2–27.	Axonal outgrowth forming a neuroma	45
2–28.	Nociceptor activation of alpha$_1$ adrenoreceptors	47
2–29.	*Failed* opioid modulation of pain in the dorsal root ganglion	48
3–1.	Young man pulling a fishnet	61
3–2.	Intrafusal muscle spindle	61
3–3.	Spindle system functional	63
3–4.	Higher cortical control of the spindle system	64
3–5.	Autonomic-somatic cord level interaction	65
3–6.	Spindle system coordination of muscular length rate of contraction and degree of tension	66
3–7.	Proprioceptive autonomic control of neuromuscular function	67
3–8.	Musculotendinous mechanism	68
3–9.	Influence of peripheral afferents on the spindle system	69
3–10.	Interneuronal role in pathophysiology of spasticity	70
3–11.	Nociceptive transmission to the dorsal horn of the cord	77
3–12.	Twitch characteristics	79
5–1.	The intervertebral disc	104
5–2.	Collagen fibers of the nucleus pulposus	105
5–3.	Annulus fibrosus	106
5–4.	Annular fiber angulation under various forces	107
5–5.	Change in shape of nucleus and angulation of annular fibers from compression	108
5–6.	The zygapophyseal joints (facets)	108
5–7.	Neural contents of the intervertebral foramen	110
5–8.	Dural and arachnoid sheaths of the nerve root	111
5–9.	Innervation of the recurrent nerve of Luschka	111
5–10.	Innervation of a vertebral functional unit	112

5–11.	Muscular deceleration-acceleration of the flexing spine	114
5–12.	Faulty lifting technique	115
5–13.	Perturber influence on neuromusculoskeletal control	116
5–14.	Tridimensional forces in trunk flexion and lifting	117
5–15.	Lumbar motion monitor (LMM)	120
5–16.	Perturber effect on normal neuromusculoskeletal function	121
5–17.	Pelvic angulation in a musician	124
5–18.	Variations of lumbosacral angle dependent on the sacral rotation	128
5–19.	Mechanisms postulated in symptomatic lordosis	129
5–20.	Confirmation of lordosis causing backache	130
5–21.	Standing test for degree of lumbar flexion and hamstring tightness	130
5–22.	Testing low back flexibility without hamstring involvement	131
5–23.	Testing lateral trunk flexibility	131
5–24.	Another test of lateral trunk flexibility	132
5–25.	Testing trunk rotational flexibility in the seated position	132
5–26.	Muscles acting on the pelvis	133
5–27.	Trunk flexor strength testing: stages	134
5–28.	Sit-back abdominal strength testing	134
5–29.	Poorly conditioned patient doing a painful situp	135
5–30.	Abdominal strength testing with bilateral leg raising	135
5–31.	Extensor muscle strength testing	136
5–32.	Lumbosacral hyperextension causing root pain from intervertebral disc protrusion	137
5–33.	Straight leg raising (SLR) test from a standing position: the dural sign	138
5–34.	Straight leg raising (SLR) test in supine and sitting positions	139
5–35.	Femoral stretch test	140
5–36.	Dermatomal areas of the lower extremity	143
5–37.	Testing myotome of L-5 root	144
5–38.	Tender myoneural junction points	145
5–39.	The Milgram test	146
5–40.	The Naffziger test	146
5–41.	The Valsalva maneuver	147
5–42.	The Kernig test	148
5–43.	Injection sites of paraspinous muscles, sacroiliac ligaments, and the sacroiliac joint	151

5–44.	Epidural injection	152
5–45.	Walking: the best exercise	154
5–46.	Walking plus	154
5–47.	Physiologic effect of walking on the intervertebral disc	155
5–48.	Concept of manipulation	157
5–49.	Spinal canal contents	159
5–50.	Mechanism of spondylolisthesis	161
5–51.	Corsetting in standing and sitting	163
5–52.	Piriformis muscle	163
6–1.	Motion at the occipito-atlas joint	172
6–2.	Occipito-atlas-axis ligaments	172
6–3.	Rotational motion of the atlas on the axis	173
6–4.	Transverse (cross) ligament	173
6–5.	Accessory atlanto-axial ligaments	174
6–6.	Emergence of the greater superior occipital nerve	175
6–7.	Greater superior occipital nerve: the C2 root	175
6–8.	Musculature of the head and neck	176
6–9.	Greater occipital nerve	177
6–10.	Relationship of vertebral artery to the lateral bodies	177
6–11.	Vertebral artery pathway	178
6–12.	Mechanical locking of rotation of C2 on C3	178
6–13.	Spindle and Golgi systems	180
6–14.	Spindle system coordination of muscle length	181
6–15.	Musculotendinous mechanism	182
6–16.	Effect of deceleration injury to neck with head turned	183
6–17.	Unilateral subluxation from excessive rotation	184
6–18.	Referred zones of cervical root levels (dermatomes)	184
6–19.	Cervical functional unit	185
6–20.	Flexion arc of a cervical unit	186
6–21.	Rotation of the cervical spine	187
6–22.	Recording range of motion	190
6–23.	Methods of movement of the vertebral segment with direct pressure (DP), right lateral (RL), or left lateral (LL) pressure on the posterior superior spine	190
6–24.	Motion of occipito-cervical and cervical spine	191
6–25.	Flexion of a functional cervical unit	191
6–26.	Cervical flexion and extension	192
6–27.	Foramenal closure in lateral flexion and rotation of the head and neck	192
6–28.	Median nerve	193
6–29.	Cervical root component of the median nerve	194
6–30.	The ulnar nerve	195

6–31.	Cervical root component of the ulnar nerve	196
6–32.	The radial nerve	197
6–33.	Sensory mapping of peripheral nerve to the hand	198
6–34.	Upper body-neck deformation from rear-end collisions	199
6–35.	Hyperextension injuries from rear-end impact	200
6–36.	Annulus tears and intervertebral disk degeneration	200
6–37.	Hemorrhage from meniscus injury	201
6–38.	Referred pain zones of zygapophyseal joints	201
6–39.	Head compression causing radicular signs and symptoms	202
6–40.	Relief of radicular symptoms with manual traction	203
6–41.	Effects of horizontal force on cervical disk	204
6–42.	Neurologic test for cord injury in the blind zone: Shimizu reflex	207
6–43.	Felt cervical collar	210
6–44.	Standard Plexiglas cervical collar	211
6–45.	Guildford cervical brace	212
6–46.	Cervical traction is applied to the supine patient causing cervical spine flexion with the angle of pull between 20° and 30°	213
6–47.	With an erect posture, the weight of the head (approximately 10 pounds) is maintained directly above the center of gravity	215
6–48.	Forward head posture of depression	216
6–49.	Distraction exercise for posture training	217
6–50.	The temporomandibular joint	218
6–51.	Trigeminal nerve	219
6–52.	Afferent areas of the trigeminal nerve	220
6–53.	Deformation of the disk during jaw opening and closing	220
6–54.	Deformation of the TMJ disk during jaw motion	221
6–55.	Lateral (external) pterygoid muscle	221
6–56.	Passive-active mobilization of the mandible	222
6–57.	Influence of posture in temporomandibular joint (TMJ) syndrome	222
6–58.	Orthosis to open mouth (principle)	223
6–59.	Forward head posture	224
6–60.	Posture exercises	225
6–61.	Exercise to decrease forward head posture	226
6–62.	Poor sitting posture	227
6–63.	Poor standing posture	228
6–64.	Neck exercises to increase flexibility	229
6–65.	Neck exercises to increase strength	230

6–66.	Neck exercises to increase strength	230
6–67.	Traction halter pressure points	231
7–1.	The supraclavicular space	240
7–2.	Scalene muscles	241
7–3.	Schematic presentation of the brachial plexus	241
7–4.	Divisions of the roots into the brachial plexus then peripheral nerves	242
7–5.	Scalene anticus syndrome	242
7–6.	Dermatomal areas of the upper extremity	243
7–7.	Adson's test	244
7–8.	Brachial plexus traction test (BPTT)	245
7–9.	Scapular elevation exercise	248
7–10.	Scapular elevation exercise and seated posture training	249
7–11.	Hyperabduction syndrome	250
7–12.	Periradicular sheath of the nerves forming the brachial plexus	251
7–13.	Schematic brachial plexus	252
7–14.	Microanatomy of sites for preganglionic and postganglionic injuries	253
7–15.	Brachial plexus pressure sign in radiculopathy	256
8–1.	Joint motion	260
8–2.	Congruity versus incongruity in joints	261
8–3.	The glenoid fossa	262
8–4.	Structure supporting the dependent humerus	262
8–5.	Spindle system control of the supraspinatus muscle	263
8–6.	Rotator cuff muscles	264
8–7.	The planes of motion of the shoulder and upper arm ...	265
8–8.	Static support of the scapula by the claviculoscapular ligaments	266
8–9.	Rotator cuff muscles at their scapular origin	267
8–10.	The internal rotators of the humerus	268
8–11.	The glenohumeral capsule	268
8–12.	Tissue relationship of the glenohumeral joint	269
8–13.	The Fibroosseous case	269
8–14.	Injury on an outstretched arm	270
8–15.	Pitching trauma	271
8–16.	Repetitive trauma: mechanisms in pitching	272
8–17.	Shoulder trauma in tennis	272
8–18.	Bowling shoulder trauma	273
8–19.	Faulty posture predisposing to cuff deterioration	274
8–20.	Stages of cuff degeneration	275
8–21.	Painful arc	276

8–22.	Shrugging abduction	276
8–23.	Drop sign of rotator cuff tear	277
8–24.	Apprehension test for capsular tear	277
8–25.	Subtle signs of adhesive capsulitis	278
8–26.	Adhesive capsulitis	279
8–27.	Pendular exercises	280
8–28.	Intraarticular injection for tendinitis	281
8–29.	One-minute break: shoulder stretch	282
8–30.	One-minute break: shoulder stretch 2	282
8–31.	One-minute break: shoulder stretch 3	284
8–32.	Internal rotator stretch with weight	285
8–33.	Overhead pulley exercises	286
8–34.	Strengthening exercise for external rotators	287
8–35.	Unilateral exercise for external rotator	288
8–36.	Intraarticular injection for brisement	288
8–37.	Anterior dislocation mechanism	289
8–38.	Four types of shoulder dislocation	290
8–39.	Kocher manipulation for shoulder dislocation	290
8–40.	Scapular elevation and circumduction	291
8–41.	Acromioclavicular meniscus	292
8–42.	Immobilization treatment of the acromioclavicular (AC) joint	292
8–43.	Sternoclavicular joint	293
9–1.	Elbow joint anatomy	296
9–2.	Bony aspects of the elbow in pronation	297
9–3.	Cubital tunnel	298
9–4.	Motor and sensory distribution of the ulnar nerve	299
9–5.	Course of the radial nerve	300
9–6.	Radial and posterior interosseous nerves	301
9–7.	Finger extensor test of the radial nerve	301
9–8.	Extensor muscles of the forearm that attach at the elbow	303
9–9.	Lateral epicondylitis: "tennis elbow"	304
9–10.	The radial nerve	305
9–11.	Radial nerve: the supinator test	306
9–12.	Abductor pollicis longus and extensor pollicis longus: test of radial nerve	306
9–13.	Manipulation treatment of tennis elbow	307
10–1.	Contents of carpal tunnel	311
10–2.	Palmar creases and their bony landmarks	311
10–3.	Transverse carpal ligaments	312
10–4.	Tenodesis action of the flexor-extensor tendons	313
10–5.	Pulley system of the metacarpalphalangeal joint	314

10–6.	The blood supply of a tendon	315
10–7.	Axoplasmic neural transport: a theory	316
10–8.	Schematic representation of a peripheral nerve	317
10–9.	Median nerve	318
10–10.	Light touch testing	319
10–11.	Postulated mechanism of paresthesia: carpal tunnel pressure changes	320
10–12.	Variants of tunnel pressures from wrist positions	321
10–13.	The effect of trauma: a vasochemical reaction	321
10–14.	A cock up splint for carpal tunnel syndrome	322
10–15.	Exercises for the forearm flexors and extensors	322
10–16.	Superficial landmarks at the palmar surface of the wrist	323
10–17.	Endoscopic release of the transverse carpal ligament ...	324
10–18.	Anatomic variations of the median nerve at the wrist ...	325
10–19.	Cross section of the wrist	326
10–20.	"Double crush": median nerve compression syndrome	327
10–21.	Axoplasmic neural transport: a theory	328
10–22.	A node of Ranvier	328
10–23.	Effect of pressure (crush) on a myelinated nerve	329
10–24.	Pronator teres median nerve compression	330
10–25.	Anterior interosseous syndrome	333
10–26.	Ulnar nerve: motor and sensory distribution	334
10–27.	Guyon's canal: the ulnar nerve tunnel	335
10–28.	Guyon's canal: entry into the hand	335
10–29.	Ulnar nerve: sensory pattern	336
10–30.	Flexor carpi ulnaris	336
10–31.	Flexor digitorum profundus	337
10–32.	Cubital tunnel ulnar nerve	337
10–33.	Trophocollagen trihelix fiber (schematic)	340
10–34.	Collagen fibers	341
10–35.	Musculotendinous mechanism	342
10–36.	Anatomic zones of tendon injuries	345
10–37.	"No man's land"	346
10–38.	Distal phalanx extensor tendon tear (mechanism)	347
10–39.	Conservative management of the mallet finger	347
10–40.	Rationale of treatment for mallet finger	348
10–41.	Plaster cast treatment of mallet finger	348
10–42.	Mechanism of extensor tendon rupture at the middle phalangeal joint	349
10–43.	Treatment of a boutonniere deformity	349
10–44.	Extensor communis tendon tear	350
10–45.	Rupture of the extensor pollicis longus	350

10–46.	de Quervain's disease: stenosing tenosynovitis of the extensor pollicis brevis and abductor pollicis longus	352
10–47.	Formation of a tendon nodule	352
10–48.	Trigger fingers (flexor tendinitis)	353
10–49.	Arches of the hand	354
10–50.	Physiologic position of the hand for immobilization	355
10–51.	Fracture healing time	356
11–1.	Congruous versus incongruous joints	363
11–2.	Joint motion: spin or rotation	363
11–3.	Angle of inclination	364
11–4.	Angle of anteversion	365
11–5.	Hydrodynamic lubrication	366
11–6.	Anterior view of the bony pelvis	366
11–7.	Hip joint	367
11–8.	Femoral capsule	368
11–9.	Cartilage of femoral head	369
11–10.	Hip range of motion	370
11–11.	Hip range of motion	371
11–12.	Hip stretch	372
11–13.	Limited motion from degenerative joint disease	372
11–14.	Composite schematic determinants of gait	373
11–15.	Gait	374
11–16.	Weight borne by the hip during stance	374
11–17.	Influence of a cane in hip joint weight bearing	375
11–18.	Lateral femoral cutaneous nerve: meralgia paresthetica	376
11–19.	Genu valgum and varum	377
11–20.	Synovial sites of inflammation in degenerative joint disease	378
11–21.	Technique and site of intraarticular injection	379
11–22.	Technique and site of intraarticular injection into the hip joint	379
11–23.	Technique of obturator nerve block	380
11–24.	Technique of hip traction	381
11–25.	Hip extensor exercises	381
11–26.	Hip flexor stretch exercise	382
11–27.	Hip extensor exercise kneeling	382
11–28.	Bedroom bicycling	383
11–29.	Forces acting on the pelvis	383
11–30.	Ligamentous support of the pelvis	384
11–31.	Pelvic ring	385
11–32.	Sites of fracture with intact pelvic ring	385
11–33.	Combined fractures within the pubic rami	386

11–34.	Combined sacroiliac and symphysis pubis separation . . .	386
12–1.	The joints of the knee	389
12–2.	The incongruity of the femorotibial joint	389
12–3.	Ligamentous support of the femorotibial joint	390
12–4.	Medial collateral ligaments	391
12–5.	Collateral ligamentous tautness	391
12–6.	Ligamentous laxity and tautness of the cruciate ligaments during flexion-extension	392
12–7.	Cruciate ligaments	393
12–8.	Effects of cruciate ligaments on flexion-extension of the knee	394
12–9.	Basis of rotation of the tibia on the femoral condyles . . .	394
12–10.	Rotational aspects of knee flexion-extension	395
12–11.	Cruciate ligament restriction	396
12–12.	Cruciate ligamentous restriction of tibial rotation	397
12–13.	Attachment of the meniscus	398
12–14.	Intrinsic circulation of the meniscus	399
12–15.	Quadriceps mechanism	400
12–16.	Posterior thigh muscles	401
12–17.	Medial aspect of the posterior knee structure	402
12–18.	Parallelogram analysis of quadriceps mechanism	403
12–19.	Facets of the patella	403
12–20.	Quadriceps mechanism	404
12–21.	Quadriceps angle	405
12–22.	Q angle measured from the tubercle	406
12–23.	Effect of Q angle on the patella	406
12–24.	Anterior knee tissues guiding patellar motion	407
12–25.	"Stop and cut" knee injury	408
12–26.	A mechanism of rotational knee injury	409
12–27.	Ballottement test for effusion	410
12–28.	Tender sites of knee pathology	411
12–29.	The drawer sign test	411
12–30.	False negative drawer sign from hamstring spasm	412
12–31.	False negative drawer sign from a torn meniscus	412
12–32.	The Lachman tests	413
12–33.	Position of the thumb in performing the Lachman test	413
12–34.	Reversed Lachman test	414
12–35.	Rotary instability test of the cruciate ligaments	414
12–36.	Hydrodynamic lubrication	416
12–37.	Microscopic structure of the meniscus	416
12–38.	Mechanism of meniscus tears	417
12–39.	External force injuring meniscus	417
12–40.	Primary meniscus tear patterns	418

12–41.	Flap tears of the meniscus	419
12–42.	Varieties of medial meniscal tears	420
12–43.	The McMurray test	421
12–44.	The Apley test	421
12–45.	Physiologic motion of the patella	422
12–46.	Patellofemoral pain clinically elicited	423
12–47.	Arthrosis for patellofemoral pathology	423
12–48.	Technique of knee aspiration	424
12–49.	Degenerative arthritis and neuroma in patellofemoral disease	425
13–1.	The three functional units of the foot	429
13–2.	The talus bone	429
13–3.	Ankle mortise and talus relationship	430
13–4.	Motion of talus within the ankle mortise	431
13–5.	Medial (deltoid) collateral ligaments	432
13–6.	Lateral collateral ligaments	432
13–7.	Relationship of medial and lateral collateral ligaments to axis of rotation of ankle	433
13–8.	Lateral collateral ligament tear	434
13–9.	Medial collateral ligament tear	435
13–10.	Inversion stress test of ankle	436
13–11.	Saggital stress test of the ankle: "drawer sign"	436
13–12.	Tilt board for proprioceptive training	437
13–13.	Tilt and lateral board for proprioceptive training	438
13–14.	Heel cord stretching exercise	438
13–15.	Talocalcaneal joint	440
13–16.	Ligamentous complex of the talocalcaneal joint	441
13–17.	The subtalar joint and tarsal canal	442
13–18.	Motion of the subtalar (talocalcaneal) joint	443
13–19.	Supination of the foot during rotation of the leg	444
13–20.	Tender areas in foot strain	444
13–21.	Jogger's foot pain	445
13–22.	Mechanism of foot strain	446
13–23.	Pronation	447
13–24.	Sites of pain in the region of the heel	448
13–25.	Nerve to the abductor digiti quinti muscle	448
13–26.	Mechanism of plantar fascia on the longitudinal arch	449
13–27.	Effects of toe motion on the plantar fascia	449
13–28.	Mechanism of plantar fasciitis	450
13–29.	Technique of plantar fascial injection	450
13–30.	Shoe modification for the plantar fascial heel spur	451
13–31.	Transverse tarsal joints	452
13–32.	Transverse arches	453
13–33.	Longitudinal arch	454

13–34.	The foot and ankle during gait	455
13–35.	Splay foot	455
13–36.	Morton's syndrome	456
13–37.	Morton's neuroma	457
13–38.	Compartments containing interdigital neurovascular bundles	457
13–39.	Entrapment of an interdigital nerve	458
13–40.	March fracture	459
13–41.	Hallux valgus conditions	460
13–42.	Concepts of etiology of hallux valgus	461
13–43.	Hallux rigidus	462
13–44.	Range of motion	463
13–45.	Muscular action on the phalanges	463
13–46.	Hammer toe	464
13–47.	Tear of the gastrocsoleus	465
13–48.	Shoe inserts and pads to minimize pressure sites	466
13–49.	Shoe modification to correct heel valgus	467
13–50.	Molded orthotic device	468
13–51.	Shoe modification in treatment of metatarsalgia	468
14–1.	Axoplasmic neural transport: A theory	473
14–2.	Axonal growth forming a neuroma	474
14–3.	Neuronal pathways of pain	475
14–4.	Central dorsal column concept of reflex sympathetic dystrophy	476
14–5.	Postulated neurophysiologic mechanism of sympathetic maintained pain	477
14–6.	Development of reflex sympathetic dystrophy "frozen shoulder-hand-finger syndrome"	478
14–7.	Innervation of the leg and foot	480
14–8.	Sensory patterns of the lower extremity	481
14–9.	Arterial supply of the leg and foot	482
14–10.	Technique of causal and epidural block	486
15–1.	Concept of sustained muscle contraction from pain memory	491
15–2.	Minnesota Multiphasic Personality Inventory	498
15–3.	Emory University Pain Clinic "Pain Estimate Chart"	501
17–1.	Neuromusculoskeletal mechanism	518
17–2.	Perturber influence on neuromuscular mechanisms	518
17–3.	Neuromuscular mechanism of lumbosacral function	519
17–4.	Neuromusculoskeletal mechanism: Flexion-extension and obliques	520
17–5.	Normal and excessive forces on the musculoskeletal system	521
17–6.	Sequence of tissue damage creating nociceptors	522

17–7.   The spindle system   523
17–8.   Neurologic pathways of nociception   524
17–9.   Spinal and supraspinal motor centers   525
17–10.   Forces influencing normal neuromusculoskeletal
          function   526

CHAPTER 1

Concepts of Pain and Impairment

Soft tissues have long been considered as the major source of pain and disability, but have not been adequately defined. Soft tissues constitute the site of impairment leading to disability and pain. They need clarification because their presence and significance present conflicting evidence in terms of delineation and their implications in syndromes associated with pain and disability.

The biologic and mechanical nature of soft tissues forms the basis of their function and thus similarly affects their malfunction when disease or trauma causes impairment. These soft tissues are composed of tendons, ligaments, joint capsules, muscles with their fascial coatings, blood vessels, and nerves.

CONNECTIVE TISSUE

Dense connective tissue consists of complex cells and fibers within a supporting matrix. The enclosed fibers include collagen, elastin, and reticulum, which undergo mechanical alteration in their function. They form the four fundamental tissues of the body:

1. Epithelial tissue (skin) provides protection, secretion, and absorption.
2. Muscular tissue allows the contraction that results in motion.
3. Nervous tissue manifests irritability and conductivity.
4. Connective tissue gives support, aids nutritional function, and provides defense.

All four of these tissues are subserved in their precise function by a nerve supply—somatic and autonomic—that initiates function and supplies sensation.

Connective tissue is the major component of soft tissue. By definition, it **connects** all other components of soft tissue in their functional role. Connective tissue includes muscles, tendons, ligaments, adipose tissue, bone, cartilage, blood, and lymph for the purpose of support, nourishment, and defense of the enclosed organs. Virchow in the 19th century called collagen, the major component of soft tissue, "body excelsior" or "inert stuffing."

Connective tissue is formed (Fig. 1–1) from the mast cell that forms the ground substance and from the fibroblast that forms the cellular components.

Connective tissue may be grouped as follows:

I. Connective tissue proper
    A. Loose connective tissue: forms many spaces in which are contained:
        1. Collagen fibers, whose arrangement determines the tensile strength of the tissue
        2. Elastin fibers, the percentage of which determines the elasticity of the tissue
        3. Reticular fibers, which act in the role of support

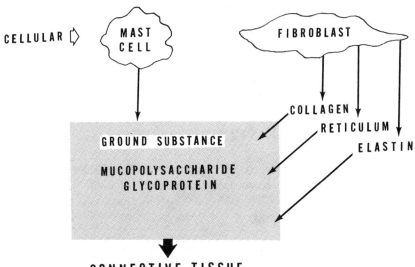

Figure 1–1. Formation of connective tissue. The mast cell secretes the ground substance, which contains mucopolysaccharide. This matrix ultimately contains collagen, reticulum, and elastin, all of which are derived from fibroblasts.

II. Special connective tissue
  A. Mucous
  B. Elastic
  C. Reticular
  D. Adipose
  E. Pigmented
III. Cartilage
IV. Bone
  V. Blood vessels

Dense Connective Tissue

Connective tissue has the following **functional** characteristics:

1. Provides support for specialized organs.
2. Provides pathways for nerves, blood vessels, and lymphatics.
3. Facilitates movement between adjacent structures.
4. Forms bursal sacs to minimize friction and pressure.
5. Forms bands, pulleys, and check ligaments to restrain or limit motion.
6. Promotes circulation of arterioles, capillaries, veins, and lymphatics.
7. Furnishes sites of attachments of muscles.
8. Aids in repair of injured tissues through formation of scar tissue.
9. Forms fat storage space for conservation of heat and metabolites.
10. Contains histiocytes for defense against bacteria and immune reactions.
11. Participates in tissue nutrition through migration of fluids.

Regular connective tissue consists of cells, ground substance, and fibers that include collagen, elastin, and reticulum. The mechanical behavior of connective tissue depends on:

1. Physical properties of the collagen, elastin, and reticular fibers.
2. Architectural arrangement of these fibers.
3. Size and type of collagen fibers.
4. Proportion of collagen to the other fibers.
5. Maturity of the collagen fibers.
6. Composition and hydration of the ground substance.

Collagen

Collagen is a major component in connective tissue and deserves special consideration. It is a tropocollagen molecule, arranged in a trihelix chain of amino polypeptides (Fig. 1–2), in which every third residue is glycine. These

PEPTIDE
CHAIN

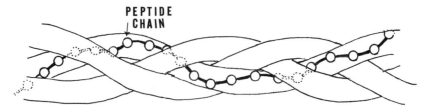

Figure 1–2. Tropocollagen trihelix fiber (schematic). This type I collagen molecule is composed of peptide chains that include two α_1 and one α_2 peptide chains in which every third molecule is a glycine amino acid. The three intertwining peptide chains form a trihelix collagen fiber. (Modified from Alberts, B, Bray, D, Lewis, J et al: In Molecular Biology of the Cell. Garland, New York, 1983, p. 694.)

chains have a curled configuration (Fig. 1–3). In its normal state, it has a specific curl that loosens under tension and contracts when totally relaxed. **Physical tone** is maintained within the fiber. In the tendon, which has collagen fibers arranged in a parallel architecture, the tone is determined by the respective tone of the extrafusal muscle fibers to which the tendon is attached.[1] In each anatomic site containing collagen fibers, the tone varies according to the sites of attachment and their function.

Several types of collagen currently are identified as types I, II, III, IV, and V with each having subclasses.[2] Tendons and ligaments contain mostly type I collagen (see Fig. 1–1). The composing atoms are chemically bonded within its matrix containing glycosaminoglycans, proteoglycans, and glycoproteins (Fig. 1–4).

Physical stress on collagen influences the collagen's organization and thus its function. Increase in stress increases it production and its organization, whereas decreased stress also adversely influences its organization, resulting in a weakening.[3]

The mechanical behavior of stress is illustrated in Figure 1–3 which shows the uncurling and physiologic elongation from tensile stress with **recovery** to its original length on release of the stress. **Creep** is the slow elongation of collagen following constant or repeated stress with limited recovery, while yet retaining physiologic limits. The many factors that influence recovery and creep will be discussed later in this chapter.

Temperatures influence the viscoelastic properties of collagen. This factor has been studied as related to tendons. Increased temperature raises creep; temperatures above 40°C cause permanent structural damage when combined with significant tension from stress and strain.

Injured connective tissue is repaired by an accumulation of inflammatory cells with stimulation of microphages and formation of fibroblasts that synthesize collagen. Fibroblasts also create fibrous tissue, thus forming a *scar.*

Fibroplasia forming fibrous tissue and increasing collagen demands that

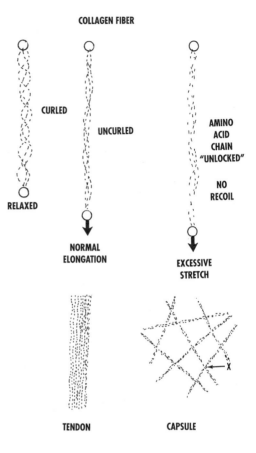

Figure 1–3. Collagen fibers. Each collagen fiber is a trihelix chain of amino acids bound together electrochemically. They uncurl to their physiologic length upon elongation. They recoil when the elongation force is released. If the collagen fiber is elongated past its physiologic length, the amino acid chains become disrupted and the fiber can no longer regain its resting length. A tendon consists of parallel bands of collagen fibers. In a capsule, collagen fibers crisscross and glide over each other at their points of intersection (*X*). The capsule depicted here elongates as far as each collagen fiber permits.

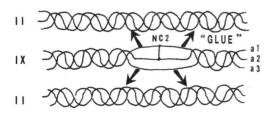

Figure 1–4. The role of type IX collagen in cartilage. Types II, IX, X, and XI collagen fibers predominate in cartilage. Genetically determined type IX has been hypothesized as being the *glue* that holds the type II fibers together. Degradation leading to degenerative changes has been thought to represent *ungluing* of the collagen, which weakens the structure of the cartilage. The cause of the ungluing remains unknown.

passive elongation be applied to ensure proper collagen remodeling, thus indicating a well-organized collagen, because tension controls the direction and alignment of collagen fiber bundles.[4-7] After scar has **matured,** the size, shape, and direction of the collagen fibers will be established, as will also the percentage of less flexible fibrous tissue.

In nontraumatized tissues, change in stress or motion results in significant alterations in the compliance, strength, and length of dense connective tissue.[8] Immobilization, implying repeated failure to elongate the fiber, causes a significant loss of dense connective tissue strength. A loss of 80% of dense connective tissue strength in muscle was found after 4 weeks of immobilization, 50% in collateral ligaments of the knee and 39% in the knee cruciate ligament.[8] Immobilization admittedly causes more rapid loss of strength than a loss of length and flexibility, but both losses occur.

Tendons

Tendons consist of fibroblasts within a large extracellular matrix that they synthesize. Fibroblasts are usually the sole cellular component of adult tendons.[9,10] Collagen is the major component of the extracellular matrix accounting for approximately 86% of the dry weight of the entire tendon.[11]

Muscle

Muscle contraction results from myofilaments sliding past one another.[12] Thin and thick filaments are bound by cross bridges (Fig. 1–5). During a contraction, the filaments do not change length but slide past one another. The thin filaments (actin) slide further into the A bands and move further out upon elongation. Contraction is a chemical reaction between ATPase and ATP in the presence of calcium.

The basis for discussion of contraction and elongation must emphasize its clinical importance in neuromusculoskeletal physiology.[13]

Muscle function is a major component of soft tissues in neuromusculoskeletal function. Several types of contraction must be understood: concentric, eccentric, isometric, isotonic, and anisotonic:

Concentric contraction producing motion through shortening. The internal force in the muscle exceeds the external force of resistance.[14]

Eccentric contraction occurs when an already shortened muscle lengthens while continuing to maintain tension.

Isometric contraction has no external movement as the external resistance equals internal force.

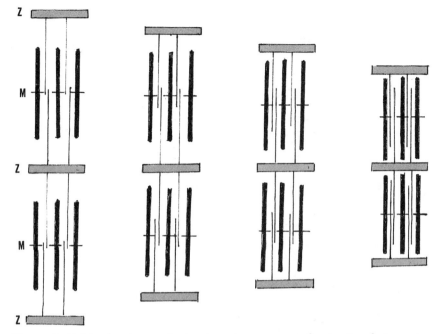

Figure 1–5. Muscle microscopic structure. A sarcomere is the structure between two Z lines. Thin filaments attach to the Z line, whereas thicker fibers attach to the M lines. In the left figure the muscle is fully elongated and the figure to the right is fully contracted. The thin fibers glide along the thick fibers during contraction.

Isotonic contraction occurs when internal contraction and external force are equal.

Anisotonic contraction occurs during motion. It is either concentric (positive work) or eccentric (negative work).

Muscle dysfunction, a cause of soft tissue injury, may result from loss of elongation resulting from fascial contracture or muscle tendon shortening arising from immobilization or faulty and inappropriate neuromuscular contraction.[15] Fatigue is a major factor in soft tissue dysfunction, which may be central or peripheral, although neuromuscular transmission failure does not appear to be a major cause of fatigue of voluntary efforts.[16–19]

Because soft tissue function is a **neuro**musculoskeletal function, the neurologic portion (Fig. 1–6) also plays a vital role and is influenced by trauma.[20] In neural functional disorders, the precise site of injury and the resultant mechanical distortion and ischemia of the offended nerve must be ascertained.[21] **Neuropraxia** refers to a local nerve conduction block with a discrete demyelination without loss of axonal continuity or Wallerian degeneration (Fig. 1–7).

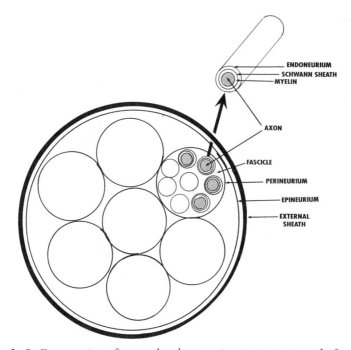

Figure 1–6. Cross section of a peripheral nerve. A nerve is composed of numerous axons grouped within a fascicle. Each axon is surrounded by myelin, enclosed within a Schwann sheath. These sheaths are coated with endoneurium made up of longitudinal collagen sheaths. A perineurium sheath contains these fascicles in bundles. Numerous fascicles are bound by epineurium, which are totally covered by an external sheath.

This nerve injury must be differentiated from a rapidly reversible physiologic block wherein symptoms are transient and residual symptoms are not present. Neuropraxia causes local demyelination with displacement of the nodes of Ranvier (Figs. 1–8 and 1–9). Regeneration of the nerve undergoes specific stages (Fig. 1–10).

After axonometic nerve injury, the cell bodies located in either the dorsal root ganglion (sensory) or the anterior horn of the spinal cord (motor) undergo chromatolysis, which involves cell body swelling, proliferation of glial cells, eccentric displacement of the nerve cell nucleus, and loss of Nissl substance arrangement.[22]

Acute nerve compression is usually attended by profound muscle wasting and some sparing of sensation.[23,24] Axonotmesis may occur without neuropraxia, which is why, for example, median nerve compression at the carpal tunnel may occur with changes visible on electromyography, but no change in the motor-sensory latencies.[25] In many patients, sensory modalities of crude and light touch and of pinprick are spared because the compression

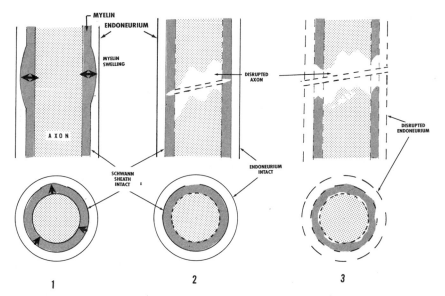

Figure 1–7. Degrees of nerve injury. (*1*) A loss of conductivity without break in continuity. The myelin sheath within an intact Schwann sheath compresses the axon (*arrows*). (*2*) Although the axon is severed, the endoneural sheath (tubule) remains intact, as may the Schwann sheath. The axon regenerates within its own tubule. (*3*) The entire fascicle, the axon, Schwann sheath, and endoneurium are disrupted. Regeneration is usually prevented by fibrosis occurring at the severed ends.

with resultant ischemia spares the small myelinated and nonmyelinated nerves.

METABOLIC EFFECTS OF INACTIVITY AND INJURY

Besides the functional impairment that results from tissue injury and inactivity, complicating metabolic changes may become more problematic than the primary disease.[26] The metabolic changes that accompany injury are compounded by inactivity, which is defined as decreased or restricted neuromuscular activity. These metabolic changes alter fluid balance, electrolyte balance, both local and general circulation, loss of nitrogen with muscle wasting, decreased resting metabolic expenditure, and loss of bone minerals.

The total body weight of adult humans has a water content of 70% a figure slightly lower in females and in the elderly. Of this amount, 55% of body weight is water in the cellular space; the remainder is within the extracellular spaces.

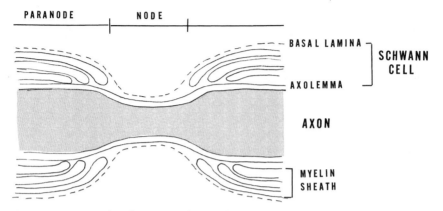

Figure 1–8. A node of Ranvier. The myelinated axon is narrowed at each node of Ranvier, which is formed by Schwann cells that invaginate to form a node with the remaining portion becoming a paranode.

Metabolic and neuroendocrine mechanisms determine the retention and excretion of water and electrolytes. During physical activity, blood volume increases approximately 10% to 19%, whereas prolonged bed rest decreases blood volume.[27,28] The maximum reduction in blood volume during bed rest occurs from the second to the sixth days of recumbency, thus indicating that little time is required for debility to occur.[29]

Deconditioning also causes an intolerance to being upright, as well as an altered response to muscular exercise. In the supine position, approximately 500 mL of blood shifts to the thorax, with an immediate decline in heart rate and a 24% increase in cardiac output. As the stroke volume increases, calculated cardiac work increases approximately 30%.[30,31]

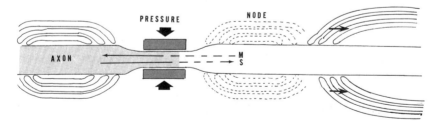

Figure 1–9. Tourniquet-induced nerve degeneration. Application of a tourniquet on a myelinated peripheral nerve causes longitudinal displacement of the nodes of Ranvier, especially at the proximal edge of the tourniquet (*pressure*). The dotted figure is the normal site of the node before pressure and the node with arrows shows the migration. Pressure on the axon causes nerve conduction deficit on the sensory (*S*) and motor (*M*) nerves (*arrows*).

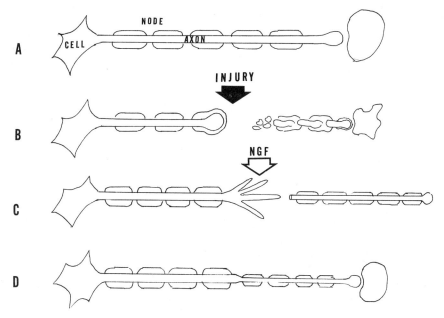

Figure 1–10. Nerve regeneration. (*A*) Depiction of a normal nerve with intact cell body, a continuous axon, and nodes of Ranvier acting on the end organ. (*B*) Injury causing degeneration of the distal axon, myelin, nodes, and end organ. (*C*) Depiction of distal nerve filaments leaving the proximal segment in search of the distal segment aided by nerve growth factor (NGF). (*D*) Union of the severed segments with the distal axon with the node as yet immature.

A well-conditioned individual responds to submaximal work load with a slow pulse and an elevated stroke volume. An unconditioned individual responds to slight or moderate work with increased heart rate and elevated blood pressure. From the decreased blood volume, the patient sustains a loss of hemoglobin, thus impairing the metabolic demands of active tissues.

Bone mass is to a significant degree determined by mechanical stimulus. Prolonged recumbency, immobilization, and flaccid paralysis cause bone atrophy resulting from hypercalciuria and negative calcium balance. Besides bone loss predisposing to stress fractures, detriment to cartilage and other connective tissues is also present.[31]

REFERENCES

1. Cailliet, R: Hand Pain and Disability. FA Davis, Philadelphia, 1994.
2. Tillman, LJ, and Cummings, GS: Biological Mechanisms of Connective Tissue Mutability. In

Currier, DP, and Nelson, RM (eds): Dynamics of Human Biological Tissues. FA Davis, Philadelphia, 1992, pp 1–44.

3. Chvapil, M: Physiology of Connective Tissue. London, Butterworth, 1967.

4. Lehman, JF, Masock, AJ, Warren, CG, et al: Effect of therapeutic temperatures on tendon extensibility. Arch Phys Med Rehabil 50:481–487, 1970.

5. Warren, CG, Lehman, JF, and Koblanski, JN: Elongation of rat tail tendon: Effect of load and temperature. Arch Phys Med Rehabil 52:481–487, 1970.

6. Rigby, BJ, Hirai, N, and Spikes, JD: The mechanical behavior of rat tail tendon. J Gen Physiol 43:265–283, 1959.

7. Van Brocklin, JD, and Ellis, DG: A study of the mechanical behavior of toe extensor tendons under applied stress. Arch Phys Med Rehabil 46:369–370, 1965.

8. Noyes, FR, Torvik, PJ, Hyde, WB, et al: Biomechanics of ligament failure. II. An analysis of immobilization, exercise, and reconditioning effects in primates. J Bone Joint Surg Am 56:1406–1417, 1974.

9. Salamon, A, and Hamori, J: Present state of tendon regeneration: Light and electron microscopic studies of regenerating tendon of the rat. Acta Morphol Hung 14:7–24, 1966.

10. Conway, AM: Regeneration of resected calcaneal tendons of the rabbit. Scand J Plast Reconstr Surg Hand Surg 5:100–102, 1971.

11. Williams, IF: Cellular and biochemical composition of healing tendons. In Jenkins, DHR (ed): Ligament Injuries and Their Treatment. Aspen, Rockville, MD, 1985, pp 43–57.

12. Huxley, HE, and Hanson, J: Changes in the cross-striation of muscle during contraction and stretch and their structural interpretation. Nature (London) 173:973–976, 1954.

13. Gordon, AM, Huxley, AF, and Julian, FJ: The variation in isometric tension with sarcomere length in vertebrate muscle fibres. J Physiol 184:186, 1966.

14. O'Connel, AL, and Gowitzke, B: Understanding the Scientific Bases of Human Movement. Williams & Wilkins, Baltimore, 1972.

15. Bouisset, S: EMG and muscle force in normal motor activities. In Desmedt, JE (ed): New Developments in Electromyography and Clinical Neurophysiology, vol 1, Karger, Basel, 1973.

16. Soderberg, GL: Skeletal muscle function. In: Currier, DP and Nelson, RM (eds): Dynamics of Human Biological Tissues. FA Davis, Philadelphia, 1992, pp 74–96.

17. Edwards, RHT: Human muscle function and fatigue. Ciba Found Symp 82:1–18, 1981.

18. Simonson, E, and Weiser, P: Physiological Aspects and Physiological Correlates of Work Capacity and Fatigue. Charles C Thomas, Springfield, IL, 1976.

19. Reid, C: The mechanism of voluntary muscular fatigue. Q J Exp Phys 19:17–42, 1928.

20. Merton, PA: Voluntary strength and fatigue. J Physiol (Lond) 128:553–564, 1954.

21. Nitz, AJ: Effects of acute pressure on peripheral nerve structure and function. In Currier, DP, and Nelson, RM (eds): Dynamics of Human Biological Tissues. FA Davis, Philadelphia, 1992, pp 205–230.

22. Lundborg, G: Nerve regeneration and repair: A review. Acta Orthop Scand 58:145–169, 1987.

23. Rudge, P: Tourniquet paralysis with prolonged conduction block: An electromyographic study. J Bone Joint Surg Br 56:716–720, 1974.

24. Trojaborg, W: Prolonged conduction block with axonal degeneration: and electrophysiological study. J Neurol Neurosurg Psychiatry 4:50–57, 1977.

25. Szabo, RM, and Chidgey, LK: Stress carpal tunnel pressures in patients with carpal tunnel syndrome and normal patients. J Hand Surg (Am) 14:624–627, 1989.

26. Long, CL, and Bonbilla, LE: Metabolic effects of inactivity and injury. In Downey, JA and Darling, RC (eds): Physiological Basis of Rehabilitation Medicine. WB Saunders, Philadelphia, 1971, pp 209–227.

27. Kjellberg, SR, Rudhe, U, and Sjostrand, T: Increase of the amount of hemoglobin and blood volume in connection with physical training. Acta Physiol Scand 19:146–151, 1949.

28. Deitrick, JE, Whedon, GD, and Shorr, E: Effects of immobilization upon various metabolic and physiological functions of normal man. Am J Med 4:3–6, 1948.

29. Fuller, JH, Bernauer, EM, and Adams, WC.: Renal function, water and electrolyte exchange during bed rest with daily exercise. Aerospace Med 41:60–72, 1970.

30. Chapman, CB, Fisher, JN, and Sproule, BJ: Behavior of stroke volume at rest and during exercise in human beings. J Clin Invest 39:1208–1213, 1960.

31. Holmgren, A, and Ovenfors, CO: Heart volume at rest and during muscular work in the supine and sitting position. Acta Med Scand 167:267–277, 1960.

32. Bassett, CAL: Effect of force on skeletal tissues. In Downey, JA and Darling, RC (eds): Physiological Basis of Rehabilitation Medicine. WB Saunders, Philadelphia, 1971, pp 283–315.

CHAPTER 2

Pain: Mechanisms, Assessment, and Management

Pain can no longer be considered merely a symptom. It is currently considered to be a disease. The evaluator's learning, expertise, or specialty will determine how the evaluator thinks about pain. To a neurologist, neurosurgeon, or neurophysiologist pain results from a neurologic abnormality. To an orthopedist pain is the result of a musculoskeletal deviation. To a psychologist or psychiatrist pain is an emotional reaction to a physical insult. The behaviorist defines pain as a process of subconsciously manipulating the environment or the injured person's relationship. Pain may be considered as *organ* language indicating the presence of organic pathology that requires specific treatment or surgical eradication.

Regardless of the interpretation of the **symptom** of pain—whether neurophysiologic, physiologic, psychologic, or behavioral—mechanical, chemical, or thermal irritation of tissue containing nociceptive receptors plays a major role in initiating the ultimate symptom of **pain.**

Pain usually originates within soft tissues in which neural pathways are stimulated. It can be stated that *pain* is considered to be an unpleasant sensation of an acute or chronic nature so differentiated by the factor of time.

NEUROANATOMIC BASIS

Pain is a warning signal that helps to protect the body from tissue damage. Pain was defined by Sherrington as a psychic adjunct to a protective reflex—the intention of the stimulus is to withdraw the affected tissue from the

14

potentially noxious (and injurious) stimuli.[1] Pain, unlike other, if not most, sensory modalities, has an essential function in survival.

The sensation of pain originates from the activation of nociceptive primary afferents by intense thermal, mechanical, or chemical stimuli. These nociceptor sites are small, free, nerve endings in body tissues; the nociceptive stimuli themselves are numerous.

Over a decade ago, it was stated that tissue damage and injury increased sensitization of the peripheral nociceptors—this was the basis for hyperalgesia at the site of injury.[2] It was also considered, at that time, that peripheral injury increased exitability in the spinal dorsal horn.[3] The clinical significance[4] of these concepts was that if the excitability of the injured tissues of the periphery was diminished, then the excitability of the central spinal horn could be similarly diminished and this, in turn, would also lessen the pain. These initial concepts are, in many ways, continuing to be documented and verified.

Pain, a sensation transmitted through the peripheral and central nervous systems until its final *interpretation* at the cortex level, has undergone many changes in its accepted neurophysiology in recent decades.

In the past, pain was considered to depend solely on the intensity of stimulation and not on stimulation of a particular pathway with specific receptors. Pain can be evoked from stimulation by a variety of different stimuli, such as excessive cold or warmth, and can be heightened by the concurrent presence of excessive noise or brightness of light. The presence of separate anatomic endings being stimulated and producing precise types of pain sensation were postulated by Frey (1894).[5] He proposed that specific nerve endings when stimulated resulted in specific pain sensations. This concept has been refuted but the notion of transmission through specific nerve fiber types is now accepted.

The nerve fiber types that are now considered to transmit sensation that ultimately will be considered *pain* are, for the most part, small myelinated A-alpha fibers and unmyelinated C fibers. This has been confirmed by recording action potentials when a painful stimulus (squeezing a muscle or injecting hypertonic saline) has been applied.[6] In a peripheral nerve block using procaine, the nerve with the smallest diameter is initially affected, resulting in the cessation of pain before sensation to touch is lost. If nerve sensation is blocked by pressure, the function of myelinated nerve fibers is diminished or lost before that of the unmyelinated nerve. Touch sensation is similarly lost before that of pain.[7]

Cutaneous A-alpha fibers respond to mechanical, chemical, and thermal stimuli. Among the chemicals currently identified as stimulating these receptors are K+, H+, histamine, bradykinin, and substance P. Hypoxia is also recognized to be a noxious stimulus to muscle tissue. Interestingly, the neural tissues of the brain are insensitive to these noxious stimuli.

In the recovery of function after injury, it is less well understood which fiber type carries specific sensation, insofar, as in recovery, awareness of pain sensation returns earlier than awareness of touch does.[8]

The *nature of pain* as a specific entity remains obscure. Identification of specific fiber types transmitting pain sensation has been physiologically ascertained; evidence exists that these painful sensations are carried within specific tracts in the spinal cord. Interruption of these tracts, however, often fails to eliminate or modify pain sensation as noted in causalgia, postherpetic neuralgia, and phantom pain, as well as in pain resulting from cancer.

In evaluating the efficacy of chordotomy in relieving chronic pain, positron emission tomographic (PET) studies[9] have indicated that high cervical cordotomy apparently works by decreasing the blood flow at the thalamic level. These PET studies have shown a significant decrease in blood flow in the anterior quadrant of the thalamus contralateral to the side of nociception. No changes were noted in the prefrontal or primary somatosensory cortices. The activity of neuronal firing in hypothalamus was decreased. These findings indicate that a peripheral mechanism activates subcentral mechanisms, probably at the thalamic level.

Paresthesia, an unpleasant sensation, although not necessarily pain, is a common symptom of diseases of the peripheral nervous system and central nervous system (CNS) that present differing concepts of pain transmission. Paresthesiae are produceable by pressure on peripheral nerves and are considered to be elicited by ischemia.

Pain-producing substances, thought to be chemicals, have become a prominent focus of pain research. Chemical mediators are released or synthesized from the damaged issue. When these mediators accumulate in sufficient quantity they activate the receptors. These become known as **nociceptor sites** and the mediators as **algogens.**

Among these chemical mediators are phospholipids that break down from arachidonic acid to form prostaglandin E (Fig. 2–1). There are also inflammatory mediators liberated from trauma called leukotrienes that do not undergo the same breakdown sequence of arachodinic acid and so are not influenced by nonsteroidal anti-inflammatory agents (NSAIAs). Trauma also causes a breakdown of blood platelets that release serotonin, which acts as a vasoconstrictor and causes local edema (Fig. 2–2). The resultant muscle *spasm* that locally accompanies trauma is possibly mediated through a neural pattern (Fig. 2–3), wherein the nociceptor impulses emanating through the dorsal root ganglia (DRG) send impulses through neuronal connections to the anterior horn cell (AHC) with resultant muscular contraction.[10] The nociceptor stimuli can emanate from the skin, the blood vessels, joint capsules, ligaments, and muscles (Fig. 2–4).

The muscle thus being involved as *recipient* of the nociceptive reaction becomes an *initiator* of nociception. This is truly a vicious cycle of pain causing muscle spasm, which in turn produces a nociceptor site of pain.

There are many other chemical nociceptive mediators other than hista-

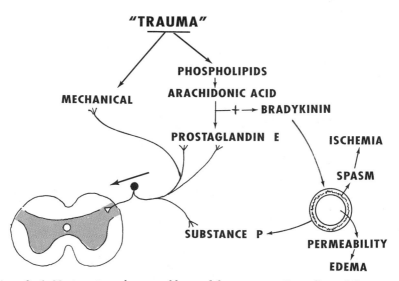

Figure 2–1. Nociceptive substances liberated from trauma. Regardless of the type of trauma, the traumatized tissues liberate breakdown products from phospholipids into aracidonic acid and will ultimately form prostaglandins. Trauma also affects the blood vessels causing spasm, edema, and the liberation of platelets that break down to free serotonin and substance P. Other kinins and toxic substances are nociceptive, thus irritating nerve endings, which ultimately cause pain.

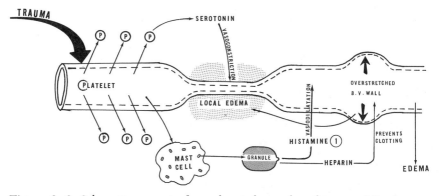

Figure 2–2. Schematic concept of vasochemical sequelae of trauma. Microhemorrhage or macrohemorrhage releases serotonin, which causes vasoconstriction and releases mast cells. The granules of mast cells release histamine, which causes vasodilitation and resultant edema formation.

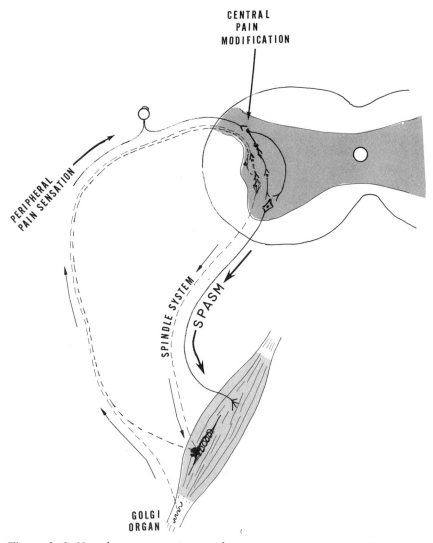

CENTRAL
PAIN
MODIFICATION

PERIPHERAL
PAIN SENSATION

SPINDLE SYSTEM

SPASM

GOLGI
ORGAN

Figure 2–3. Neural patterns causing muscle spasm in response to pain. Nociceptive impulses ascend the peripheral nerves to the dorsal horn where they become modified at the various layers of Rexed. A mononeural reflex.

mine, substance P, and the many leukotrienes that are being reported almost weekly in the research literature. Substance P, somatokinin, vasoactive polypeptides, and cholecystokinin are all present in small-diameter unmyelinated primary afferents that terminate in the superficial dorsal horn. Substance P is the most studied of these peptides and its role of exciting transmission of the fibers that convey pain is well established.[11,12] Release of substance

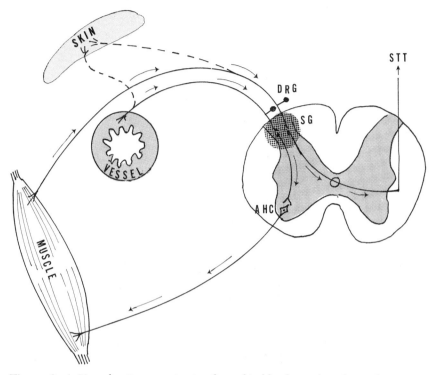

Figure 2–4. Neural patterns eminating from skin blood vessels and muscles causing spasm. The muscle held in a constant state of sustained contraction (*spasm*) liberates nociceptive substances that ascend through the dorsal root ganglion (DRG) into the substantiia gelatinosum (SG), then traverse to the spinothalamic tracts (STT) to the thalamus. A branch innervates the anterior horn cell (AHC), which causes further extrafusal muscle contraction. Muscle contraction causes ischemia with the liberation of lactic acid and substance P, thus becoming another site of sustained nociception.

P from the peripheral terminals[13] of these nerves produces the cutaneous wheal and flare so often noted in traumatic painful injury. Inhibition of this substance-P transmission and peripheral emission could enhance the therapeutic armamentarium in controlling pain.[14]

The nociceptive fibers terminate in laminae I through IV[15–17] (Fig. 2–5) of the dorsal horn, which is divided into five laminae. Areas of the dorsal horn of the spinal cord are innervated by both somatosensory and visceral autonomic fibers.

Lamina V has been identified as responding to both cutaneous and visceral nerve stimulation.[18] Strong cutaneous stimulation can effect activity of preganglionic autonomic neurons in the lateral horns of the spinal cord.[19] These connections between somatic and sympathetic (autonomous) systems are increasing in clinical significance in determination of the neurologic path-

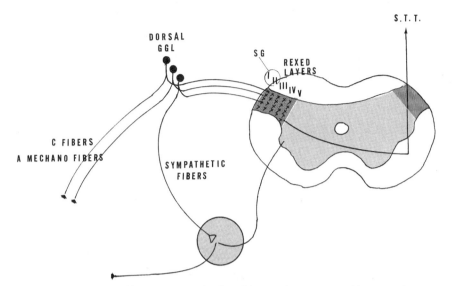

Figure 2–5. Sensory fibers entering the dorsal horn. The sensory C fibers, mechano A fibers, and sympathetic sensory afferent fibers enter the dorsal horn into the cord gray matter. The dorsal horn is divided into numerous Rexed layers with the main sensory fibers entering Rexed layers I and II, which constitutes the substantia gelatinosum (SG). Sensory impulses traverse the cord to ascend in the spinothalamic tracts (STT). One third of the unmyelinated C fibers are considered to enter the dorsal column through the motor roots of the anterior horn (not shown in this illustration).

ways of pain. Sympathetic discharges, fired over a long period of time, can initiate somatic muscular contractions, which become sites of nociception when their sustained contraction causes ischemia.

Two types of peripheral nociceptor fibers (fast and slow) have terminals in lamina V, although most terminate in laminae I to IV. The afferent nerves that transmit the impulses that will ultimately evoke the sensation of *pain* are mostly unmyelinated nerves (C fibers). Of all axons in cutaneous nerves, 80% are unmyelinated C fibers. These fibers conduct very slowly, enter the dorsal column, and immediately synapse with the neurons crossing through the anterior commissure to ascend to the thalamus through the spinothalamic tracts to the thalamus (Fig. 2–6). Of the remaining sensory nerves that can conduct noxious stimuli are myelinated nerves of small diameter. The larger diameter myelinated sensory nerves respond to innocuous mechanical stimuli such as touch, temperature, and proprioceptive stimuli.

Anatomists have demonstrated[20] that approximately one third of all afferent small diameter unmyelinated C fibers enter the cord through the anterior route. These fibers also have their cell bodies in DRG. This fact may well explain the mechanism of **muscle pain,** wherein descending motor fibers to the extrafusal fibers also carry ascending sensory fibers.

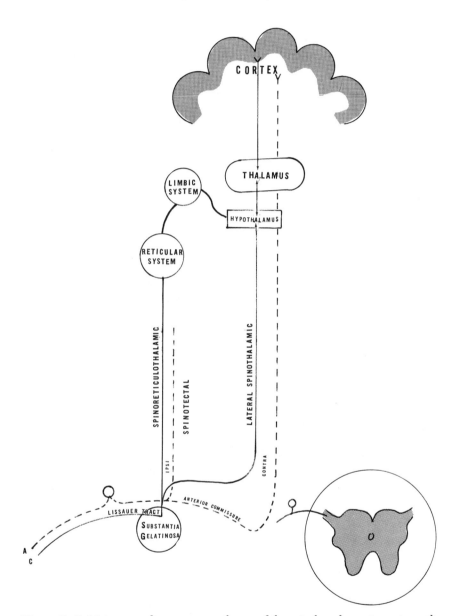

Figure 2–6. Major ascending sensory pathways of the spinal cord carrying pain mediating fibers. The major pathways for pain transmission are the spinothalamocortical systems that have spatiotemporal localization and the spinoreticulothalamic system that has no localization, but is involved in emotional (limbic) and avoidance reaction. Both ascend through the substantia gelatinosum of Lissauer's tract (now termed layers of Rexed I and II). The reticular system associates with the hypothalamic-limbic system and relates emotions with the sensation of pain.

Pain sensation is similarly transmitted through neurons of the A-delta neurons that synapse in the dorsal horn of the cord and proceed superiorly through the lateral spinothalamic tracts to the thalamus. Several sensations are transmitted through these spinothalamic tracts of which an estimated 54% are pain sensations and 46% are temperature sensations.

Unmyelinated C fibers are more numerous in the peripheral sensory fibers than are the A-delta fibers; they proceed cephalad in a different manner. The A-delta fibers have essentially one neuronal synapse, whereas the entering C fibers synapse with numerous short intersegmental neurons that ascend cephalad through multi-ascending synaptic pathways termed **MAS.** Some ascending paths are in the dorsal columns as well as in the anterolateral columns (Fig. 2–7).

There are at least two major pathways in the spinal cord that are involved in rostral projection of the pain message: the spinothalamic tract (STT) and

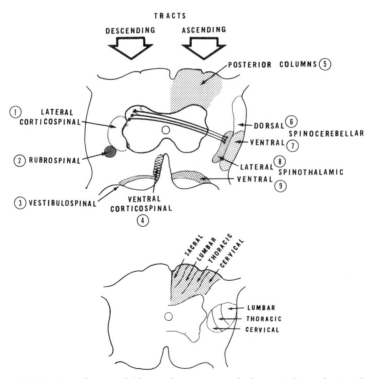

Figure 2–7. Ascending and descending tracts of the spinal cord. Besides the spinothalamic tracts (8) (9), there are numerous tracts that carry motor, sensory, and coordinating functions. All are needed for function, but not all transmit sensation or pain. (From Cailliet, R: Head and Face Pain Syndromes, ed 1. FA Davis, Philadelphia, 1992, p 187, with permission.)

the spinoreticulothalamic tract (SRTT). Both ascend within the same tract in the cord, but SRTT separates in the brain stem to synapse with neurons of the reticular system (Fig. 2–8). Activity of this latter pathway allegedly produces more diffuse and emotionally disturbing pains.[21]

Each of these tracts terminate at different sites within the thalamus. The spinoreticulothalamic tract is more medial, whereas the spinothalamic tract projects into the lateral, ventral, and caudal lobes (see Fig. 2–8). The two thalamic regions project to different cortical sites. The action of these projections remain unclear.

The speed of impulse's selectivity determines the type of pain transmitted. The A-delta fibers transmit faster and carry *sharp* pain; whereas the C fibers are slower and carry a *duller*, more enduring pain. In head and face pain, the trigeminal nerve consists of fibers that carry sharp pain. This nerve travels toward the thalamus within the lateral and trigeminal lemnisci, ending in the ventrobasal nucleus of the thalamus.

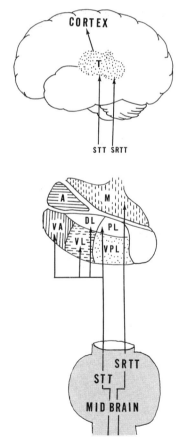

Figure 2–8. Thalamic pathways. The thalamus (T) is a large ovoid gray mass located on either side of the third ventricle. The anterior tubercle (A) is thin and lies close to the midline. The posterior portion is known as the pulvinar (P). From the cord, the ascending pathways that connect to the thalamus divide within the midbrain. They include the spinoreticulothalamic (SRTT) tract to the medial aspect of the thalamus and the spinothalamic tracts (STTs). They go directly to the lateral, ventral, and caudal regions. (A = anterior; VA = ventro anterior; DL = dorsolateral; VL = ventrolateral; PL = posterolateral; and VPL = ventroposterolateral.) From the thalamus, the pathways ascend to the cortex to as yet unknown areas of *representation*.

The ascending fibers of the multiple ascending system (MAS) synapse with neurons of the thalamocortical aspects of the thalamus (Fig. 2–9) then proceed to the reticular system (Fig. 2–10) in the midbrain, which processes diffuse fibers from all cranial nerves and upper motor-sensory brain system, including the cortex. The reticular system also relates to the hypothalamic and limbic systems, which interpose the emotions to the sensory system. The reticular system relates to another structure, the locus coeruleus (LC), located at the floor of the fourth ventricle that appears directly related to the emotions of fear and anxiety, as well as being involved in pain modulation. This area is thoroughly evaluated in this text.

The thalamus divides into two major systems: the ventrobasal and the dorsal, consisting of the lateral and posterior nuclei which receive fast conducting impulses. This system is topographically organized, meaning that received sensations relate to specific points of the face, head, and body. The neurons receiving the impulses of the MAS are not specifically organized. The latter fibers radiate to the general cerebral cortex. The limbic system is concerned with memory and emotions.

Significant findings[9] have emerged regarding the neural pathways to the thalamus as a result of percutaneous cordotomies and ultimate pathologic studies. Anterolateral cordotomy in monkeys (Fig. 2–11) produced degeneration of the ipsilateral nucleus ventralis of the thalamus. Studies made with horseradish peroxidase demonstrated that 83% of the ventrothalamic tracts terminate in the ipsilateral thalamic nuclei. Bowsher in 1983[17] demonstrated that patients who underwent cordotomy for treatment of pain had massive

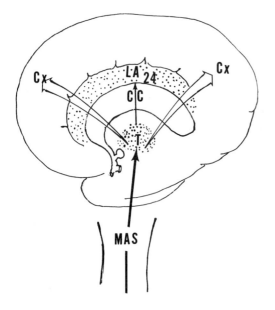

Figure 2–9. Thalamocortical projections. From the multiple ascending system (MAS) of the cord the tracts ascend to the thalamus (T) from which there are pathways to the limbic system (LA) thence to the cortical area (Cx). The limbic regions of the cingula above the corpus callosum (CC) are numbered according to the Brodmann designation (24). (*See* Fig. 51 In Gilman, S, and Winans, SS (Eds). Manter and Gatz's Essentials of Clinical Neuroanatomy and Neurophysiology, ed 6. FA Davis, Philadelphia, 1982, p. 178)

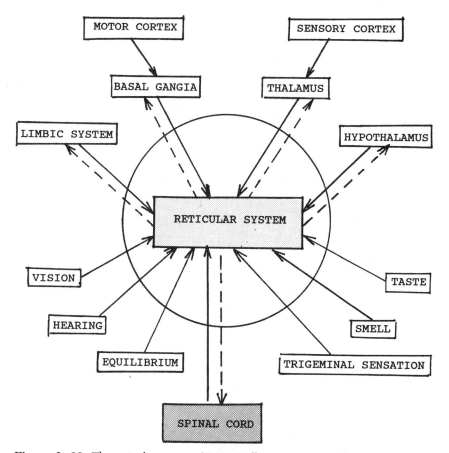

Figure 2-10. The reticular system. (From Cailliet, R: Pain: Mechanisms and Management. FA Davis, Philadelphia, 1993, p 11, with permission.)

bilateral degeneration of cells in the medial reticular formation (medulla) as well as some degeneration in the pons. He, however, reported only sparse degeneration in the thalamus.

These recent studies are significant, because the pain issues from the anteriolateral tracts (i.e., contralateral) of the cord being stimulated peripherally with noxious impulses. Because of the contralateral pathways of these ascending cord pathways, the finding that 17% of the ascending fibers are ipsilateral is considered significant. There are also direct or contralateral projections of spinothalamic tracts to the posterior thalamus and the periaqueductal gray area (PAG), the functional significance of which remains unknown.

Stimulation of the ipsilateral nucleus ventralis *does not elicit pain*, whereas stimulation of the more medial intralaminal nuclei does. The interrelationship between these two thalamic projections remains in need of greater study.

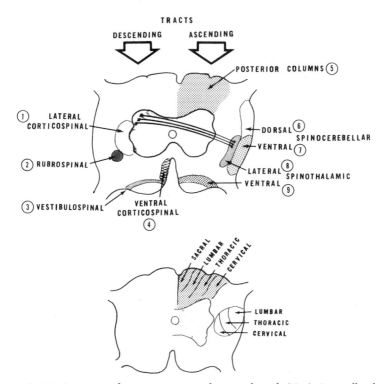

Figure 2–11. Sensory and motor tracts on the spinal cord. (*Top*) Generally, the descending tracts (1, 2, 3, 4) are for motor skills or for coordination. The ascending tracts (5, 6, 7, 8, 9) carry sensation from the periphery to the higher centers. (*Bottom*) The ascending tracts convey the sensations of pain, touch, proprioception, and discrimination for interpretation. Areas of the extremities are conveyed by the ascending (*shaded area*) and descending (lumbar, thoracic, and cervical) tracts. (From Cailliet, R: Head and Face Pain Syndromes, ed 1. FA Davis, Philadelphia, 1992, p 187, with permission.)

Cordotomy, which decreases cerebro blood flow (CBF) to the thalamus,[9] may alter the synaptic activity of the entering spinothalamic tract impulses. After successful cordotomy, CBF increases. Injecting glycerol into the trigeminal ganglion in the treatment of intractible trigeminal neuralgia has also been found to increase CBF.[22,23] This is further evidence that peripheral pain mechanisms perform with simultaneous associated central mechanisms.

The afferent fibers that enter the dorsal horn relays the information (see Fig. 2–9, marked with +) of the nociception. These are termed **projection (transmission) fibers.** This *information* is complex and originates from both nociception and non-nociception, thus also conveying other more innocuous sensations. In the dorsal roots, besides unmyelinated sensory fibers carrying nociceptor impulses, there are afferent myelinated fibers which enter the dorsal horn of the cord carrying *inhibitory* (−) impulses (Fig. 2–12).

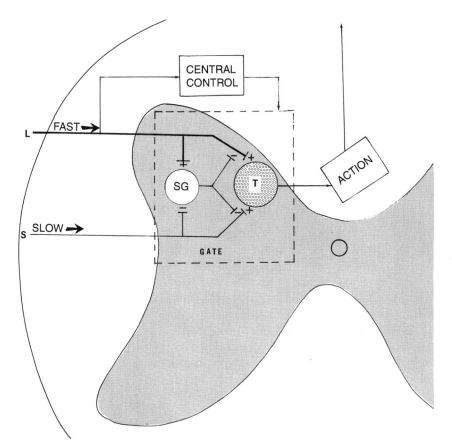

Figure 2–12. Nociceptive transmission and inhibition at the dorsal horn level. The shaded area is the dorsal horn region of the cord (the layers of Rexed of which regions I and II are the substantia gelatinosum (SG). The sensory fibers carrying nociceptive (C *neuron slow pain*) impulses activate (+) the SG, which then proceed to the fibers ascending to the reticular formation through the spinoreticulothalamic tracts and the spinothalamic tracts (STT) to the thalamus and reticular system. These impulses ultimately are interpreted as *pain*. Neuron fast fibers and mechano A neuron fast fibers enter the dorsal root and stimulate inhibitory (−) fibers (L) that modulate the severity of the slower acting C neuron fibers. The gray area is the *gate* area.

MODULATION

The large myelinated fibers as they enter the dorsal horn essentially *moderate* (inhibit) the nociceptive impulses transmitted through the unmyelinated fibers (C-fibers). This situation explains the efficacy of transcutaneous electrical nerve stimulation (TENS), which is carried by the large myelinated fibers.

If the large myelinated fibers are interrupted, the uninhibited nociceptive fiber impulses cause the pain to become more severe. This indicates that peripheral stimuli, both noxious and innocuous, reach the dorsal horn, where they are modulated. A noxious stimulus is transmitted through all the sensory fibers, both unmyelinated and myelinated. Such sensations are modulated at the cord level. The concept of pain modulation has been titled the **Wall-Melzak Gate Theory** (see Fig. 2–12). The modulation occurs at the dorsal horn level, but is now also known to occur at the dorsal root level and at more central levels in the midbrain.

Intrinsic factors in the system that modulate pain exist. The study of these increases understanding of how narcotics, analgesic drugs, and certain physical modalities work. Endogenous opioid substances are now considered to be synthesized by and within nerve cells. Substances which mimic the action of narcotics and analgesics are termed **endorphins (enkephalins).**

Fields and Levine[24] pose interesting questions that remain unanswered: Why does the brain need this pain-modulating system? When is it activated? How are its actions manifested?

Enkephalins that act at the peripheral neural sites are also present at the dorsal root ganglia, spinal cord, midbrain, hypothalamus, PAG, and the rostral medulla.[25] The first neuropeptides discovered were leucine and methionine enkephalin. They are currently classified as amino acids (glutaminic acid and aspartic acid). These amino acids act upon receptor sites (N-methyl-D-aspartic acid) (NMDA) at the dorsal horn.[20] Hyperactivity of the central receptors can be initiated by electrical stimulation of C fibers, which apparently occurs through these NMDA receptors.[22] Such hyperexcitability can be prevented by administration of antagonists (i.e., 3-[2-carboxypiperazin-4-yl]propyl-1-phosphoric acid [D-CPP] NMDA antagonists).[26] Ketamine, a noncompetitive NMDA antagonist, has been considered effective in reducing postoperative pain.[26] Drugs with activity similar to Ketamine's are now being sought. Other receptor sites are also being researched.

Other neurochemical mediators from tissue damage have been found to initiate hyperexcitability of the central nervous system—their antagonists could afford promise in pain management. Among other numerous endorphins, norepinephrine and serotonin can be added.

Serotonin (5-hydroxytryptamine) has been divided into three main families—specified as types 1, 2, and 3—each having a subtype of receptor. The dorsal raphe in the midbrain has the highest concentration of 5-hydroxytryptamine-1a receptors in the brain.

The hypothalamus may be the activation site for migraine and cluster headaches wherein the posterior thalamus, which contains cells that regulate autonomic function, is closely related to the anterior hypothalamus, which contains the suprachiasmic nuclei that serve as the principal circadian pacemaker functions in mammals. This may explain the rhythmic pattern of many types of pain, including time-related cluster headaches. This hypothalamic pacemaker is mediated by the serotonergic system: the 5-hydroxytryptamine system.[27]

The International Association for the Study of Pain (IASP)[28] has characterized neural pain mechanisms along five site axes: (1) site of pain; (2) physiologic system; (3) temporal pattern and recurrence; (4) intensity and duration; and (5) etiology.[29]

All the above neurologic mechanisms have been postulated based on the mechanism described first by Foster and Sherrington in 1897,[30] implying that all *messages* transmitted within the CNS are transduced electrically. This occurs in the numerous synapses (Fig. 2–13) along the course of the nerves wherein chemical messages are converted into chemical (metabolic) forces before they revert to electrical impulses. These *messages* are considered to be diffuseable molecules termed **neurotransmitters**.

According to this concept, the postsynaptic neuron integrates thousands of signals by depolarization at the synapse with generation of an action potential. This constituted the "neuron theory" of Waldeyer and Cajal.[31] In Luciani,[32] Golgi partially refuted their findings and offered his *reticular network theory*, terming his concept **functional syncytium. Syncytium** is itself defined[33] as "a group of cells in which the protoplasm of one cell is continuous with that of adjoining cells."

A more provocative concept of neural transmission has been proposed[34] which questions the accuracy of the concept of electrical continuity of presynaptic and postsynaptic transmissions. This has been highlighted by electron microscopic studies. This concept as proposed accepts transmission within the neural network (as described by Waldeyer and Cajal) but it also postulates diffusion of electrochemical signals through the extracellular medium.

Figure 2–13. The synapse. The wiring transmission (WT) functions by electrical stimulations of the preganglionic bulb (PR), which is charged with numerous vesicles (V) containing acetylcholine. When released across the synaptic space (SS), they cause depolarization of the postganglionic membrane (PS), thus causing electrical-chemical direct neurotransmission. (From Cailliet, R: Pain: Mechanism and Management, ed 1. FA Davis, Philadelphia, 1993, with permission.)

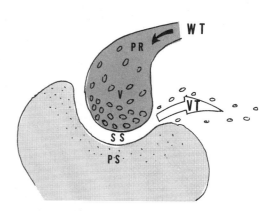

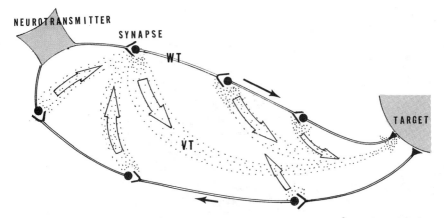

Figure 2–14. Neurotransmission: wiring transmission versus volume transmission (schematic). Direct neurotransmission resembling a direct wire transmission (WT) is depicted as going directly to its specific receptor (*dark arrows*), albeit through synapses. Chemical neurotransmitters allegedly *leak* at each synapse and enter the interstitial spaces and chemically find their receptors. This transmission goes in afferent and efferent directions (*white arrows*).

This finding both supports Golgi's concept and does not refute the ultimate transmission of impulses through the CNS, the hypothalamus, and the thalamus. It does, however, question the medium through which transmission occurs. The former system is termed **wiring transmission** (WT), the latter **volume transmission** (VT) (Fig. 2–14).

Signals are conducted electrically and chemically through the extracellular fluid. Anatomic direct pathways cannot be identified, although the signal release site and the target can be (Fig. 2–15). The WT system fails to support

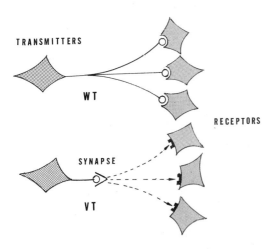

Figure 2–15. Wire transmission versus volume transmission. The wiring transmission (WT) indicates a specific connection from the neurotransmitter to its specific receptor organ. In the volume transmission (VT), the chemical neurotransmitters leave the synapse and are free to find a receptor wherever and however numerous as they are. VT and WT do not replace each other; they merely enhance each other.

morphologic coupling between neurotransmitter release sites and receptor sites (Fig. 2–16). The presynaptic nerve is thought to couple with numerous postsynaptic receptors, which may lead to the use of the term **transmitter-receptor mismatch.** [35,36]

The VT concept relies on a specific target's being present to accept the specific transmitted impulse being admitted through an ill-defined transmission system. According to this system concept, *coding* must exist.[37] The efficacy of VT over WT has been computed to state that VT transmits at a lower speed of transmission and has a higher degree of divergence; but because it relies on a limited number of transmission lines (axons) and limited number of switches (synapses), it functions with significantly lower biologic cost. The type of energy used in the process of transmission has not yet been ascertained.

Proof of the presence of VT transmission has been the finding that a complex neuropeptide such as NPY (neuropeptide Y) injected through microcannulae into the striatum was able to reach distances longer than 1 mm at a dosage sufficient to make it an active neurotransmitter. Its ultimate presence initiates sustained modulation of CNS receptors, thus creating a *syndrome response.*[38,39]

Principles of *analgesia* resulting in insensitivity to pain without loss of consciousness is affected at all levels of the CNS and affected by a *descending pain control system.*[40]

Stress has been invoked as influencing pain perception both objectively

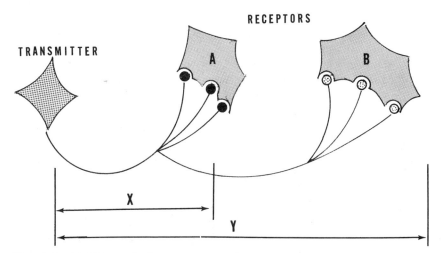

Figure 2–16. "Mismatched" transmitters and receptors: a concept. Mismatching neurotransmitters and receptors are schematically postulated. The distance a neurotransmitter must go varies. Distance X to receptor A obviously transmits the *message* faster than to receptor B at a distance of Y. Receptor A allegedly has a greater affinity than does receptor B, which explains the transmission.

and subjectively. Two neuroendocrine systems have been asserted to be in-volved in the coping mechanism against stress: the hypothalamopituitary-adrenocortical and the hypothalamosympathoadrenocortical. The roles of these two systems are mediated by medullary-pontine catecholamine neurons and by corticotropin-releasing hormone (CRH) neurons.[41,42] The intricacy of these transport systems causes somatic visceral responses to stress to involve several neuronal systems of transportation triggering syndrome responses. Both the WT and the VT systems are involved.

The older concept of a single isolated system of afferent transmission re-lating to pain mechanisms is therefore no longer tenable. This concept was oversimplistic and more recent studies of systems involving *another* now have evolved to answer such perplexing questions as why pain returns after a surgi-cal lesion of ascending pathways has been successfully performed for the relief of pain.

The basis of the *psychophysiologic* aspect of pain is clearer as to the mechanism whereby chemical substances and hormones subsequently re-leased affect receptor sensitivity. Systemic opioids and epidural administration that are effective at the cord level now allude to a VT transmission, as well as providing an effect through the WT system.

ROLE OF THE CEREBRAL CORTEX IN PAIN PERCEPTION

A provocative theory in the role of the brain in perceiving pain has been offered by Melzack.[43] He questions the more prevalent theory that holds that the brain acts as a passive receptor of information from the outside. He does not question the current concepts of transmission but indeed accepts them. *How* the brain interprets the external impulses is his central concern.

The direct ascent of sensation to the brain was postulated by Descartes in the 17th century (Fig. 2–17).[44] He held that the brain was the center of sensa-tion and further postulated that pain was transmitted to the brain by means of small threads running from the skin to the brain. The emphasis was on the pe-riphery: receptors, fibers, nociceptive and other peripheral substances and pathways of the cord, the midbrain, and finally the cortex. This theory did not explain why paraplegics and quadriplegics *feel* their bodies without any trans-mission from nerves. Melzack postulated that "the brain can generate every quality of experience which is normally triggered by sensory input."[45]

Although stimulation from the periphery can initiate sensory patterns; it cannot produce them. Melzack postulates that patterns (pain) are present in the brain *substrate* with genetic specifications modified by experience. This substrate is composed of a widespread network of neurons between the thala-mus and the cortex termed a **neuromatrix.** The repeated cyclic processing and synthesis of the impulses surging through the neuromatrix form a **neu-**

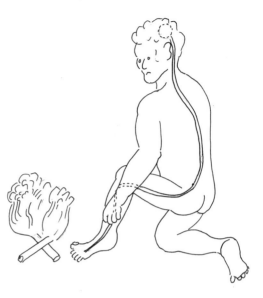

Figure 2–17. Kneeling man perceiving pain (Descartes). The kneeling figure of Descartes (1596–1650) depicts a burning sensation irritating the filaments of a nerve in the foot, which then ascends to the brain through filaments of that nerve. (René Descartes' illustration from "De l'homme." Modified by the author.)

rosignature. A sentient neural hub converts the flow of these neurosignatures into a flow of *awareness* which in its turn activates an action neuromatrix; that is, a pattern of movements influenced by awareness: in this instance, pain.

The neuromatrix reflects patterns felt and experienced as a *whole body*. Melzack states: "We do not learn to feel qualities of experience: our brains are built to produce them." This concept is consistent with the molecular concept of neural activity postulated by Black,[46] according to which environmental regulators effect changes in existing genetically encoded molecular structures.

Black's molecular concept gives insight into how the brain understands sensation from the periphery. He and Melzack both postulate that the human body as a whole is encoded in molecular structures within the CNS that is being constantly modified by external impulses.

Since the advent of PET, a test that ascertains the precise area of CBF, the region of the brain activated by peripheral stimulation can be determined. Evidence now exists that the frontal lobe is involved after a noxious electrical stimulus. Painful peripheral heat application also activates the anterior cingulate gyrus (a portion of the limbic system), as well as the primary and secondary somatosensory cortices, thus suggesting their participation in pain perception. The primary cortices are known to be involved in mechanoreception. Hormones have also been implicated in pain perception. Hormones produced by endocrine glands have been known to act upon distant organs, including the brain (Fig. 2–18).

Neurotransmitters have been termed **paraneurons** because their secretions are substantially similar to hormones. Hormones, structurally, are proteins or polypeptides, similar to adrenocorticosteroids (ACTH), thyroxine, beta endorphin, and steroids. The latter compounds exert their effect in a

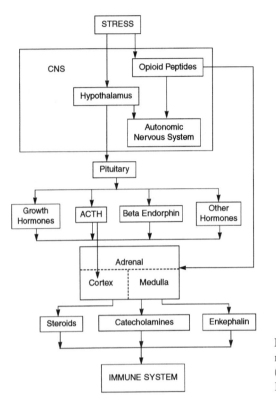

Figure 2–18. Sequence of neurohormonal aspects of stress. (Modified from Shavity et al: J Immunol 135:8368, 1985.)

tonic manner over a long period, whereas paraneurons act phasically in durations of milliseconds.

Tonic hormones are elevated in response to various physical and psychic stresses.[47,48] Their neuroanatomic site of action lies within the limbic midbrain and the ascending reticular system.

Not yet fully understood is the relationship of pain to *chronobiology*, that is, circadian rhythms. The identification of the central role of the hypothalamus in the regulation of circadian rhythms has raised the possibility that neural pathways pass temporally through the supraoptic nuclei (SON) to the hypothalamus.[49] Destruction of the SON has interrupted the circadian cycle in the rat. It is known that patients with depression have disruption of their regulation of the sleep-wake cycle attributable to dysfunction of the circadian rhythm.[50]

CHRONIC PAIN MECHANISMS

Acute pain relates to *recurrent pain* and ultimately can become *chronic pain*. Any pain that lasts longer than 3 months has been considered chronic, but that arbitrary distinction of duration is now varied. Some pain states are considered as chronic after shorter periods, and some pain of longer duration is arbitrarily considered chronic, although it is not so labeled.

The process by which acute or recurrent pain becomes chronic requires an understanding of the mechanisms of pain already discussed. The concept that pain is a specific sensation and that its intensity is proportional to the degree of tissue (noxious) damage is no longer tenable. Pain is a sensory experience influenced by attention, expectancy, learning, anxiety, fear, and distraction.

Selection and modification of the sensory component of noxious transmission is neurologically accepted (see Fig. 2–6) but the receptive system of the dorsal horn and every higher level is directly influenced by the same conditions that influence pain (Fig. 2–19).

As stated, emotions do affect the peripheral ventral mechanisms of pain transmission through the limbic system, which affects the descending tracts to the dorsal horn of the cord and ascending tracts to the thalamus (lateral spinothalamic tracts and spinoreticulothalamic tracts), then to the cortex (Fig. 2–20).[51] These emotions are basically divisible into three categories: (1) per-

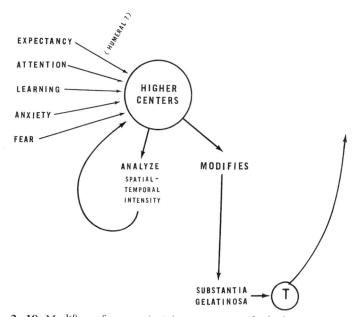

Figure 2–19. Modifiers of sensory (pain) transmission. The higher centers that interpret pain as a sensation are modified by humeral factors that involve expectation, attention, learning, anxiety, and fear. These factors modify and analyze sensation in the gray matter level (SG) of the cord, at the thalamus-hypothalamus (T), and at the cortical level.

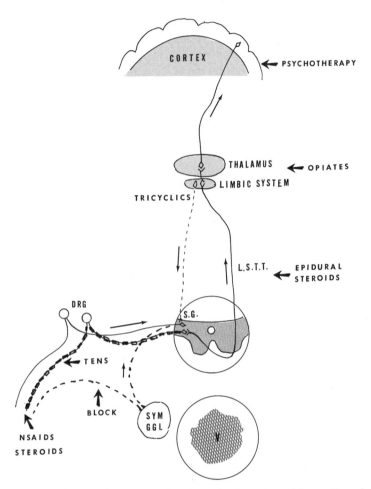

Figure 2–20. Pharmacologic sites of action of pain pattern interruption. Aspirin, steroid, and nonsteroid sites of action are at the peripheral areas of noxious tissue injury. The myelinated nerves respond to TENS. The sympathetic nerves transmitting pain respond to sympathetic blocks. The lateral spinothalamic tracts (LSTTs) are the site of epidural steroids and analgesic agents, and the thalamus is the site of opioid effectiveness. Psychotherapy influences the interpretation of pain at the level of the cortex. Tricyclic drugs and other antidepressants affect the descending tracts to the dorsal root (substantia gelatinosum [SG]) as well as at the dorsal root ganglia (DRG).

ceptual information locating the site of the noxious insult; (2) motivational tendency that indicates a need for reaction by the patient; and (3) cognitive information based on previous information.[52]

    Perceptual information implies the significance of the tissue damaged and its sequelae. Motivational causes, that is, fight or flight, and cognitive information involve previous experiences and their sequelae. Anxiety, anger, depression, and other emotions are involved. Treatment must consider and attack all such sources of pain.

Pain is modulated by chemical substances, which are secreted by nerve cells (endorphins) which can be experimentally blocked by naloxone. This finding has shed much light on pain caused by trauma, stress, anxiety, and depression and has clarified the inhibition of pain within the CNS.

Chronic pain has for too long been viewed by the medical profession as an organic-psychogenic dichotomy. It must now be considered as a complicated synthesis of biologic, psychologic, behavioral, and neurohormonal-chemical factors.

PAIN MEDIATED THROUGH THE SYMPATHETIC NERVOUS SYSTEM

Most of the nervous system is under voluntary control and is concerned with activation of the skeletal muscle system. It also transmits sensory impulses from the periphery for feedback information during neuromuscular activities and for interpretation of noxious stimuli. A division of the sympathetic nervous system controls the activities of smooth muscles, cardiac musculature, and glandular secretion. This is the autonomic nervous system (ANS) which is not under voluntary control. The role of noxious sensory transmission by the ANS currently remains unconfirmed.

The functional anatomy of the ANS is well documented (Fig. 2–21)[53] as regards its sensory and motor functions.

The ANS consists of the central portion at the cortical, midbrain, spinal cord, and peripheral levels. The peripheral portion consists of preganglionic and postganglionic efferent and afferent fibers. In this section, only the relationship of the ANS to the sensation of *pain*, will be emphasized.[53]

The ANS fibers transmit visceral sensations such as nociception, nausea, and satiation. The concept[54] that the ANS was restricted to an efferent function has been refuted. To accept the fact that function can be maintained by merely efferent nerve input denies that normal function, albeit a reflexive one, requires *feedback* through afferent fiber function.

The peripheral efferent pathways of the ANS, unlike the single fiber of the somatic nervous system to the skeletal muscle fibers, consist of two neuronal connections: primary presynaptic (preganglionic) and a secondary postsynaptic (postganglionic) (Fig. 2–22). The cell bodies of the axons start as groups located in the brain stem and spinal cord. As they proceed toward their peripheral destinations, they pass through various ganglia at which points they synapse to new fibers that eventually proceed to the effector organs (Fig. 2–23).

Preganglionic fibers leave the brain stem and spinal cord at three levels:

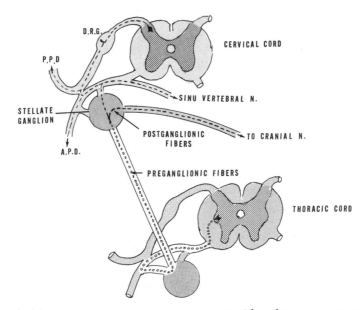

Figure 2–21. Autonomic nervous system: anatomic. The white preganglionic fibers originate from the intermediolateral horn cells of the thoracic cord and ascend to the stellate ganglia where they synapse with the postganglionic gray fibers. There are sympathetic fibers that accompany the somatic within the anterior primary divisions (APD) and the posterior primary divisions (PPD) of the nerve roots. Sensory nerve roots enter the dorsal column through the dorsal root ganglia (DRG). Sympathetic nerves carry the sensation of pain (paresthesia) and are motored to the blood vessels, sweat, and pilatory glands.

cranial outflow, thoracolumbar outflow, and *sacral outflow.* The cranial and sacral portions form the **parasympathetic system** in contradistinction to the thoracolumbar which is the **sympathetic system.**

Cranial outflow consists of the nucleus of Edinger-Westphal, the nucleus of Perlia, and the dorsal motor nucleus of the vagal system originating within the midbrain, the pons and the medulla. They proceed to synapse in the following ganglia: the *celiac, oculomotor, pterygopalatine, submandibular,* and *otic.* These, in turn, divide into the facial nerve and the glossopharyngeal nerve to innervate facial structure.[3]

The other parasympathetic system is the sacral outflow (S2, S3, S4) forming the pelvic nerve (N. erigentes). None of these segments contribute to the ANS. They form the *parasympathetic system* as distinguished from the *sympathetic system.*

The function of neurons is considered to be the axonal transport of protein along the length of the nerve fiber (Fig. 2–24). This transported protein

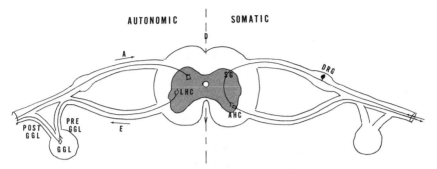

Figure 2–22. Autonomic compared with somatic. The *left side* depicts the autonomic nervous system with the afferent A (*arrow*) entering the gray matter of the cord dorsal (D) and the efferent (E) (*arrow*) originating at the lateral horn cell (LHC). The efferent fibers are preganglionic (pre GGL); after leaving the autonomic ganglion (GGL), they become the postganglionic fibers (post GGL). The somatic (*right side*) afferent enters the dorsal root ganglion (DRG) and then enters the cord at the substantia gelatinosus (SG). The efferent (motor) fibers originate from the anterior horn cells (AHC) from the ventral (V) aspect of the gray matter.

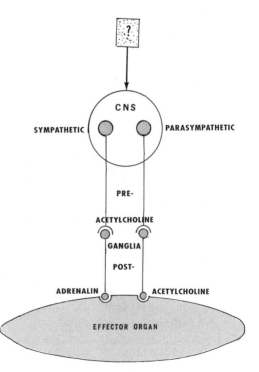

Figure 2–23. Transmission sequence of the peripheral autonomic nervous system. The box (?) represents the transmitter substance from numerous sources that initiate autonomic impulses in the sympathetic central nervous system (CNS). Acetylcholine is liberated at the termination of the preganglionic and the postganglionic fibers upon the effector organ, whereas the sympathetic postganglionic fibers release adrenalin upon the effector organ.

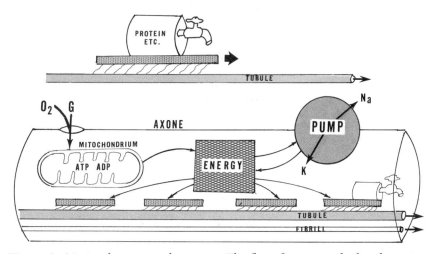

Figure 2–24. Axoplasmic neural transport. The *flow* of protein and other derivatives begin with the entry of glucose (G) into the fiber. Glycolysis and phosphorylation occur (O₂) in the mitochondria through metabolism of adenosine-triphosphate (ATP), which creates the energy to the sodium pump. This pump regulates the balance of sodium (Na) and potassium (K) and determines nerve activity. The transport *filaments* (tubule and fibrill) move along the axon by oscillation and carry the nutritive protein elements along the nerve pathway. (Data from Ochs, S: Axoplasmic transport: A Basis for Neural Pathology. In Dyck, PJ, Thomas, PK, Lambert, EN (eds): Peripheral Neuropathy. WB Saunders, Philadelphia, 1975, pp 213–230.)

tissue depends greatly on an adequate blood supply. Pressure on the nerve axon causes blood vessel impairment and thus also impairs axonal transportation.

The terminals of the parasympathetic system liberate acetylcholine and so are termed **cholinergic.** The postganglionic sympathetic fibers (except those connected to sweat glands) liberate epinephrine-like substances. Many organ systems receive supply from both sympathetic and parasympathetic systems with opposing action, wherein the effect depends upon the receiving organ.

The preganglionic fibers of the sympathetic division leave the spinal cord along with other motor fibers of the ventral root but soon separate from those of the ventral roots to form **white rami communicantes** (Fig. 2–25). These fibers pass on to the ganglia, which are long, ganglionated chains of nerve fibers extending along either side of the vertebral column throughout its entire length. Many of these white rami terminate in ganglia, although some do not synapse at these sites but instead proceed onwards to synapse within the ganglia of the specific organ system (celiac or mesenteric). The postganglionic fibers, after synapse, form plexi that envelop the large blood vessels supplying the viscera. One example is that the lower fibers forming the hypogastric

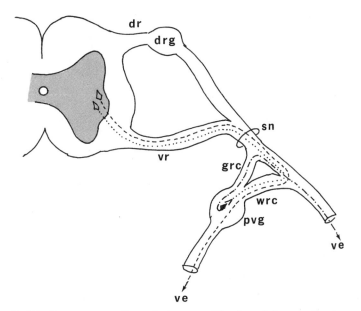

Figure 2–25. Components of a spinal nerve. The lateral horn cells, from which emerge the autonomic nerves, are located in the gray matter of the cord. The dorsal root ganglia (drg) is the site of the emergence of the somatic nerve (dr).The afferent autonomic nerves emerge through the ventral root onto the spinal nerve (sn), which then proceeds to the paravertebral ganglia (pvg). The preganglionic fibers enter the ganglia through the white ramus communicans (wrc) where some proceed without synapse and others synapse to reenter the spinal nerve through the gray ramus communicans (grc). These fibers proceed down the primary division of the nerve root. (ve = visceral efferent nerves.)

plexus which enters the pelvis and innervates the rectum, bladder, and reproductive organs.

Postganglionic fibers are unmyelinated and so are termed **gray rami communicantes.** Each spinal nerve receives a gray ramus fiber which innervates specific blood vessels and sweat glands in its region. A major function of the sympathetic nervous system that can cause a generalized bodily reaction is its supply to the adrenal gland, which liberates epinephrine in addition to other epinephrine secreted at its terminals.

The medulla of the adrenal gland is innervated by preganglionic fibers that do not synapse in any intervening ganglia. This involvement of the nerve supply in the glandular system of the body explains the association of epinephrine secretion resulting from rage, fear, anger, and reaction to exposure to cold. It also explains the cardiac reaction related to pulse rate and blood pressure, dilation, and constriction of the coronary blood vessels, bronchioles of the pulmonary system, and even to contraction of the spleen in releasing red blood cells to the body.

In 1933 Cannon and Rosenbleuth[55] postulated that there must be two classes of *sympathin*: one excitatory and the other inhibitory. This thesis has now been proven, whereas norepinephrine is the principal postganglionic sympathetic transmitter and epinephrine, in smaller doses, is liberated at the sympathetic nerve endings.

Epinephrine acts on two separate types of receptors termed **alpha** and **beta.** Activation of alpha receptors produces effects blocked by ergotamine and also affects vasoconstriction, uterine contraction, and pupillary dilatation. Beta activation causes vasodilitation, cardiac acceleration, and relaxation of the bronchioles. In comparing action, epinephrine works equally on both receptors,[56] whereas norepinephrine acts almost exclusively on alpha receptors. The process by which epinephrine and norepinephrine are deactivated after release remains unknown.[57] The term **adrenergic blockade**[58] implies blocking the catecholamine neurohumeral transmission system at any of its sites of action. It originally was considered to be destroyed by the enzyme amine oxidase with reserpine initially recognized as the blocking agent. These agents either inhibit synthesis, storage, or release.

Control of the final common pathway of sympathetic release is currently believed to be the Locus Coeruleus (LC).[58,59] The LC is a small band of neurons[60] located at the base of the fourth ventricle within the brain substance. The fourth ventricle is a (Fig. 2–26) cavity bordered ventrally by the pons and dorsally by the cerebellum. It is connected to the third ventricle by the aqueduct of Sylvius and caudally to the central canal of the medulla. The floor, known as the *rhomboid fossa*, is formed by the dorsal surfaces of the pons,

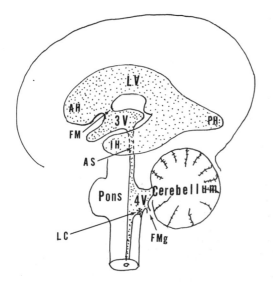

Figure 2–26. The ventricular system of the brain. A schematic illustration of the ventricular system of the brain containing the spinal fluid. (LV = lateral ventricle; ASH = anterior horn; PH = posterior horn; IH = inferior horn; FM = foramen of Monro; 3V = third ventricle; AS = aqueduct of Sylvius; 4V = fourth ventricle; FMg = foramen of Magendie; LC = site of locus coeruleus neurons.)

medulla oblongata, and the lateral boundaries of the floor by the cerebellar peduncles. Within this area, the LC is located.

The LC is composed of many neurons containing the highest density of norepinephrine within the neurons of the brain.[61] When stimulated, the LC liberates norepinephrine to the cerebrum,[62] limbic system, brain stem, and spinal cord, which tends to create symptoms of anxiety and fear. When ablated, there is an attenuation of these emotions[63]: the *alarm system* role of the LC.[64] The LC may be the *final pathway* for the manifestation of psychologic stress, physical trauma, immune imbalance, and even viral infection, causing a sympathetic-parasympathetic nervous system imbalance.[65]

In a state of anxiety, the LC remains on *constant alert* with resultant depletion of the postganglionic presynaptic sympathetic endplates leading to a condition termed **sympatheticotonia.** This is considered prevalent in many disease states,[65] some of which are involved in chronic pain states.

Stimulation of the LC, in animals, has raised questions as to whether the adjacent nonadrenogenic neurons in the region of the fourth ventricle are stimulated or ablated, thus causing the reaction attributed to specific LC neurons. This site of action has also been questioned by norepinephrine's blocking of the postsynaptic norepinephrine release by propranolol, a beta blocker.[66]

The presence of anxiety has been invoked in the mechanism of acute and chronic pain. Darwin[67] in 1872, in a discussion of fear merging with terror, described physiologic changes involving the sympathetic nervous system. Epinephrine was implicated as the stimulating factor.[68] Failure of infusion of epinephrine to induce emotional symptoms caused Cannon[69] to postulate CNS mechanisms. The limbic system was considered as also being involved.[70]

Besides the involvement of the LC in anxiety, other areas of the parietal lobe of the brain have also been implicated. Brodmann area 24 of the cortical region has been related to the control of the emotions, as well as affective response to pain.[71] This area receives ipsilateral projections from the ventral border of the thalamus, which has been implicated in the reception of nociceptive impulses. Neurosurgical resection of this cortical area in patients with intractible pain has allowed the patient to continue to acknowledge pain but to "complain less."[72]

Studies[73] have determined that temporal and spatial features of pain occur in the parietal area of the brain and that an emotional reaction to pain occurs in the limbic region of the frontal lobes.

There are two neuroendocrine systems: the hypothalamopituitary-adrenocortical and the hypothalamosympathoadrenomedullary. Both affect stress in the transmission of pain.[74] A corticotropin-releasing hormone (CRH) may be the main chemical that triggers the neuroendocrine response to stress,[74] which is mediated through the VA and VT systems acting upon its target.[75]

A reason formerly given for the delay in recognizing pain as emanating from the autonomic system was "its lack of neurotomal distribution of symptomatology."[76] Review of the mechanisms of the autonomic nervous system in dealing with pain has clarified the problem.[77-79]

Leriche[80] electrically stimulated the cervical sympathetic trunk between the occiput and the middle ganglion. This provoked painful anxiety, but without dermatomal distribution. Such stimulation produced severe pain in teeth in the lower jaw and behind the ipsilateral ear.

In patients suffering from spinal cord severance (quadriplegics) or those under the effects of spinal anesthesia, constriction of the arteries caused pain. Considering arteries to be *sensitive*, the researchers alluded[80] that this phenomenon was a "sympathalgia." These *zones*, termed **topographic,** were considered to be the region of the vascular area supplied and were associated by vasomotor, sudomotor, and trophic changes.[81]

Three indications suggest the relevance of sympathetic nervous system involvement in pain.

1. Neuropathic pain is frequently exacerbated by stimuli, such as a startle reflex or other acute emotional activities that evoke sympathetic discharges. It has been questioned whether a sympathetic discharge exacerbates or maintains the pain.[1] Hu and Zhu[82] demonstrated that nociceptors discharging after prolonged noxious stimulation (thus being alogenic), are further excited by sympathetic discharge and norepinephrine discharge. This finding also helps to explain that although the sympathetic nervous system may exacerbate and prolong the pain, it may not necessarily begin nor mediate it.

2. Neuropathic pain is frequently accompanied by signs and symptoms that indicate abnormal sympathetic activity, such as excessive vasomotor reactions or sweating. In this respect, a causalgic hand that is pale, cold, and cyanotic (usually considered as evidence of sympathetic vasoconstriction) may actually result from circulating catecholamines *caused by* vasoconstriction. The opposite sign, a hot, erythematous, causalgic hand usually considered to be sympathetically caused by vasodilatation may in fact be erythematous because of antidromic vasodilatation resulting from C-fiber nociceptor sensitization.

3. Relief from pain has often been achieved by interrupting the sympathetic nervous system by chemical or surgical means. This is true in some, and in fact in many, cases, but it is not true in all. Some think this interruption, whether surgical or chemical, may interrupt contiguous afferent nerve fibers running along the sympathetic fibers.

What has indicated a sympathetic influence in the provocation of pain is the finding that a regenerating axon from an injured or severed nerve forms **spouts**[83] (Fig. 2–27), which develop sensitivity to norepinephrine which has been created by the alpha-adrenergic receptors that release further discharges on exposure to norepinephrine. Stimulation of these damaged nerves that

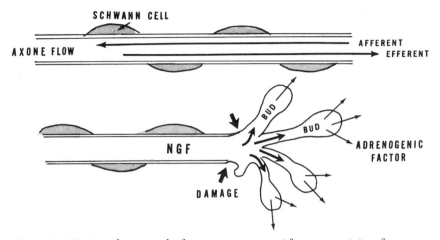

Figure 2–27. Axonal outgrowths forming a neuroma. After a nerve injury from compression or partial to total severance, the nerve growth factor (NFG) stimulates the nerve to advance distally and form "buds," which create more endings than the normal nerve shown in the upper drawing. By virtue of the greater secretion of adrenogenic factors, the nerve becomes more sensitive to adrenogenic agonists and transmits a greater number of potential pain fiber impulses to the spinal cord. (From Cailliet, R: Pain: Mechanisms and Management. FA Davis, Philadelphia, 1993, p 38, with permission.)

have formed spouts further liberate norepinephrine,[84] which results in firing of the nerve. Injury to a nerve that severs axons of the nerve[85] creates norepinephrine receptors at the terminal endings of the nerve, thus indicating that peripheral connections exist.

Nociceptors released in response to prolonged continuing noxious stimuli are further intensified by exposure to norepinephrine. This implies that a connection must exist between the afferent nociceptor reaction to noxious stimulants and sympathetic efferents.[86]

There may be local discharge of peptides in the area of tissue innervated by the injured nerve, which sends antidromic impulses that release further afferent peptides to the periphery: a domino concept. All these findings, however, fail to clarify whether the resultant pain is caused by, or is only a sequela of, abnormal sympathetic impulses.

The question has been raised[87] of the reason for performing a sympathectomy in an extremity that demonstrates hyposympathetic activity. Relief of pain from sympathetic intervention is also questioned, because not all patients with identical conditions respond favorably to sympathetic interruption. The possibility has been raised that sympathectomies may also interrupt the primary afferent axons located in the region of the ganglion. Morphine, injected into the dorsal root ganglion,[88] alleviates pain with no evidence of sympathetic blockage. Patients who have sympathectomies performed in the treatment of Raynaud's phenomenon often develop causalgia after the procedure.

HYPERALGESIA IN REFLEX SYMPATHETIC DYSTROPHY

In patients who are experiencing pain considered to be mediated through the autonomic nervous system also experience superficial sensitivity termed hyperalgesia.

Hyperalgesia has been attributed to activation of peripheral adrenergic receptors (alpha-1 and alpha-2) in the involved area.[89] A provocative paper[90] has asked the question "Is nociceptor activation by alpha-1 adrenoreceptors the culprit in sympathetically maintained pain?" This article postulates that after trauma in the peripheral tissues at the end organs of the nociceptors, norepinephrine is released from the sympathetic terminals, which activates these nociceptors and causes the sensation of pain[91] (Fig. 2–28).

After sympathectomy, stimulation of the peripheral (not the central) cut end reproduces the pain.[92] Anesthetic blockage of the sympathetic ganglion abolishes hyperalgesia, as does regional intravenous quanethidine, which depletes peripheral catecholamines. These factors indicate that hyperalgesia is dependent or markedly influenced by sympathetic innervation of the painful (peripheral) part and that therapy should address this peripheral aspect of the pain.

Intradermal injection of norepinephrine restores the hyperalgesia in reflex sympathetic dystrophy (RSD) whereas intradermal epinephrine does not cause hyperalgesia in normal skin. Phenoxybenzamine,* a nonspecific alpha-adrenergic antagonist, relieves hyperalgesia.

Hyperalgesia is apparently directly related to activation of adrenergic receptors: especially alpha-1 and alpha-2 adrenergic receptors. Addressing these receptors topically with antagonists should afford relief to the patient and this has proven to be a fact with local application of clonidine.†

Clonidine is an alpha-adrenergic blocking agent that works by activating presynaptic adrenergic autoreceptors, resulting in a reduction of amount of epinephrine released.[89] No alpha-adrenergic antagonist is commercially available, but clonidine is available as a transdermal patch and has been highly effective in that form.

---

*Phenoxybenzamine hydrochloride: Dibenzyline Hydrochloride (SK-Beecham). Capsule 10 mg, daily times four: increased to 10 mg daily until desired dosage.

†Clonidine hydrochloride: Antepres (Parke Davis). Transdermal system 2.5, 5.0, and 7.5 mg that delivers 0.10, 0.20, and 0.30 mg/day for 1 week.

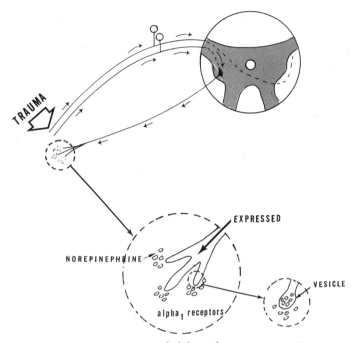

Figure 2–28. Nociceptor activation of alpha₁ adrenoreceptors. Trauma causes the sympathetic nerves going to the area to express norepinephrine, which is contained within the vesicles. The liberated norepinephrine reacts with alpha receptors to create symptoms of causalgia.

Peripheral alpha-1-adrenergic receptors are apparently active in sympathetically maintained pain and are initiated after injuries.[93,94] Before intervention of the innervation to the anticipated injured part, local administration of appropriate medications should be given. This route should also always be considered in conjunction with other, more centrally directed, modalities.

Does *failed* natural opioid modulation in regional sympathetic ganglia cause reflex sympathetic dystrophy? This question was raised by Hannington-Kiff.[95] Following this concept, the *plasticity* of the dorsal root ganglia, the spinal horn cells, and the wide dynamic range cells increase from repeated or intensive nociception from the periphery.[96–98] The normal modulating opioid radicals contained within dorsal root ganglia also increase to prevent excessive sympathetic activity. This increased activity affects the blood vessels, sweat glands, and hair follicles, as well as other areas with sympathetically controlled activities.

Normally the opioid radicals equal the norepinephrine activity with "modulation." The theory behind this is that when increased norepinephrine within the gland is not balanced with commensurate opioid radical activity and excess (Fig. 2–29) bombardment of the spinal horn cells, the wide-dynamic range and lateral horn cells result.

Although sympathetic mediated pain has been considered, RSD or its equivalent is so prominent in soft tissue injuries, all of Chapter 14 is devoted to it.

The diagnosis of RSD, because it is related to dysfunction of the autonomic nervous system in its pathomechanics, is suggested by:

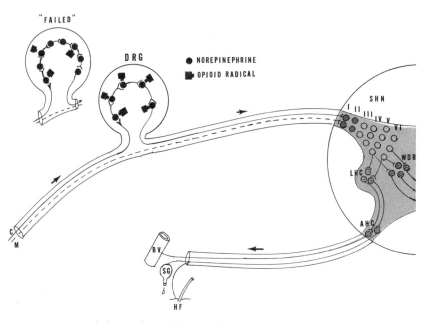

Figure 2–29. *Failed* opioid modulation of pain in the dorsal root ganglion. Opioid radicals in the normal dorsal root ganglion (DRG) modulate the norepinephrine contained within the small saccules in the ganglion. Normally, afferent impulses from C fibers (C) transmitting nociceptive impulses to the spinal cord nuclei (SHN) impinge on Rexed layers I and II. These impulses react with wide dynamic range (WDR) cells in the cord (Rexed layer VII) with impulses going cephalad to the lateral spinothalamic tracts (*arrows*). Fibers connect the Rexed layer cells with lateral horn cells (LHC) that innervate the sympathetic fibers to blood vessels (BVC), sweat glands (SG), and hair follicles (HF). Repeated or intense nociceptive impulses increase (plasticity) the number of norepinephrine cells within the DRG, which increases sensitivity to even mechanoreceptor (M) impulses, causing allodynia. In failed opioid modulation (*upper left drawing*), the epinephrine cells are increased and the opioid radical are proportionately decreased. Therefore, bombardment to SHN is increasing the number of WDR cells.

1. Pain is out of proportion to the injury sustained.
2. Pain described as "neuralgic" or "dysesthetic" with terms such as **burning, numbness, tingling,** and **itching** often being used by patients.
3. Pain may be confined to a neurologic dermatomal area, but usually is more diffuse and less precise.
4. Pain is usually restricted to a distal peripheral limb; although there may be some variation involving the face or the tongue.
5. Usually there are no objective lesions.
6. Superficial non-noxious stimuli, such as touch, air, and vibration accentuate the pain.
7. Significant and often inappropriate behavioral responses accompany the pain leading to seclusion and withdrawal.

The physical findings of the involved extremity in RSD will be discussed in Chapter 14 as will their various stages.[99] Of some significance is that relief of this pain can be obtained from sympathetic intervention.[100]

There has been a great deal of discussion regarding reflex sympathetic dystrophy, including an editorial in the journal *Pain*.[101] There are variations in RSD from a single symptom to the "full-blown syndrome" with all the manifestations of dystrophy, including osteoporosis and increased uptake seen on radioisotope scan.[102]

In the presence of only minimal symptoms, and with findings short of full-blown dystrophy, the diagnosis of RSD is often overlooked. Janig[103] addressed this quandry when he was a member of an IASP committee devoted to determining a consensus definition of RSD. It was concluded that RSD pain did not need to be of "burning" quality but did need to be associated with "abnormalities of sensation," that is, abnormality of motor function, blood flow, sweating, and trophic changes in the involved skin and the deep tissues of the involved extremity.

This final definition was as vague as that of the term **syndrome.** The *abnormalities* required were not specifically defined nor was a listing of which abnormalities were diagnostic for RSD. Janig[104] later proposed three types of RSD:

1. Algodystrophy which includes pain and *all* features of dystrophy in what was called *full-blown syndrome*.
2. Dystrophy without pain.
3. Sympathetically maintained pain (SMP) (without dystrophy).

Essentially, Janig's definitions were those diagnostic of RSD accompanied by vasomotor trophic changes which were unexplained by any other cause.

Relief of the pain by a sympathetic nerve block presented another variant to acceptance of these three classifications. Relief by local analgesic sympathetic block was previously considered earlier as necessary for a specific diagnosis of RSD.[105] This raised the question as to whether a diagnosis of RSD could be entertained if a sympathetic block was *not* effective. This in turn raised another question as to whether the anesthetic agent used in a sympathetic block has any affect on the somatic nerves in the vicinity of the injection and whether or not the anesthetic agent (e.g., lidocaine) has a systemic effect.

There are RSD-like syndromes, such as nerve-damaged tissues, that can benefit from systemically administered lidocaine. There are also conditions of nerve damage resulting in pain and allodynia with skin temperature changes and resultant atrophy, yet without any involvement of the sympathetic system.[106,107] Lidocaine given intravenously[108] has relieved neuropathic pains.

The *specific* sensory abnormalities mentioned in the IASP definition without clarification have been studied[109] and include heat-induced hyperalgesia, low-threshold A-beta–mediated or high-threshold mechanical allodynia, and slow temporal summation of mechanical allodynia.

Further classification of the findings mandatory for an accurate diagnosis remain to be clarified.

A provocative (i.e., it raises clinical questions) research paper[110] appeared discussing vasomotor changes resulting in peripheral nerve injuries resembling RSD. There was in it reference made to the article by Wakisaka, Kajander, and Bennett[111] who had created a laboratory model for RSD. Skin temperature changes were described by these researchers in plantar skin, following a mechanical constriction applied to a rat's sciatic nerve that deviated from the expected sympathetic vasomotor reaction.

Loose ligatures were applied to the sciatic nerve at the thigh, thereby causing swelling and constriction of the nerve. Morphologic studies of the nerve at this site revealed loss of large myelinated nerves but sparing of the unmyelinated nerves. Sprouting, indicating regeneration, occurred within days at these injured nerve sites. This was considered to be an ideal model of RSD, because the afflicted rats showed behavior consistent with pain.

The common belief vasoconstrictive activity occurring in painful neuropathies (e.g., cold or hot skin reaction attributed to sympathetic flow) was questioned.[112]

In the rats in the Wakisaka-Kajander-Bennett study, the skin in the region of the constricted nerve remained hotter than normal for 10 days and colder than normal for the remaining 3 to 4 weeks after constriction. During the initial reaction, the noradrenergic innervation of the plantar skin blood vessels appeared normal. When the skin became colder, norepinephrine neuropeptide Y and dopamine-b-hydroxylase were absent. These findings were considered to imply that skin temperature was not necessarily correlated to sympathetic activity.[113]

The unitary reaction of the sympathetic nervous system, described in most physiology textbooks is brought into question as being different from severe stress in normal conditions and whether it is dependent on the target organs being regulated by the sympathetic CNS. There is no basis for the expectation of *generalized* sympathetic tone from sympathetic intervention.

The use of human cutaneous blood vessels as a target organ is complex. Blood vessels of the hands and feet have a noradrenergic supply in normal ambient temperatures. The blood flow through these vessels is directly related to sympathetic activity: cooling occurs from adrenergic constriction, and warming occurs from decreased sympathetic activity. Which arterial vessels — precapillary arterioles, postcapillary capacitance vessels, or arteriovenous anastamosis — receive significant specific sympathetic innervation is not known. Vasodilatory mechanism remains unclear.[114]

Changes in environmental temperature affect the smooth muscles of the blood vessels and alter the reaction of sympathetic nerve control.[115] Whether cutaneous blood vessels are properly reinnervated after denervation is also not clear,[116] nor is the effect of *adaptive supersensitivity* following denervation.[117]

To evaluate the dystrophic aspects of RSD as attributable to vasomotor activity also remains if not controversial, at least unproven. The clinical diagnosis of causalgia in everyday practice is rare and the dystrophic aspects of RSD seen in clinical practice are not frequently recognized nor appropriately evaluated nor treated.

The criteria for diagnosing RSD remain imprecise, the pathophysiology unclear, and the therapeutic approach ambiguous. A tentative diagnostic criteria has, however, been proposed:

> "RSD is a descriptive term referring to a complex disorder or group of disorders that may develop as a consequence of trauma affecting the limbs, with or without obvious nerve lesion. RSD may also develop after visceral diseases and central nervous system lesions or, rarely, without an obvious antecedent event. It consists of pain and related sensory abnormalities, abnormal blood flow and sweating, abnormalities in the motor system and changes in structure of both superficial and deep tissues ("trophic changes"). It is not necessary that all components are present. It is agreed that the name "reflex sympathetic dystrophy" be used in a descriptive sense and does not imply specific underlying mechanisms."[118]

A psychophysiologic model of RSD can be proposed based only on limited clinical experience but more precise experimental and objective clinical studies are needed to explain precisely the neurophysiology of RSD. The recent finding of an animal model will enhance clarification of central and peripheral components, neuroeffector transmission, neurovascular aspects of affected blood vessels, mechanisms of the nociceptors, and their identification and effect upon the vascular smooth muscles. After greater clarification of neural mechanisms, meaningful diagnostic criteria will ensue, as well as development of appropriate physiologic therapy.

CHRONIC FATIGUE SYNDROME

In many neuromusculoskeletal painful states a chronic fatigue syndrome (CFS) occurs, which aggravates the disability and delays recovery. The basis for CFS remains obscure.

A concept has been proposed by Cheu and Findley[119] regarding the pathophysiology of CFS as being closely related to sympathetic mediated pain which theory deserves evaluation, because pain has a sympathetic nervous system component.

The Cheu and Findley concept posits five phases:

1. An inciting event which stimulates the posterior thalamus which is responsible with sympathetic action (fight or flight). These inciting incidents are claimed to be (a) viral; (b) immune imbalance congenital or secondary to infection; (c) caused by psychologic stress over a prolonged time; or (d) resulting from physical trauma.

   These inciting factors that initiate an *inflammatory* nociceptor process,[120] that is, the presence of nociceptors or algogens, have been cited but suffice it that they include an accumulation of lymphoid cells which release vasodilator substances (i.e., histamine, serotonin, bradykinin, arachidonic acid metabolites, and platelet activating factors). As well as initiating vasomotor reaction, they also depolarize other primary afferent nerve fibers that release substance P, K^+, H^+, arachidonic acid, prostaglandin,[121] bradykinin, serotonin, and histamine. In the presence of inflammation,[122] these nociceptors cause hyperalgesia and myalgia.[123]

2. Progressive sympathetic output (over the parallel parasympathetic output from the posterior thalamus) causes an imbalance and a preponderance of sympathetic output. It is assumed by the authors of standard neurophysiologic textbooks that stimulation of the sympathetic nervous system produces general physiologic responses rather than discrete localized effects (although this conclusion has been questioned). Preganglionic fibers supply the medulla of the adrenal glands. Pain and other strong emotional reactions (e.g., fear, rage, stress) evoke sympathetic activity, and consequent adrenal reaction.

3. The progressive sympathetic preponderance reaches the postganglionic presynaptic and terminal autonomic nerves to *leak* norepinephrine from the vesicles that store catecholamines. Acetylcholine and norepinephrine are the principal transmitter agents involved in transmission at synaptic junctions between preganglionic and postganglionic neuron and autonomic effectors.[124] Norepinephrine is the chemical transmitter at most sympathetic postgangion endings.

Norepinephrine and its methyl-derivatives are secreted by the adrenal glands after stimulation from higher centers. The anatomic pathways connecting supraspinal regions with autonomic outflows have not been clearly demonstrated.[125] Autonomic control of the cardiovascular phenomenon must be situated below the mesencephalic region, because transection at this level does not interfere with these functions.[125] The most important controlling area appears to be at the rostral end of the medulla. There must be other centers in the spinal cord, because *recovery* after section of midbrain centers occurs. Stimulation of the anterior hypothalamus was initially considered to discharge only parasympathetic impulses effectively but later studies[125] claim that it is the dorsomedial nucleus of the thalamus that has influence over the autonomic system.

Adrenergic division of the autonomic nervous system is determined by the chemical liberated by stimulation. Postganglionic sympathetic neurons are generally considered to be adrenergic except for those of vasodilators and sweat glands. Some secretions of norepinephrine by adrenergic neurons are preceded by liberation of acetylcholine by these neurons. Sympathetic and parasympathetic *balance* appears precarious. A preponderance of sympathetic outflow can have a significant impact on the patient's lifestyle and daily activities.

Stimulation of the adrenal medulla releases epinephrine in a 4:1 ratio with norepinephrine and catecholamine into the circulation which is agonistic (i.e., it enhances) to receptors in cell membranes and thus stimulates their activity. Agonism is also termed **up regulation**[64]; it increases the ability to initiate activities. The number of receptors in cell membranes obviously increases the activities of the membranes stimulated. Receptor regulation depends on protein synthesis. Excessive agonism over a prolonged period decreases the number of receptors, thus providing the term **down regulation.**

Continued sympathetic preponderance causes depolarization from the CNS with resultant *leak* of norepinephrine from the peripheral vesicles that store catecholamine. This decreases the sensitivity of the alpha-2 receptors and never reaches the alpha-1 receptors.

The adrenogenic receptors, alpha-1, predominate at the postsynaptic effector sites of smooth muscles and glands. Alpha-2 receptors are cholinergic as well as adrenogenic in their function. If stimulated, these receptors *decrease* the release of norepinephrine. Beta-1 and beta-2 exert their effects upon cardiac muscle and gastrointestinal musculature with the latter (beta-2) reducing calcium influx. They are therefore seen as inhibitory in function.

A delicate balance occurs in which a continued sympathetic preponderance (*up regulation*) in the system responds with an increase in receptors or their sensitization with greater sympathetic activity. An example of this is seen in hyperthyroidism—the number of beta-adrenogenic receptors increases with chronic tachycardia and other signs of hyperthyroidism. Any drug that inhibits or modulates the preponderance of agonists causes an upset in this balance which must be understood more clearly.

Synthesis of catecholamine is accelerated by acute sympathetic discharge by decreasing the norepinephrine level. Chronic stimulation increases the production by enzymic activity of dopamine into norepinephrine. Seventy percent of norepinephrine is retaken up into the presynaptic nerve endings. What is not retaken and remains free is inactivated by mitochondrial monoamine oxidase (MAO). This balance and attendant possible imbalance indicate the sensitivity of alpha and beta receptors vying for control of sympathetic activity. This also partially explains pharmacologically the therapeutic benefit of antidepressant medication in the treatment of chronic pain.

Patients with endogenous depression have up-regulated alpha-2 regulators with depression of catecholamines, which is a current concept and an explanation of why tricyclic antidepressants (e.g., MAOs) are effective. Patients with CFS[124] are claimed to have down-regulated alpha-2 and up-regulated alpha-1 receptors, the therapy for which is also aided by tricyclics, although with a different period of administration. This varying of time factors is postulated by Cheu and Findley as a possible tool for differential diagnosis between CFS and depression.

All currently accepted aspects of pain as related to disability and impairment resulting from **soft tissue pathology** have been elucidated. Many more will emerge as further clinical studies and research continue. The remainder of this book discusses individual entities involving soft tissue pain according to their precise anatomic sites. This discussion of the mechanisms of **pain** will hold true for all subsequent topics covered in this book.

REFERENCES

1. Sherrington, CS: The Integrative Action of the Nervous System. Yale University Press, New Haven, 1906.
2. Woolf, CJ: Evidence for a central component of post-injury pain hypersensitivity. Nature 306:686–688, 1983.
3. Dunner, R: Neuronal plasticity and pain following peripheral tissue inflammation or nerve injury. In Bond, M, Charlton, E, and Woolf, CJ (eds): Proceedings VIth World Congress on Pain, Pain Research, and Clinical Management, Vol 5. Elsevier, Amsterdam, 1991, pp 263–276.
4. Wall, PD: The prevention of postoperative pain, Pain, 33:289–290, 1988.
5. Frey, M von. Beitrage zur Sinnesphysiologie des Schnerzsinns. Ber. sachs Ges. Wiss. meth. phys. Gl: 46, 185, 196 and 283–296, 1894.
6. Zellerman, Y: Touch, pain and tickling: An electrophysiological investigation on cutaneous sensory nerves. J Physiol (Lond) 95:1–28, 1939.
7. Sinclair, DC and Hinshaw, JR: A comparison of the sensory disocciation produced by procaine and by limb compression. Brain 73:480–498, 1950.
8. Napier, JR: The return of sensibility in full thickness skin grafts. Brain 75:147–166, 1952.
9. DiPiero, V, Jones, AKP, Iannotti, F, et al: Chronic pain: a PET study of the central effects of percutaneous high cervical cordotomy. Pain 46:9–12, 1991.

10. Dubner, R: Specialization in nociceptive pathways: Sensory discrimination, sensory modulation and neuronal connectivity. In Fields, HL, Dubner, R, and Cervero, F (eds): Advances in Pain Research and Therapy, Vol 9. Raven Press, New York, 1985, pp 111–133.

11. Hokfelt, T, Johannsson, O, Ljungdahl, A, et al: Peptidergic neurones. Nature 284:515–521, 1980.

12. Hunt, SP, Kelly, JS, Emson, PC, et al: An immunohistochemical study of neuronal populations containing neuropeptides or gamma-aminobutyrate within the superficial layers of the rat dorsal horn. Neuroscience 6:1883–1898, 1981.

13. Brimijoin, S, Lundberg, JM, Brodin, E, et al: Axonal transport of substance P in the vagus and sciatic nerves of the guinea pig. Brain Res 191:443–457, 1980.

14. Gamse, R, Holzer, P, and Lembeck, F: Decrease of substance P in primary afferent neurones and impairment of neurogenic plasma extra-vasation by capsaicin. Br J Pharmacol 68:207–213, 1980.

15. Light, AR and Perl, ER: Reexamination of the dorsal root projection to the spinal dorsal horn including observations on the differential termination of coarse and fine fibers. J Comp Neurol 186:117–132, 1979.

16. Fields, HL and Basbaum, AI: Brainstem control of spinal pain-transmission neurons. Annu Rev Physiol 40:217–248, 1978.

17. Bowsher, D: Pain mechanisms in man. Res. Staff Phys 29(12):26–34, 1983.

18. Selzer, M and Spencer, WA: Convergence of visceral and cutaneous afferent pathways in the lumbar spinal cord. Brain Res 14:331–348, 1969.

19. Aihara, Y, Nakamura, H, Sato, A and Simpson, A: Neural control of gastric motility with special reference to cutaneo-gastric reflexes. In Brooks C, et al. (eds): Integrative Functions of Autonomic Nervous System. Elsevier, New York, 1979, pp 38–49.

20. Davies, SN and Lodge, D: Evidence for involvement of N-methylaspartate receptors in "wind-up" of class 2 neurones in the dorsal horn of the rat. Brain Res 424:402–406, 1987.

21. Melzack, R and Casey, KL: Sensory motivational and central control determinants of pain. In Kenshalo, DR (ed): The Skin Senses. Springfield, Ill., Charles C Thomas, 1968, pp 423–443.

22. Salt, TE and Hill, RG: Pharmacological differentiation between responses of rat medullary dorsal horn neurons to noxious mechanical and noxious thermal cutaneous stimuli. Brain Res 263:167–171, 1983.

23. Trans Dinh, YR, Thural, C, Serrie, A, et al: Glycerol injection into the trigeminal ganglion provokes a selective increase in human cerebral blood flow. Pain 46:13–16, 1991.

24. Fields, HL and Levine, JD: Pain mechanisms and management. West J Med 141:347–357, 1984.

25. Fields, HL and Basbaum, AI: Brainstem control of spinal pain-transmission neurons. Annu Rev Physiol 4:451–462, 1978.

26. Woolf, CJ and Thompson, SWN: The induction and maintenance of central sensitization is dependent on N-methyl-aspartic acid receptor activation: Implications for the treatment of post-injury pain hypersensitivity states. Basic Section. Pain 44:293–299, 1991.

27. Raskin, NH: Serotonin receptors and headache. N Engl J Med 325:353–354, 1991.

28. Mersky, H: Classification of chronic pain: Description of chronic pain syndromes and definitions. Pain 16:(suppl 3):S1–S225, 1986.

29. Melzak, R: Psychological Concepts and Methods for the Control of Pain. Advances in Neurology, vol 4. Raven Press, New York, 1974, pp 275–280.

30. Fulton, JF: Physiology of the Nervous System. Oxford University Press, London, 1943, p 52.

31. Kandel, ER: Brain and behavior. In Kandel, ER and Swartz, JH (eds): Principles of Neural Science, Edward Arnold, London, 1983, p 4.

32. Luciani, L: Fisiologia dell'Uomo. Societá Editrice Libraria, Milan, 1912, p 239

33. Thomas, CL (ed): Taber's Cyclopedic Medical Dictionary, ed 15. FA Davis, Philadelphia, 1985.

34. Francesco Agnati, L, Tiengo, M, Ferraguti, F, et al: Pain, analgesia, and stress: An integrated view. The Clin J Pain 7 (Suppl 1):S23–S37, 1991.

35. Kuhar, MJ: The mismatch problem in receptor mapping studies. Trends Neurosci 8:190–1, 1985.

36. Zoli, M, Agnoti, LF, Fuxe, K, and Bjelke, B: Demonstration of NPY transmitter receptor mismatches in the central nervous system of the male rat. Acta Physiol Scand 135:201–202, 1989.

37. Swartz TW, Fuhlendorff J, Langeland N, et al: Y1 and Y2 receptors for NPY. The evolution of PP-fold peptides and their receptors. In Mutt, V, Fuxe, K, Hokfelt, T, and Lundberg, JM (eds): Neuropeptide Y. Raven Press, New York, 1989, pp 103–114.

38. Agnati, LF, Zoli, M, Merlo Pich, E, et al: Aspects of neural plasticity in the central nervous system, VIII. Theoretical aspects of brain communication and computation. Neurochem Int 16:479–500, 1990.

39. Agnati, LF, Zoli, M, Merlo Pich, E, et al: NPY receptors and their interactions with other transmitter systems. In Mutt, V, Fuxe, K, Hokfelt, T, and Lundberg JM (eds): Neuropeptide Y. New York: Raven Press, 1989, pp 103–114.

40. Nieuwehuys, R (ed): Chemoarchitecture of the Brain. Springer-Verlag, Berlin, p 36.

41. Kurosawa, M, Sato, A, Swensen, RS, Takahashi, Y: Sympatho-adrenal medullary functions in response to intracerebroventricularly injected corticotropin-releasing factor in anaesthetized rats. Brain Res 367:250–257, 1986.

42. Ehlers, CL, Henrikson, SJ, Wang, M, et al: Corticotropin releasing factor produces increases in brain excitability and convulsive seizures in rats. Brain Res 278:332–6, 1983.

43. Melzack, R: Central pain syndromes and theories of pain. In Casey, KL (ed): Pain and Central Nervous System Disease. Raven Press, New York, 1991, pp 59–75.

44. Descartes, R: Treatise of Man. (trans, Thomas Steele Hall) Harvard University Press, Cambridge, Mass, 1972. [The Traité de l'Homme was published posthumously—and—imperfectly—in 1662.]

45. Melzack, R: Phantom limbs, the self and the brain (The D.O. Hebb Memorial Lecture). Can J Physiol 30:1–14, 1989.

46. Black, IB: Information in the Brain: A Molecular Perspective. A Bradford Book. MIT Press, Cambridge, Mass., 1991.

47. Kalin, NH and Dawson, G: Neuroendocrine dysfunction in depression: Hypothalamic-anterior pituitary systems. Trends Neurosci 9:261–266, 1986.

48. Ganong, W: The stress response: A dynamic overview. Hosp Prac 23(6):155–190, 1988.

49. Moore, RY: The suprachiasmic nucleus and the organization of a circadian system. Trends Neurosci 5:404, 1982.

50. Moore-Ede, MC, Sulzman, FM, and Fulle CA: The Clocks that Time Us: Physiology of the Circadian Timing System. Harvard University Press, Cambridge, Mass., 1982.

51. Barinaga, M: Watching the brain remake itself. Science 266:1475–1476, 1994.

52. Halbreich, U and Rose, R: Hormones and Behavior. Raven Press, New York, 1987.

53. Bennett, GJ: The role of the sympathetic nervous system in painful peripheral neuropathy. Pain 45:221–223, 1991.

54. Goldman, S and Newman, SS: Manter and Gatz's Essentials of Clinical Neuroanatomy and Neurophysiology, ed. 7. FA Davis, Philadelphia, 1987.

55. Cannon, WB and Rosenblueth, A: Studies on conditions of activity in endocrine organs XXIX. Sympathin E and Sympathin I. Am J Physiol 184:557–574, 1933.

56. Ahlquist, RP: A study of adrenotrophic receptors. Am J Physiol 153:586–600, 1948.

57. Lenman, JAR: Clinical Neurophysiology. Blackwell Scientific Publications, Oxford, 1975, pp 250.

58. Gennaro, AR, Chase, GD, Marperosian, AD (eds): Adrenergic and Adrenergic Neuron Blocking Drugs. Remington's Pharmaceutical Sciences, Mack, Easton, PA, 1990, p 898.

59. Redmond, DE and Huang, YH: II. New Evidence of the locus coeruleus norepinephrine connection with anxiety. Life Sci 25:2149–2162, 1979.

60. Swanson, LW: Ultrastructural evidence for central monoanemic innervation of blood vessel in the paraventricular nucleus of the hypothalamus. Brain Res 110:338–56, 1976.

61. In Nashold, BS, Wilson, WP, Slau B, et al (eds): Advances in Neurology, vol 4. Raven Press, New York, 1974.
62. Kerr, FWC: Neuroanatomical substrates of nociception in the spinal cord. Pain 1:325–356, 1975.
63. Sladek, JR and Walker, P: Brain Res 134:359–366, 1977.
64. Redmond, DE and Huang, YH: New evidence for a locis coreculeus norepinephrine connection with anxiety. Current Concepts, Life Sciences. 25:2149–2162, 1979.
65. Korr, IM: Sustained Sympathicotonia as a Factor in Disease (1978). In Korr, IM (ed): The neurobiologic mechanisms in manipulative therapy. New York, Plennum Press, 1978, pp 229–268.
66. Nobin, A and Bjorkland, A.: Acta Physiol Scand 388(suppl): 1–40, 1973.
67. Darwin, C: The Expression of Emotion in Man and Animals. Philosophical Library, New York, 1975, p 134.
68. Eliot, TR: J Physiol 32:401–467, 1905.
69. Cannon, WB, and Rosenbleuth, A: Studies on conditions of activity in endocrine organs. XXIX Sympathin E and Sympathin I. Am J Physiol 184:557–574, 1933.
70. Papez, JW: Proposed mechanisms of emotion. Arch Neurol Psychiat 38:725–744, 1937.
71. MacLean, PD: Psychosomatic Med 11:338, (1949); Papaez JW.: Arch Neurol Psychiat 38: 725, 1937; Vogt, BA, Reosene, DL and Pandya, DN: Science 204–205, 1979.
72. Foltz, EL and Lowell, EW: J Neurosurg 19:89, 1962; Hurt, RW and Ballantine, HT: Clin Neurosurg, 21, 334 (1973).
73. Talbot, JD, Marrett, S, Evans, AC, et al: Multiple representations of pain in human cerebral cortex. Science 251:1355–1358, 1991.
74. Goldstein, S and Halbreich, U: Hormones and stress. In Nemeroff, C and Loosen, P (eds): Handbook of Clinical Psychoneuroendocrinology. John Wiley, New York, 1987, pp 460–469.
75. Dunn, A and Berriodge, C: Is corticotropin-releasing factor a mediator of stress response? In Koob, G, Sandman C, and Strand, F (eds): A Decade of Neuropeptides. New York Academy of Sciences, New York, 1990, 579, 183–191.
76. Palkovits, M.: Organization of the stress response at the anatomical level. Neuropeptides and brain function. Prog Brain Res 72:47–55, 1987.
77. Bonica, JJ: Anaesthesiology 29:793, 1968.
78. Laux, W: Akt. Fragen Psychiat Neurol 3:138, 1966.
79. Head, H: Sensibilitutsstorungen der Haut bei visceralen Erkrankungen. Hirschwald-Verlag, Berlin, 1988.
80. Leriche, R.: Schmerzchirurgie. Joh. Ambrosius Barh Verlag, Leipzig, 1958. (Translation into German of La Chirurgie de la Douleur) Masson, Paris, 1959.
81. Gross, D: Pain and autonomic nervous system. In: Advances in Neurology. vol 4. Raven Press, New York, pp 93–103.
82. Hu, S and Zhu, J: Sympathetic facilitation of sustained discharges of polymodal nociceptors. Pain 38:85–90, 1989.
83. Devor, M and Janig, W: Activation of myelinated afferents ending in a neuroma by stimulation of the sympathetic supply in the rat. Neurosci Lett 24:43–47, 1981.
84. Sato, J and Perl, FR: Peripheral nerve injury causes cutaneous nociceptor to be excited by activation of catecholamine receptors (abstr). Soc Neurosci 16:1072, 1990.
85. Levine, JD, Coderre, TJ, Basbaum, AI: The peripheral nervous system and the inflammatory process. In Dubner, R, Gebhart, GF, and Bond, MR (eds): Pain Research and Clinical Management, vol 3. Proceedings Vth World Congress on Pain. Elsevier, Amsterdam, 1988, pp 33–43.
86. Wakisaka, S, Kajander, KC, and Bennett, GJ: Abnormal skin temperature and abnormal sympathetic vasomotor innervation in experimental painful peripheral neuropathy. Pain 46, 1991.
87. Schott, GD: Mechanisms of causalgia and related clinical conditions. Brain 109:717–738, 1980.

88. Shir, Y and Seltzer, Z: Effects of sympathectomy in a model of causalgiform pain produced by partial sciatic nerve injury in rats. Pain 45:309–320, 1991.

89. Davis, KD, Treede, RD, Raja, SN, et al: Topical application of clonidine relieves hyperalgesia in patients with sympathetically maintained pain. Pain 47:309–317, 1991.

90. Campbell, JN, Meyer, RA, and Raja, SN: Is nociceptor activation by alpha-1 adrenoreceptors the culprit in sympathetically maintained pain? Am Pain Soc 1(1):3–11, 1992.

91. Janig, W: Can reflex sympathetic dystrophy be reduced to an alpha-adrenoreceptor disease? APS Journal 1(1):16–22, 1992.

92. Walker, AE and Nulsen, F: Electrical stimulation of the upper thoracic portion of the sympathetic chain in man. Arch Neurol Psychiatr (Chicago) 59:559–560, 1948.

93. Starke K: Alpha-adrenoreceptor subclassification. Rev Physiol Biochem Pharmacol 88: 199–236, 1981.

94. Roberts, W and Elardo, SM: Sympathetic activation of A-delta nociceptors. Somatosens Mot Res 3:33–44, 1985.

95. Hannington-Kiff, JG: Does failed natural opioid modulation in regional sympathetic ganglia cause reflex sympathetic dystrophy? Lancet 338:1125–1127, 1991.

96. Cook, AJ, Woolf, CJ, Wall, PD, and McMahon, SB: Dynamic receptive field plasticity in rat spinal cord dorsal horn following C-primary afferent input. Nature 325:151–153, 1987.

97. Dubusisson, D, Fitzgerald, M, and Wall, PD: Ameboid receptive fields of cells in laminae 1, 2, and 3. Brain Res 177:376–378, 1979.

98. Woolf, CJ and Fitzgerald, M: The properties of neurones recorded in the superficial dorsal horn in rat spinal cord. J Comp Neurol 221:313–328, 1983.

99. Cailliet, R: Reflex sympathetic dystrophy. In Cailliet, R (ed): Shoulder Pain, ed 3. FA Davis, Philadelphia, 1991, pp 227–252.

100. Wang, JK, Johnson, KA, and Ilstrup, DM: Sympathetic blocks for reflex sympathetic dystrophy. Pain 23:13–17, 1985.

101. Fields, HL: Editorial comment. Pain 49:161–162, 1992.

102. Kosin, F, McCarty, DJ, Sims, J, and Genant, H: The reflex sympathetic dystrophy syndrome. Am J Med 60:321–331, 1976.

103. Janig, W: Experimental approach to reflex sympathetic dystrophy and related syndromes. Pain 46:241–245, 1991.

104. Janig, W: Pathophysiology of reflex sympathetic dystrophy: some general considerations. In Stanto-Hicks, M, Janig, W, Boas, RA (eds): Reflex Sympathetic Dystrophy. Kluwer, Boston, 1990, pp 42–54.

105. Evans, JA: Reflex sympathetic dystrophy. Surg Gynecol Obstet 82:36–43, 1946.

106. Wall, PD and Gutnick, M: Ongoing activity in peripheral nerves: the physiology and pharmacology of impulses originating from a neuroma. Exp Neurol 43:580–593, 1974.

107. Tanelian, DL and MacIver, MB: Analgesic concentrations of lidocaine suppress tonic A-delta and C-fiber discharges produced by acute injury. Anaesthesiology 74:934–936, 1991.

108. Rowbotham, MC, Reisner-Keller, MB, and Fields, HL: Both intravenous lidocaine and morphine reduce the pain of postherpetic neuralgia. Neurology 41:1024–1028, 1991.

109. Price, DD, Long, S, and Huitt, C: Sensory testing of pathophysiological mechanisms of pain in patients with reflex sympathetic dystrophy (Clinical Section). Pain 49:163–173, 1992.

110. Shir, Y and Seltzer, Z: Effects of sympathectomy in a model of causalgiform pain produced by partial sciatic nerve injury in rats. Pain 45:309–320, 1991.

111. Wakisaka, S, Kajander, KC, and Bennett, GJ: Abnormal skin temperature and abnormal sympathetic vasomotor innervation in experimental painful peripheral neuropathy. Pain 46:299–313, 1991.

112. Janig, W: Experimental approach to reflex sympathetic dystrophy and related syndromes (guest editorial). Pain 46:241–245, 1991.

113. Janig, W: The sympathetic nervous system in pain: physiology and pathophysiology. In Santon-Hicks, M (ed): Pain and the Sympathetic Nervous System. Kluwer, Dordrecht, 1990, pp 17–89.

114. Cassell, JF, McLachlan, EM, and Sittiracha, T: The effect of temperature on neuromuscular transmission in the main caudal artery of the rat. J Physiol 397:31–44, 1988.

115. Janig, W, and Koltzenburg, M: Sympathetic activity and neuroeffector transmission changes after chronic nerve lesions. In Bond, MR, Charlton, JE, and Woolf, CJ (eds): Pain Research and Clinical Management. Proceedings VIth World Congress on Pain. Elsevier, Amsterdam, 1991, pp 365–371.

116. Fleming, WW and Westfall, DP: Adaptive supersensitivity. In Trendelenburg, U and Weiner, N (eds.): Catecholamines I. Handbook of Experimental Pharmacology, vol 90/I. Springer-Verlag, Berlin, 1988, pp 509–559.

117. Janig, W, Blumberg, H, Boas, RA, and Campbell, JN: The reflex sympathetic syndrome. Consensus statement and general recommendations for diagnosis and clinical research. In Bond, MR, Charlton, JE, and Woolf, CJ (eds.): Pain Research and Clinical Management. Proceedings VIth World Congress on Pain. Elsevier, Amsterdam, 1991, pp 373–376.

118. Price, DD, Bennett, GJ, and Raffii, A: Psychophysiological observations on patients with neuropathic pain relieved by sympathetic block. Pain 36:273–288, 1989.

119. Cheu, J and Findley, T: Pathophysiology of the Chronic Fatigue Syndrome (CFS), UMDNJ, Kessler Institute, 1988, Personal correspondence.

120. Rubin, E and Farber, JL: The gastrointestinal tract. In Rubin, E and Farber, JL (eds.): Pathology. JB Lippincott, Philadelphia, pp 628–721, 1988.

121. Chahl, LA: Pain induced by inflammatory mediators. In Beers, RF and Bassett, EG (eds.): Mechanisms of Pain and Analgesic Compounds. Raven Press, New York, 1979, p 273.

122. Perl, ER: Pain and nociception. In Smith, D (ed): Handbook of Physiology, 1984, pp 915–975.

123. Schaible, HG and Schmidt, RF: Effects of an experimental arthritis on the sensory properties of fine articular afferents units. J Neurophysiol 54:1109–1122, 1985.

124. Chusid, JG: The autonomic nervous system. In (ed): Correlative Neuroanatomy and functional Neurology, ed 14. Lange Medical Publ., Los Altos, 1970, p 154.

125. Campbell, HJ: Autonomic Mechanisms In (ed): Correlative Physiology of the Nervous System, Academic Press, New York, 1965, p 155.

126. Gennaro, AR (ed): Remington's Pharmacological Sciences, ed 18. Mack Publ. Co. Penna. 1990 pp 718–721.

CHAPTER 3

The Muscle Component of Soft Tissue Function and Pain

The muscle component of the neuromusculoskeletal system is so significant that it deserves a separate chapter. All biologic function depends on a well-coordinated neuromuscular system. Deficiencies in this system result in impaired function, pain, and disability.

The front cover of the book *Multiple Muscle Systems*[1] (Fig. 3–1) depicts a young man pulling a fishnet. This is a complex task requiring intricate balance and eye-hand coordination. All musculoskeletal components of the body are implicated. Over the last decades, a better understanding has been developed between neural function and biomechanical movement and function.

Once a movement is contemplated, a neural strategy is developed within the central nervous system (CNS) (Fig. 3–2).

The ultimate function is accomplished by precise neuromuscular activities that have significant feedback mechanisms assuring coordination, effort saving, and painless activities. Neuromuscular control of these systems is fundamental to accomplish almost any purpose.

The spindle system has become the central focus in this complex neuromusculoskeletal system.[2]

SPINDLE CELL: GAMMA SYSTEM

Although this system has been studied thoroughly in the neurophysiologic laboratory for centuries, it is only now beginning to have significant clinical significance.

The question has been asked "Are our muscles sentient? Do they per-

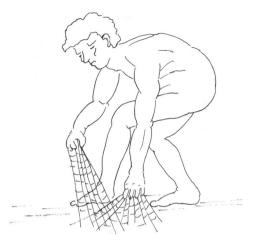

Figure 3–1. Young man pulling a fishnet. This complex task against external forces and precise load transmission throughout the body demands precise body balance and eye-hand coordination. (Modified from cover of Multiple Muscle Systems. Winters, JM and Woo, S L-V. (Eds). Springer-Verlag, New York, 1990.)

ceive motion as well as pain?"[3] We have pain signals from muscles, but do muscles signal what is "going on" as in impulses from skin and joint capsules? Are there kinesthetic sensations from muscles? In 1900, Sherrington reviewed the concept of "muscle sense"[4] implying the presence of "specific sense organs in muscle, tendons and joints."[5]

Receptors that lead to conscious perceived sensation are termed **exteroceptors**. Those not responsible for conscious sensation, yet still having primary motor function are termed **proprioceptors**. Sensory receptors exist in and around those joints primarily located within ligaments, which stabilize the

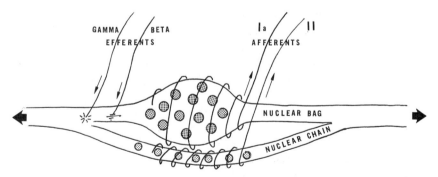

Figure 3–2. Intrafusal muscle spindle. The intrafusal spindle system has motor fibers through the gamma and beta efferent that control the length of the spindle. The sensory feedback from the spindle is transmitted through the Ia and II afferent fibers. As the fiber is lengthened (*arrows*), the system is stimulated by changes in the bag and the chain. Sensory impulses indicate the force speed and duration of the elongation. The spindle system is "reset" by the motor fibers for the next muscular extrafusal fiber contraction.

joints. Proprioceptors within muscles are *stretch* receptors within spindle cells and Golgi tendon organs.

The muscle spindle is made up of so-called **intrafusal muscle fibers** of which there are two types: nuclear bags and nuclear chains (see Fig. 3–2). There are typically two nuclear bag fibers and three to five nuclear chains per spindle. The spindle is about 2 to 3 mm long and about 0.15 mm wide. Smaller muscles with finer dexterity have a greater density of spindles per muscle than do the grosser muscles of the trunk and extremities. Because spindle muscles attach to both ends of the extrafusal muscle to which they are appended, they undergo the same changes in length as extrafusal fibers do. They act essentially as a *sophisticated strain gauge*.[5]

Another muscle-tendon proprioceptor is the Golgi tendon organ, which is located in the junction between the muscle and its tendon fibers. There are only one third to one half as many Golgi organs as there are spindle fibers. These organs are contained within an elastic capsule entered by nerve fibers. When the capsule is stretched, these nerve endings are distorted, thus sending barrages of impulses to the cord. The Golgi organ being placed in series with the extrafusal fibers is a *force transducer* measuring muscle tension.

Nerve axons extend from the organs to the cord, carrying information. Termed **afferents**, they are named based on their size, that is, I, II, and so on, depending on their axon diameters and relative conduction velocities. They carry information *from* spindle organs (Ia) and Golgi tendon organs (Ib) (Fig. 3–3).

The Ia nerve endings wrap around the central portion of both nuclear bags and nuclear chains. Group II afferents have smaller axons that terminate within the spindle organs. Higher cortical control of the spindle system (Fig. 3–4) has been well documented in neurophysiologic studies.[6] There are autonomic as well as somatic nerve fiber innervations of the spindle system but the postulated autonomic-somatic relationship at the cord level has not yet been confirmed (Fig. 3–5).

When an activated muscle is stretched (i.e., elongated) by the action of an outside agency, it contracts more forcefully than it would have before being stretched. Elongation of extrafusal fibers also stretches the spindle system equally (in an intrafusal manner), and sends an instant message to the cord through the Ia fibers.

The spindle system coordinates the length of the muscle spindle which is under alpha motor neuron fiber control (Fig. 3–6). The reflex also simultaneously controls the gamma system (Fig. 3–7).

These organ impulses make *inhibitory* connections with their *homonymous* motoneurons and *excitatory* connections with their *antagonistic* motoneurons.[6] This action invokes a reciprocal agonist-antagonist action; that is, the antagonist relaxes commensurate with the agonistic activity. Because this reflex involves only one synapse between the axon of Ia and the motor neuron A, the reaction is instantaneous.

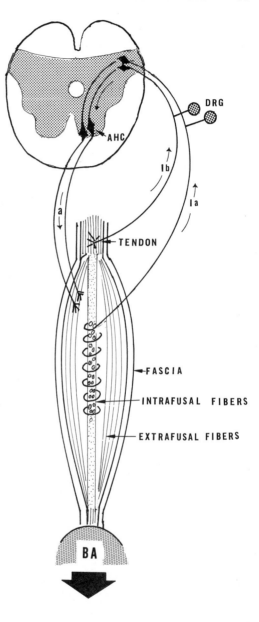

Figure 3–3. Spindle system function. The spindle system (intrafusal fibers) lies parallel to the extrafusal muscle fibers. When stretched, they signal the cord by way of the Ia fibers from the spindle and the Ib fibers from the Golgi tendon through the dorsal root ganglion (DRG). The impulses received in the gray matter have an internuncial connection with the contiguous anterior horn cells (AHC) that motor (a fiber) the extrafusal muscle fibers causing an appropriate muscular contraction. The fascia elongates to its physiologic limit. The muscle tendon is attached to the bony attachment of the vertebral bodies (BA).

Muscle tension activated by muscle contraction markedly increases this tension by inhibition of the homonymous motoneurons through the Ib fibers from the Golgi organs (Fig. 3–8). This action *protects* against overloading and also prevents any such rapid rise in tension that might tear muscle or tendon.

The stretch reflex is capable of making automatic corrections in muscle

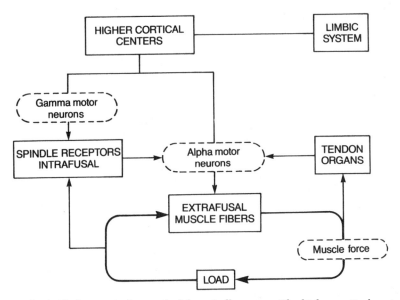

Figure 3–4. Higher cortical control of the spindle system. The higher cortical centers implement the muscular activity to perform the action. A feedback system correlates this activity. The load of the action determines the effort needed. The limbic system is one of the pathways of the perturbers (emotional) that may impair correlated action.

tone to oppose the action of outside disturbances along its length. It will, however, impair fine coordination of normal voluntary motion when control of these reflexes is commanded only by the higher centers that invoke numerous synapses. The shortening of the extrafusal fibers (under alpha control) slackens the intrafusal fibers and causes the Ia afferent activity to stop impairing muscular function. The motor control of the intrafusal fibers comes into play, thus negating this unwanted action. Impairment of this activity is being extensively studied in neuromusculoskeletal impairments.

Free nerve endings in muscles have been suggested as sources of nociception[7]; these A-alpha or group II fibers are now renamed groups I to IV.[8] They lack a corpuscular receptive structure and are typically located in the walls of the arterioles and surrounding connective tissue. No specific neuropeptide has been identified in muscle-free ending nociception. Under experimental conditions, many group III and group IV muscle afferents can be activated by deformation of muscle, such as seen in a forceful stretch.

Painful muscles apparently become *silent*, or inhibited, whereas muscles protective of an inflamed joint undergo spasm.[7] A muscle becomes silent, when inflamed compensatory muscles become involved, because the prime mover has failed to contract. Exercises to *strengthen* a muscle determined to be weak in clinical testing will fail because the function prime mover is appar-

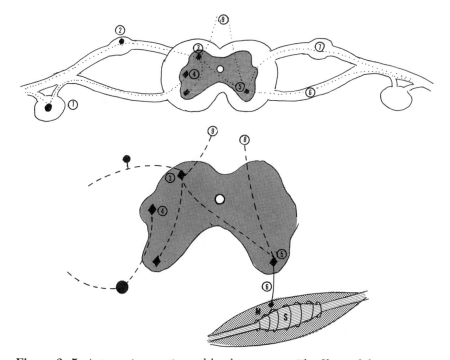

Figure 3–5. Autonomic-somatic cord level interaction. The fibers of the autonomic and somatic nervous system at the cord level are shown: (*1*) the stellate ganglion; (*2*) the dorsal root ganglion; (*3*) sensory fiber nuclei within the gray matter; (*4*) motor cells of the autonomic nervous system; (*5*) anterior horn cell (somatic motor efferent); (*6*) motor fibers (efferent) to the muscles; (*7*) somatic sensory (afferent) fibers; (*8*) internal neuronal connections of the autonomic system; and (*9*) the cortical upper motor neuronal connections. The connection (*8*) remains unproven. (From Cailliet, R: Pain: Mechanisms and Management. FA Davis, Philadelphia, 1993, p 86, with permission.)

ently taken over by accessory muscles. Cocontraction of antagonist muscles also impairs adequate contraction of *paretic* muscles.

Contribution of the sympathetic efferent activity in nociception remains controversial. Although many autonomic factors accompany local muscle tissue lesions; their mechanism remains to be confirmed.

After a tissue lesion, a state of subthreshold sensitization may result for a prolonged period.[9] This fact may account for the persistence of trigger areas long after an injury. Such persistent lesions may also result from ruptures in the sarcoplasmic reticulum because of the release of calcium from their intracellular stores. This calcium release causes sliding of the myosin and actin filaments, thus causing contraction without electrical activity, but attendant high-oxygen use causes hypoxia. Hypoxia is followed by a drop in intracellular

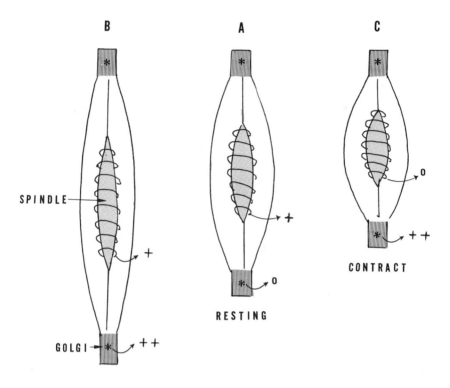

Figure 3–6. Spindle system coordination of muscular length rate of contraction and degree of tension. (A) depicts resting muscle, which by its intrinsic elongation, activates the spindle system. (B) shows activity engendered in the Golgi organ by passive stretch, but no spindle activity. In the actively contracted muscle (C), the spindle is relaxed and the Golgi is strongly activated. The spindle and Golgi coordinate muscular action. (From Cailliet, R: Pain: Mechanisms and Management. FA Davis, Philadelphia, 1993, p 88, with permission.)

adenosine triphosphate, which is required as an energy source by the calcium pump (see Fig. 2–24). If the activity of the pump is impaired, the intracellular calcium level remains elevated and the actin-myosin filaments are permanently activated thus causing *functional contracture* (trigger point), and chronic pain.

These neurophysiologic concepts explain many aspects of muscle pain in itself, are also significant in cervical and low back pains and in entrapment syndromes, which are discussed in subsequent chapters. The role of referred muscle pain as noted in trigger points in *Chronic Musculoskeletal Pain Syndromes* (CPMS), such as myofascial pain and temporomandibular dysfunction syndrome, remains unexplained.

Muscle tension develops when a muscle stretches—it consists of two

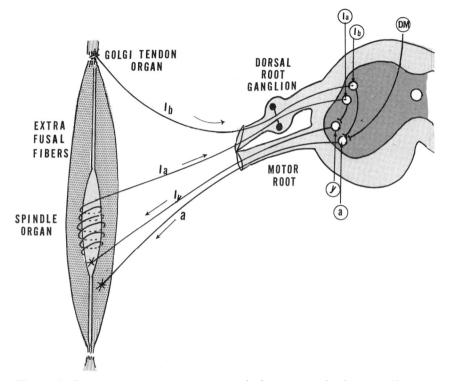

Figure 3–7. Proprioceptive autonomic control of neuromuscular function. The spindle system (intrafusal) of the muscle is innervated by Ia, Iy, and a fibers that originate in the gray matter of the cord. The Golgi tendon organ is also innervated by Ib fibers that ascend through the dorsal root ganglion. These two systems *inform* the cord of the strength and duration of the neuromuscular activity being accomplished.

components: *intrinsic* muscle stiffness and *reflex-mediated* muscle stiffness. The former is determined by the mechanical viscoelastic properties of the actomyosin bounds of the muscle; the latter by the excitability of the alpha-motoneuron pool and stretch-evoked activity in the primary muscle spindle afferents. After an insult to the neuromusculoskeletal system, there is a subsequent immediate *protective spasm*, which is essentially a reflex-mediated muscle stiffness that, if not relieved, becomes a prolonged stiffness of the viscoelastic system, possibly providing a basis for chronic pain and impairment.

The concept of muscle *spasm* as a protective mechanism: pain-tension-spasm: to protect the injured part[10] has generally been accepted, yet scientifically unproven. This concept has recently been challenged,[11] because muscles considered as under spasm were electrically silent.

Headley[11] considered these muscles as essentially *shut down*, creating a *functional contracture*[12] prevented by elongation. Such muscles were considered as *trigger* sites, because when relieved, elongation of the muscle in

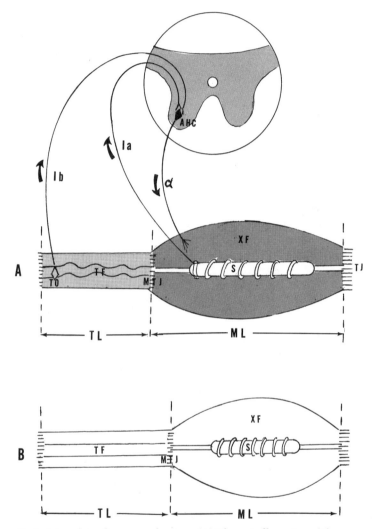

Figure 3–8. Musculotendinous mechanism. (A) The spindle system (S) measures the length of the muscle (ML), and the tendon organs (Golgi) (TO) monitor the tension. Stretching of the spindle system activates the Ia fibers, whereas stretching the tendon organs activate the Ib fibers. These influence the anterior horn cell (AHC), which activates motor fiber through alpha fibers to the extrafusal muscle fibers (XF). (B) When the extrafusal fibers contract, the muscle shortens (ML) and the tendon elongates (TL) to the degree that the tendon fibers can elongate. The tendon fibrils (TF) uncoil. Excessive muscular contraction can tear the musculotendinous juncture (MTJ).

"spasm" could be immediate. This action was attributed to gamma-motoneuron *inhibition* that occurred 5 to 15 minutes after onset of inflammation.[13] This inhibition is essentially fusiform.

The degree of activity of a homonymous muscle determined by the size and velocity of the stretch upon both static and dynamic fusiform afferents within the spindle system.[14,15] Spindle-system activity is regulated by descending commands (Fig. 3–9), but is also influenced by reflux receptor afferents from the skin, joints, and muscles. These latter reflexes may increase the activ-

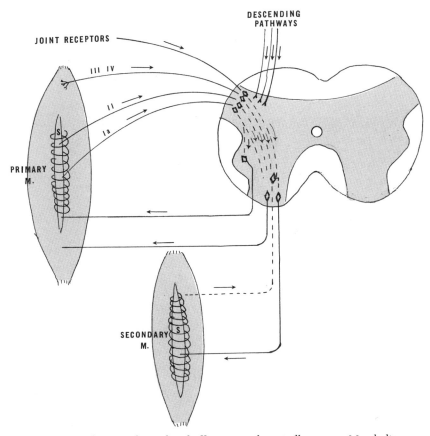

Figure 3–9. Influence of peripheral afferents on the spindle system. Metabolites produced from static muscle contraction stimulate groups III and IV, which activate alpha-motoneurons that project to primary and secondary muscles. These afferents increase the sensitivity of the spindle causing greater discharge on alpha-muscle fibers and increases their stiffness. Group II fibers act preferentially on dynamic alpha motor neurons with excess activity on extensor rather than flexor muscle fibers. Increases in potassium, lactic acid, and arachidonic acid enhance discharge of group III and IV afferents.

ity of the fusiform neurons, which in their turn increase discharge of spindle afferents, thus increasing muscle stiffness in both the homonymous and in distant muscles.[16]

Central control of the spindle system through descending pathways has been well documented[17] in upper motor neuron disease such as spasticity from stroke (Fig. 3–10), but the influence of peripheral factors have been minimally discussed in the literature. Significant disagreement exists as to whether there is a coactivation of alpha and gamma motoneurons in active movement with overemphasis on upper motor neuron control.[15,16]

In assuming greater peripheral control, the spindle system is seen not only as a receptor but also as a vital step in the gamma motor system where it

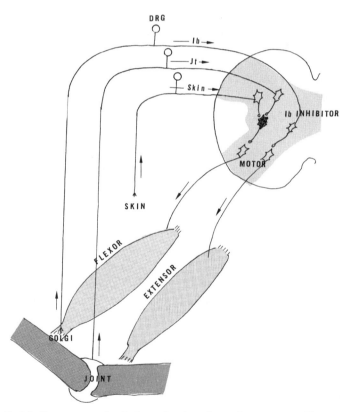

Figure 3–10. Interneuronal role in pathophysiology of spasticity. Afferent impulses from Golgi tendon organs provide a negative feedback (inhibitor) effect on muscle tension. Spasticity occurs when the inhibitory fibers are dissociated within the cycle and the motor units become hyperirritable, from impairment of the descending pathways.

integrates signals from peripheral receptors. The alpha motoneuron is influenced by ascending pathways to the spindle system, but is also significantly modified by signals from the muscle, skin, and joint efferents.

Some studies[18] of knee injuries have concluded that activation of stretch and tension-sensitive mechanoreceptors within the anterior cruciate ligament of the knee exerts effects on the static and dynamic sensitivities of the muscles acting at the knee joint. One study supports the hypothesis that articular receptors contribute, through the gamma muscle spindle system, to regulation of joint stiffness and stability in joints.[19]

In the shoulder, restricted and painful motion of the capsule of the glenohumeral joint causes apparent weakness of most motions. A reflex inhibition occurs that is relieved when the capsule regains full range of motion and becomes pain free.

This hypothesis is based on results of micro-electrode recording of dynamic and static alpha cells.[20] Gamma motoneurons from muscle group type I were found to be nonresponsive. Muscle group II afferents act preferentially on *dynamic* gamma motoneurons, whereas muscle group III afferents influence *static* motoneurons. Obviously, a different muscle type, whether dynamic or static, is stimulated by different afferent impulses from the contracting muscle.

Both group II and III afferents evoke excitatory and inhibitory effects. Flexor cells respond more forcefully to excitatory impulses than extensor cells do. Stimulation of different joint structures, such as capsules and ligaments, change the primary muscle spindle efferent system as do skin afferents. These facts imply the effect of joint and skin structures on reflex motoneuron activity in diagnosis and therapy.

Group III and IV muscle afferents differ in their response to chemical and mechanical stimuli. Increased potassium concentration, lactic acid, and arachidonic acid cause increased activation of group III and IV afferents.

Muscle stiffness is therefore increased by various chemical and mechanical effects upon muscle afferents. This action explains, in part, the prominence of muscle stiffness in the small muscles of the neck and the jaw—closing muscles rich in muscle spindles.

A second positive feedback loop (see Fig. 3–9) shows that this cycle evokes response in a secondary muscle, which may then undergo a similar response thus producing *secondary* muscle stiffness or *referred pain.*

The effect of the descending pathways' modifying alpha fusiform neurons partially explains the effect anxiety and stress have upon muscle stiffness. Occupational muscle pain may also result from the conflict between motor control of postural muscular activity and that needed for rhythmic movement or skilled manipulations, that is, slow-twitch versus fast-twitch muscles.[21]

Muscle pain caused by prolonged muscle contraction develops into ischemia with resultant activation of the secondary loop. Referred pain and trigger point response, as well as protective spasm from tissue injury, probably result from this development.

Many soft-tissue injuries with prominent muscle stiffness and pain may ultimately be explained by these neurophysiologic studies which may come to explain symptoms and justify treatment modalities such as manipulation, trigger point intervention, and precise corrective exercises.

The pathophysiologic mechanisms discussed transmit through the dorsal root ganglia as do the nociceptive impulses preceding the sensation of pain. Treatment of painful musculoskeletal conditions should take this fact under consideration because *function* and impairment must be addressed as much as relief of pain. Acute pain usually subsides, but residual impairment with resulting disability presents the greatest concern in most musculoskeletal disorders.

Physical therapy aimed at relieving pain is also directed at exercise intending to minimize functional impairment. Precise exercises directed at slow-twitch and fast-twitch fibers, both dynamic and static, need careful evaluation and research. Trigger points in hyperactive painful muscles are now better understood when results from monopolar needle electromyograms (EMGs)[22] have shown activities mediated through sympathetic activated intrafusal loops. Understanding the spindle system of neuromuscular action will need further clinical implementation.

FIBROMYALGIA SYNDROMES

Muscle physiology and pathology have been discussed earlier in this chapter. Much current research is concerned with the fibromyalgia syndrome (FS): "a syndrome characterized by chronic pain widely distributed through all the skeletal muscles and soft tissues." Study of its pathomechanics and neuropathology have not yet provided a sound physiologic basis for successful treatment. All neuromuscular painful syndromes, whether acute or chronic, probably have a fibromyalgic component.

This condition was first written about by Hippocrates[23] but only in the last 150 years has there been significant attention paid to it as a clinical entity. Froriep[24] recognized areas of muscle *hardness* ("Muskelharten") that, when palpated, elicited pain. Beard[25] later described the syndrome which he called neurasthenia. The term *fibrositis* first appeared in the literature in 1904.[26] Since then, there have been numerous other diagnostic terms used to describe the condition.[27]

The International Association for the Study of Pain (IASP)[28] has codified the diagnosis under the heading of **Primary Fibromyalgia Syndrome** (PFS), considering the condition as *generalized myofascial syndrome*. The IASP classified these chronic musculoskeletal pain syndromes "without identifiable cause" as follows:

1. PFS as fibrositis or diffuse myofascial pain syndrome; primary diffuse fibrositis syndrome.
2. Myofascial pain syndrome (MPS) as specific myofascial pain syndrome.
3. Temporomandibular pain and dysfunction syndrome (TMPDS).

Diagnostic criteria are based on subjective evidence of long-standing musculoskeletal pain, fatigue, sleep disturbance, and the clinical findings of reproducible tender points (TP). The standard diagnostic criteria determined by Yunus and co-workers[29] are the most widely accepted. These criteria are divided into *obligatory, major, and minor* groupings necessary for the diagnosis to be confirmed. No objective diagnostic studies have led to a specific diagnosis.

Obligatory criteria include:

1. Generalized aches and pains or prominent stiffness, involving three or more anatomic sites for a period of at least 3-months' duration.
2. Absence of traumatic injury,* structural rheumatic disease, infectious arthropathy, endocrine-related arthropathy, and abnormal laboratory test results.

Major criterion: 3 or more typical and consistent tender points.
Minor criteria include:

1. Symptoms modulated following physical activity.
2. Symptoms altered by weather or atmospheric changes.
3. Symptoms aggravated by anxiety or stress.
4. Poor sleep.
5. General fatigue or tiredness.
6. Anxiety.
7. Chronic headaches.
8. Irritable bowel syndrome.
9. Subjective swelling.
10. Numbness: non-radicular and nondermatomal.

Smythe,[30] a pioneer in the research into fibrositis postulated the following findings for diagnostic purposes:

1. Widespread aching of longer than 3-months' duration.
2. Local tenderness present at 12 of 14 possible specific sites.

---

*"Absence of traumatic injury" is not accepted by the author because "trauma" is usually, if not universally, present.

3. Skin roll tenderness over the upper scapular region.
4. Disturbed sleep with morning fatigue and stiffness.
5. Normal estimated sedimentation rate (ESR), serum glutamate ox-aloacetate transaminase levels, rheumatoid factors' test, antinuclear factors (ANFs), muscle enzyme levels, and positive sacroiliac radiographs.

Obviously, these diagnostic criteria are subjective; they seem actually to mandate that there are no abnormal organic test results other than those sleep abnormalities objectively ascertained.[31]

Pathophysiology

Abnormalities of musculature have been implicated, as well as abnormal histologic findings from biopsies. None remain fully reproducible or confirmatory. Yunus[32] has speculated that all histologic abnormalities observed could result from ischemia or from microspasm of the musculature.

The nociceptors located in the muscles, tendons, and perivascular sites are the thin myelinated A-alpha and non-myelinated C fibers discussed in Chapter 2. Sensitization of these nerve endings are seen in *inflammation* caused by endogenous algesic chemical substances such as bradykinin, prostaglandins, leukotrienes, potassium ions, serotonin, and interleukin-1.[33,34]

Simultaneous administration of two of the above algesic substances has been shown to have potentiating effect at the nociceptor sites.[35] When preceded by either serotonin or prostaglandin E_2, the effect upon the receptor of bradykinin is enhanced by 10 minutes. It has also been demonstrated that bradykinin stimulates synthesis of prostaglandin from arachidonic acid so that the interplay of these algesic agents results in *inflammatory* response.

These substances affect local microcirculation, causing not only vasoconstriction or vasodilatation, but also increasing vascular permeability, which results in extravasation and edema. Ischemia of the involved tissues results in pain. The irritating effects of algogens cause *spasm*, which in turn enhances ischemia.

Hypoxia of the muscle allegedly decreases the intramuscular levels of adenosinotriphosphate and phosphocreatine which accounts for the pain.[36] Compromised capillary microcirculation in a *fibrositic* trapezius muscle has been found[37] to be diminished after ultrasound treatment, compared with the increase produced in normal muscle. Electromyographic studies have failed to reveal specific abnormalities that can be considered diagnostic although characteristic fatigue in the fibrositis muscle groups has been demonstrated.[38]

Muscle strength evaluated by B 2000 Isostation (Isotechnologies, Hillsborough, NC) has shown *weakness* in involved muscles when compared with contralateral *normal* muscle,[39] but the objectivity of this conclusion can be questioned as to the amount of *effort*[40] expended in the use of a painful muscle.

Although sleep disturbance in patients with fibromyalgia has been thoroughly described, it does not yet clarify the neurophysiologic basis for the syndrome.[41]

Metabolic abnormalities creating algogens in FS are promising. Serotonin (5-hydoxytryptamine), a central nervous system (CNS) neurotransmitter, is being studied. Serotonin is converted from the essential amino acid, tryptophan, when it crosses the blood-brain barrier. The source of serotonin is considered to be in the raphe nucleus in the brain stem.[42] It is well documented that depletion of serotonin decreases non-REM sleep,[43,44] as well as causes symptoms of depression. The relationship of tryptophan to symptoms of FS has been questioned,[45] but recently,[46] FS patients have been found to have lower than normal levels of tryptophan, as well as six other amino acids.

Therapeutic benefit from the use of tricyclic drugs (amitriptyline, imipramine, cyclobenzaprine) in FS enhances the postulate of their action being the blocking of serotonin reuptake at the synaptic cleft.[44] The precise role of serotonin itself has not yet been confirmed.[47]

Catecholamines have also been implicated in producing FS symptoms. Catecholamines are described as "biologically active amines, epinephrine and norepinephrine, derived from amino acid tyrosine. They have marked effect on the nervous and cardiovascular systems, metabolic rate, temperature and smooth muscle."[48] Serotonin is described "as a chemical (5-hydroxytryptamine) present in platelets, gastrointestinal mucosa, mast cells and carcinoid tumors. Serotonin is a potent vasoconstrictor. It is thought to be involved in neural mechanisms important to sleep and sensory perception."[48] All these have been found to be involved in FS.

Patients with FS have been determined[49] to have higher than normal urinary norepinephrine levels. In studies making this assertion, elevated levels were also found in patients with a high level of anxiety. These high levels incidentally were not found in patients exhibiting depression.

Substance P, a neuropeptide considered to be an algogen ("causing pain"),[49] has been found to exist in virtually all neuronal structures of the CNS: the spinal and trigeminal ganglia, the substantia gelatinosa (Rexed layers I and II) of the dorsal horn of the cord as well as in higher brain centers.[49] Their elevation or depression in the spinal fluid of patients with FS has had varying results.[50,51]

Endorphins, another group of neuropeptides, have been studied in the possible mechanism of FS pain. Endorphins are endogenously produced opioid substances of complex chemical structure and action. They are located in the same regions of the CNS as substance P, in peripheral nerve endings, the dorsal horn of the cord, midbrain, brain stem, and the thalamus. There is speculation that endorphins modulate the transmission of pain by inhibiting substance P.

Studies were conducted[52] suggesting that physical fitness decreases the perception of pain based on endorphin levels. Yunus,[53] however, found no difference in serum endorphin levels between patients with FS and normal controls.

Similarity of FS to rheumatoid arthritis, Raynaud's syndrome, hypothyroidism, and Sjögren's syndrome[54] has postulated involvement of the immune system. A 30-month follow-up of patients with FS, however, showed no patients had developed systemic disease.[55] Recent interest in the chronic fatigue syndrome and its relationship to FS is being explored with promise.[56]

A model for the fibromyalgia syndrome[57] was proposed with the muscle being the end organ responsible for the syndrome with microtrauma to muscle causing the symptoms. Perturber interruption of normal coordinated activities was considered as *trauma*.

In this proposed FS model, sleep impairment affects the growth hormone,[58] which depends on slow-wave sleep. When such sleep is deprived, suboptimal secretion[59] of growth hormone has a negative effect on protein metabolism. This may delay healing after microtrauma. Microtrauma also impairs muscle glycogen storage by causing fatigue.[60]

An interesting sequence of pathophysiologic mechanisms bringing all these concepts together has been proposed,[61] in which the syndrome is a complex interaction of nociceptive and neuropathic activity, with dysregulatory CNS function enhanced by psychosomatic mechanisms.

In this concept the sensory C fibers also have a neurosecretory function.[62] Neuropeptides released at the peripheral endings of C fibers cause vasodilatation and increase capillary permeability with extravasation. These peptides stimulate mast cells related to the immune system. They also release serotonin and histamine,[63] which act on local tissues causing *neurogenic inflammation*. Neurogenic inflammation was observed to be elevated in patients with fibromyalgia.[64]

Fifty years ago, neurogenic inflammation was termed **axon reflex** by Lewis,[65] reflecting it caused local vasodilatation from an increase in the microcirculation of the regional muscle.[66]

In cases diagnosed as fibromyalgia, substance P levels in cerebrospinal fluid (CSF) were found to be high,[67] which was considered to indicate an increased production of substance P in the afferent C fibers.

Abnormal posture causing hypertonus in many muscles may be a cause rather than a consequence of fibromyositis.[68] This is evident by the benefit derived from biofeedback in patients with low back pain, even though abnormal results from EMG examinations have not been found in these types of patients.[69]

A *central* mechanism is postulated in this muscular hypertonus.[70,71] Although unconfirmed, it is accepted that algogens reaching the CNS are further processed in the ultimate conscious perception of pain. Dysfunction of this process may result in the symptoms of fibromyalgia.[34,72] This dysfunction may be chemically based because it has been shown that substance P levels in the CSF are abnormally high in patients with fibromyalgia,[73] which causes overactivity of excitatory transmission. The associated sleep disorder in fibromyalgia is also evidence that there is impairment of the CNS.

Dysfunction may occur at the dorsal horn level,[74,75] or within the descending controls (Fig. 3–11) upon the dorsal horn from the periaqueductal gray (PAG) (*see* Chapter 2).[76] Serotonin synthesis has a definite chemical action on this descending system.[77] A proposed deficiency of serotonin has promoted the use of L-tryptophan, a precursor of 5-HT,[78] in treating chronic pain.

Management of Fibromyalgia Syndromes

From the possible mechanisms of the above models, it appears that management of FS requires modifying sleep, regaining conditioning, and controlling all neuromuscular perturbers. As the pain is considered to be within the muscles, all modalities including heat, massage, ice, spray and stretch, exercise, posture, biofeedback, meditation, and hypnosis can be used.[79]

Sleep abnormalities must be addressed by the use of tricyclic drugs. Mus-

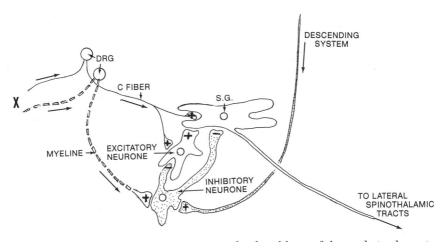

Figure 3–11. Nociceptive transmission to the dorsal horn of the cord. A schematic version of nociceptive transmission to the dorsal horn is presented. *X* is the noxious stimulus that is transmitted through afferent C fibers and myelinated large diameter fibers. In the substantia gelatinosa (SG) of the dorsal horn, the impulses go to and activate (+) the transmission cell of the SG. Impulses from the myelinated fibers activate the inhibitory neurons (−), which modulate the projection cell. Ultimately, the impulses are transmitted to the lateral spinothalamic tracts where they ascend to the thalamus. The descending tracts also modulate the impulses arriving at the transmission cells.

cle relaxants (e.g., cyclobenzamine) may enhance relaxation. Antidepressants have possible value and their use should be explored.

Because FS is considered a benign self-limited entity, explanation and reassurance from the physician are therapeutic. Permanent functional disability must be avoided. Because most soft tissue injuries have a muscular component, all the above aspects of fibromyalgia may be considered in evaluating and treating these specific conditions.

One article summarized fibromyalgia as "a chronic disorder of muscle pain, muscle stiffness and poor muscle endurance which varies from day to day but remissions are rare."[80]

The statistics regarding recovery were bleak. Only 32% of patients were able to resume full-time work and 55% resumed only part-time work.[81] Only a single person during an 8-year follow-up was free from symptoms. Muscle strength and endurance in comparison with those of healthy controls were markedly reduced.

That selective *dysfunctional muscles* cause fatigue and possibly even fibromyalgia has recently been postulated.[82] Static work loads using a small specific muscle group of slow-twitch fibers develop fatigue. If not given frequent rest periods, albeit for only a few seconds, they fatigue rapidly.[84] Once fatigued, they require longer periods of *rest* to recover.

The choice of a specific motor unit to perform a specific job is *centrally* decided. That specific motor unit becomes selectively incorporated into a *motor plan*. Continually using a single motor plan overloads the motor units within that plan and the precise motor unit becomes inhibited (i.e., *shut off*), initiating compensatory movement patterns. Any unit that is *shut off* may become the site of fibromyalgia.

This concept may have an implication in the development of carpal tunnel syndrome and low back pain syndrome, as well as in fibromyalgia.

A review of basic physiology may be instructive in this regard. There is specialization among muscle fibers understood since the *white meat* and *dark meat* of fowls were identified.[85] Muscle types were originally classified based on their metabolic characteristics, whether oxidative or glycolytic, but these were later found to be influenced by activity and training.

Slow-twitch fibers (type I) and fast-twitch fibers (type II) were ultimately found to be stable under normal innervation (Fig. 3–12). That they depend on their innervation is proven in that if the nerve to a fast-twitch muscle is transplanted into a slow-twitch muscle fiber, the new host muscle assumes the characteristics of the muscle previously supplied.[86]

Fast-twitch and slow-twitch fibers have their own force-velocity relationships with a greater rate of shortening in the fast-twitch fibers, but both fibers develop the same amount of force.

Motor unit recruitment patterns[87] depend on the size and the component parts of the motor unit. Type I have slow oxidation, a low threshold of recruitment, and generate low forces. This can be determined electromyographically

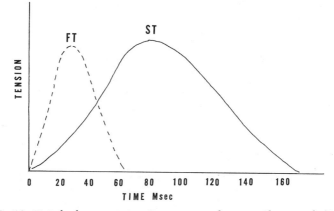

Figure 3–12. Twitch characteristics: Contraction-relaxation. Slow-twitch (ST) type I and fast-twitch (FT) type II muscle curves are depicted in milliseconds.

and can be influenced by biofeedback. The order of recruitment also influences the force. Low force units recruit early, fire regularly, and fatigue little. These units are termed *tonic*.

Type II units recruit later, fire irregularly, exert higher forces, and fatigue rapidly. *Fatigue* is any decrement in performance resulting from a previous activity and may be defined as the inability to carry out the assigned task in the assigned manner. The basis of fatigue is analyzed in aerobic terms.

Recruitment can best be defined as: repetitive equal stimuli applied to presynaptic fibers producing postsynaptic discharges of gradually increasing magnitude and frequency, thus *recruiting* surrounding neurons in a temporal relationship.[88]

Training modifies muscular activity with regard to strength, endurance, and coordination. This cannot be thoroughly discussed in this book but numerous references to the topic exist in the literature. Its evaluation by electromyography is also now scientifically possible.[89]

REFERENCES

1. Winters, JM and Woo, S L-V (eds): Multiple Muscle Systems: Biomechanics and Movement Organization. Springer-Verlag, New York, 1990.
2. Boyd IA, Eyzaguirre, C, Matthews, PBC, and Rushworth, G (eds): The Role of the Gamma System in Movement and Posture. Association for the Aid of Crippled Children, New York, 1964.

3. Matthews, PBC: Where does Sherrington's "Muscular Sense" originate? Muscle, joints, corollary discharges. Annu Rev Neurosci 5:189–218, 1982.
4. Sherrington, CS: 1990. Joint position sense. In Shafer, EA (ed): Textbook of Physiology, vol 2. Pentland, Edinburgh and London, 1900.
5. McMahon, TA: Reflexes and motor control. In: Muscles, Reflexes and Locomotion. Princeton University Press, Princeton, 1984, pp 144–148.
6. Schmidt, RF: Motor systems. In Schmidt, RF (ed): Fundamentals of Neurophysiology. Springer-Verlag, New York, 1985, pp 162–164.
7. Mense, S: Nociception from skeletal muscle in relation to clinical muscle pain. Pain 54:241–289, 1993.
8. Lloyd, DPC. Neuron patterns controlling transmission of ipsilateral hind limb reflexes in cat. J Neurophysiol 6:293–315, 1943.
9. Nakamura-Craig, M and Gill, BK: Effect of neurokinin A, substance P and calcitonin gene-related peptide in peripheral hyperalgesia in the rat paw. Neurosci Lett 124:49–51, 1991.
10. Cailliet, R: Pain: Mechanisms and Management. FA Davis, Philadelphia, 1993.
11. Headley, BJ: Muscle Inhibition. Phys Ther Forum, Nov 1, 24–26, 1993.
12. Travell, J and Simon D: Myofascial Pain and Dysfunction. The Trigger Point Manual, vol 1. Williams & Wilkins, Baltimore, 1992.
13. Menses, S and Skepper, P: Discharge behavior of feline gamma-motoneurones following induction of an artificial myositis. Pain 46:201–210, 1991.
14. Houk, JC, Crago, PE, and Rymer, WZ: Function of the spindle dynamic response in stiffness regulation—a predictive mechanism provided by non-linear feedback. In Taylor A Prochazka (ed): Muscle Receptors and Movement. Macmillan, London, 1981, p 299.
15. Johansson, H: Reflex integration in the gamma (γ) motor-system. In Boyd, JA and Gladden, MH (eds): The Muscle Spindle. Macmillan, London, 1985, p 297.
16. Johansson, H and Sojka, P: Pathophysiological mechanisms involved in genesis and spread of muscular tension in occupational muscle pain and in chronic musculoskeletal pain syndromes: A hypothesis. Med Hypotheses 35:196–203, 1991.
17. Gladden, GMH and Murphy, P: Static and dynamic fusiform neurones and their reflex control In: Boyd, IA and Gladden MH (eds): The Muscle Spindle. Macmillan, London, 1985, p 243.
18. Johansson, H, Lorentzon, R, Sjolander, P and Sojka, P: The anterior cruciate ligament: A sensor acting on the gamma-muscle spindle systems of muscle around the knee joint. Neuro-Orthopedics 9:1–23, 1990.
19. Johansson, H, Sjolander, P, and Sojka, P.: Fusiform reflexes in triceps surae muscle elicited by natural and electrical stimulation of joint afferents. Neuro-Orthopedics 6:67–80, 1998.
20. Appleberg, B, Hulliger, M, Johansson, H and Sojka, P: Actions on gamma neurone elicited by electrical stimulation of group III muscle afferent fibers in the limb of the cat. J Physiol (Lond) 335:275–292, 1983.
21. Edwards, RHT: Hypothesis of peripheral and central mechanisms underlying occupational muscle pain and injury. Eur J Appl Physiol 57:275–281, 1988.
22. Hubbard, DR and Berkoff, GM: Myofascial trigger points show spontaneous needle EMG activity. Spine 18:1803–1907, 1993.
23. Hippocrates. The Medical Works of Hippocrates. Chadwick, J and Mann WN (transl), Blackwell, Oxford, 1950.
24. Simons, DG: Muscle pain syndromes, part 1. Am J Phys Med 54:289–311, 1975.
25. Beard, GM: A Practical Treatise on Nervous Exhaustion (Neurasthenia). William Wood, New York, 1880.
26. Gowers, WR: Lumbago: its lesions and analogues. Br Med J 1:117–123, 1904.
27. Cailliet, R: Head and Face Pain. FA Davis, Philadelphia, 1992, pp 100–124.
28. International Association for the Study of Pain Subcommittee of Toxonomy: Chronic pain syndromes and definition of pain terms. Pain (Suppl 3):S1–S225, 1986.
29. Yunus, MB, Masi, AT, Calabro, JJ, et al: Primary fibromyalgia (fibrositis) clinical study of 50 patients with matched normal controls. Semin Arthritis Rheum 11:151–171, 1981.

30. Smythe, HA: "Fibrositis" as a disorder of pain modulation Clin Rheum Dis 5:823–832, 1979.
31. Moldofski, H: Sleep and musculoskeletal pain. Am J Med 81:(suppl 3A):85–89, 1986.
32. Yunus, MB and Kalyan-Ramon, UP: Muscle biopsy findings in primary fibromyalgia and other forms of nonarticular rheumatism. Rheum Dis Clin North Am 15:115–134, 1989.
33. Berberich, P, Hoheisel U, Mense, S, and Skeppar, P: Fine muscle afferent fibers and inflammation: Changes in discharge behaviour and influence on gamma-motoneurones. In: Schmidt, RF, Schaible, H-G, Vahle-Hinz, C (eds): Fine Afferent Nerve Fibers in Pain. VCH-Verlag, Weinheim, pp 165–175, 1987.
34. Diehl, B, Hoheisel, U and Mense, S: Histological and neurophysiological changes induced by carrageenan in skeletal muscle of cat and rat. Agents Actions 25:210–213, 1988.
35. Mense, S: Sensitization of group IV muscle receptors to bradykinin by 5-hydroxytryptamine and prostaglandin E2. Brain Res 225:95–105, 1981.
36. Bergtsson, A and Hendriksson, KG: The muscle in fibromyalgia: a review of Swedish studies. J Rheumatol 16(Suppl 19):144–149, 1989.
37. Klemp, P, Staberg, B, Korsgard, J., et al: Reduced blood flow in fibromyotic muscles during ultrasound therapy. Scand J Rehab Med 15:721–723, 1982.
38. Hagsberg, M and Kvarnstrom, S: Muscular endurance and electromyographic fatigue in myofascial shoulder pain. Arch Phys Med Rehabil 65:522–525, 1984.
39. Jacobsen, S and Danneskiold-Samsen, B: Isometric and isokinetic muscle strength in patients with fibrositis syndrome Scand J Rheumatol 16:61–65, 1987.
40. Ferraccioli G, Ghirelli L, Scita F, et al: EMG-biofeedback training in fibromyalgia syndrome. J Rheumatol 14:820–825, 1987.
41. Moldoksky, H, Scarisbrick, P, England, R, and Smythe, H: Musculoskeletal symptoms and non-REM sleep disturbance in patients with 'fibrositis syndrome' and healthy subjects. Psychosom Med 37:341–351, 1975.
42. Morgane, PJ: Serotonin twenty five years later: monamine theories of sleep. Psychopharmacol Bull 17:13–17, 1981.
43. Moldofsky, H: Rheumatic pain modulation disorder: the relationship between sleep, CNS serotonin and pain. In Critchley, M and Friedman A (eds): Headache: Physiopathological and Clinical Concepts. Raven Press, New York, 1982, pp 51–57.
44. Bowden, CL, Michalek, J, Fletcher, F, and Hester, GA: Imipramine receptor density on platelets of patients with fibrositis syndrome: correlation with disease severity and response to therapy (abstr). Arthritis Rheum 30:S63, 1987.
45. Moldofsky, H and Warsh, JJ: Plasma tryptophan and musculoskeletal pain in non-articular rheumatism. Pain 5:65–71, 1978.
46. Russell, IJ, Michalek, JF, Vipraio, GA, et al: Serum amino acids in fibrositis/fibromyalgia syndrome (abstract). Arthritis Rheum 32:S24, 1989.
47. Rice, JR: 'Fibrositis' syndrome. Med Clin North Am 70:455–468, 1986.
48. Thomas, CL: Taber's Cyclopedic Medical Dictionary, ed 15. FA Davis, Philadelphia, 1985.
49. Feldman, RS and Quenzer, LF: Fundamentals of Neuropsychopharmacology. Sinauer, Sunderland, MA, 1984.
50. Almar, BGL, Johansson, F, Von Knorring, L, et al: Substance P in CSF of patients with chronic pain syndromes. Pain 33:3–9, 1988.
51. Vaeroy, H, Halle, R, Forre, O, et al: Elevated CFS levels of substance P and high risk incidence of Raynaud's phenomenon in patients with fibromyalgia: new features for diagnosis. Pain 32:21–26, 1988.
52. McCain, GA: Role of physical fitness training in fibrositis/fibromyalgia syndrome. Am J Med 31:(Suppl 3A):73–77, 1986.
53. Yunus, MB, Denko, CW and Masi, AT: Serum beta-endorphin in primary fibromyalgia syndrome: a controlled study. J Rheumatol 13:183–189, 1986.
54. Goldenberg, DI: Fibromyalgia syndrome: an emerging but controversial condition. JAMA 257:105–115, 1987.
55. Dinerman, H, Goldenberg, DL, and Felson, DT: A prospective evaluation of 118 patients

with fibromyalgia syndrome: prevalence of Raynaud's phenomenon, Sicca syndrome. ANAs low complement and IG deposition at the dermal-epidermal junction. J Rheumatol 13:368–373, 1986.

56. Cheu, JW and Findley, T: Integrated Parallel-Cycle Model of Chronic Fatigue Syndrome. Univ Med Dent New Jersey, 1991: personal communication: publication pending.

57. Bennett, RM: Beyond Fibromyalgia: Ideas on Etiology and Treatment. J Rheumatology 16(Suppl 19):185–191, 1989.

58. Friden, J, Sjostrom, M and Ekblom, B: A morphological study of delayed muscle soreness. Experientia 37:506–507, 1981.

59. Newham, DJ, Mills, KR, Quigley, BM, and Edwards, RHT: Ultrastructural changes after concentric and eccentric contractions. Clin Sci 64:129–131, 1982.

60. Nimmo, MA and Snow, DH: Time course of ultrastructural changes in skeletal muscle after 2 types of exercise. J Appl Physiol 42:910–913, 1982.

61. Zimmermann, M: Pathophysiological Mechanisms of Fibromyalgia, Clin J Pain 58(Suppl 1):S15, 1991.

62. Chahl, LA, Szolcsanyi, J, and Lembeck, F (eds): Antidromic Vasodilitation and Neurogenic Inflammation. Akademiai Kiado, Budapest, 1984.

63. Lembeck, F and Gamse, R: Substance P in peripheral sensory processes. In: Porter, R and O'Connor, M (eds): Substance P in the nervous system. Ciba Found Symp 91:35–49, 1982.

64. Littlejohn, GO, Weinstein, C and Helme, RD: Increased neurogenic inflammation in fibrositis syndrome. J Rheumatol 14:1022–1025, 1987.

65. Lewis, T: Pain. Macmillan, London, 1942.

66. Ohlen, A, Lindbom, L, Hokfelt, T, et al: Effects of substance P and calcitonin gene-related peptide on the skeletal muscle microcirculation. In Henry, JL, Couture, R, Cuello, AC, et al (eds): Substance P and neurokinins. Springer Verlag, New York, 1987, pp 192–194.

67. Duggan, AW and North, RA: Electrophysiology of opioids. Pharmacol Rev 35:219–281, 1984.

68. Flor, H and Turk, DC: Etiological theories and treatments for chronic back pain. I. Somatic models and interventions. Pain 19:105–121, 1984.

69. Zidar, J, Backman, E, Bengtsson, A, and Henriksson, KG: Quantitative EMG and muscle tension in painful muscles in fibromyalgia. Pain 40:249–254, 1990.

70. Devor M.: Central changes mediating neuropathic pain. In Dubner, R, Gebhart, GF, Bond, MR, (eds): Proceedings of the Vth World Congress on Pain. Pain Research and Clinical Management, vol 3. Elsevier, Amsterdam, 1988, pp 114–128.

71. Zimmermann, M: Central nervous mechanisms modulating pain-related information: interaction with peripheral input. In Casey, KL (ed): Pain and Central Nervous System Disease: The Central Pain Syndromes. Raven Press, New York, 1991, pp 183–199.

72. (as reference 30) Smythe, HA: Fibrositis: a disorder of pain modulation. Clin Rheum Dis 5:823–832, 1979.

73. Vaeroy, H, Helle, R, Forre, O, et al: Elevated CFS levels of substance P and high incidence of Raynaud's phenomenon in patients with fibromyalgia: New features for diagnosis. Pain 32:21–26, 1988.

74. Willis, WD: Control of nociceptive transmission in the spinal cord. Springer Verlag, Berlin, 1982.

75. Zieglgansberger, W: Central control of nociception. In Mountcastle, VB, Bloom, FE and Geiger, SR (eds.): Handbook of Physiology—The Nervous System IV. Williams & Wilkins, Baltimore, 1986, pp 581–645.

76. Basbaum, AI and Fields, HL: Endogenous pain control systems: Brain stem spinal pathways and endorphin circuitry. Annu Rev Neurosci 7:309–338, 1984.

77. Carstens, E, Fraunhoffer, M and Zimmerman, M: Serotonergic mediation of descending inhibition from midbrain periaqueductal gray, but not reticular formation, of spinal nociceptive transmission in the cat. Pain 10:149–167, 1981.

78. Seltzer, S, Marcus, R, and Stoch, R: Perspectives in the control of chronic pain by nutritional manipulation. Pain 11:141–148, 1981.

79. Vecchiet, L, Giamberardino, MA and Saggini, R: Myofascial pain syndromes: Clinical and pathophysiological aspects. Clin J Pain 7(Suppl 1):S16–S22, 1991.

80. Felson, DT and Goldenberg, DL: The natural history of fibromyalgia. Arthritis Rheum 21:1522–1526, 1986.

81. Cathey, MA, Wolf, F, and Kleinheksel, SM, et al: Functional disability and work status in patients with fibromyalgia. Arth Care Res 1:1–14, 1988.

82. Bengtsson, A, Backman, E, Lindblom, B and Skogh, T: Long-term follow-up of fibromyalgia patients: Clinical symptoms, muscular function, laboratory tests—an eight-year comparison study. J Musculoskeletal Pain, 2(2): 1994.

83. Stokes, M, Edwards, R, and Cooper, R: Effect of low frequency fatigue on human muscle strength and fatigability during subsequent stimulated activity. Eur J Appl Physiol 59:278–283, 1989.

84. Jorgensen, K, Fallentin, N, Knrogh-Lund, C, and Jensen, B: Electromyography and fatigue during prolonged low-level static contractions. Eur J Appl Physiol 57:316–321, 1988.

85. DeLateur, BJ and Lehmann, JF: Therapeutic exercises to develop strength and endurance. In Kottke, FJ, Lehmann, JF (eds): Krusen's Handbook of Physical Medicine and Rehabilitation, ed 4. WB Saunders, Philadelphia, 1990, pp 480–519.

86. Knuttgen, HG (ed): Neuromuscular Mechanisms for Therapeutic and Conditioning Exercise. University Park Press, Baltimore, 1970, pp 31–53.

87. Henneman, E: Peripheral mechanisms involved in the control of muscle. In Mountcastle, VB (ed): Medical Physiology, ed 13. CV Mosby, St. Louis, 1974.

88. Campbell, HJ: Correlative Physiology of the Nervous System. Academic Press, New York, 1965, pp 103–104.

89. Lehman, JAR: Integration and analysis of the electromyogram and related techniques. In Walton, JN (ed): Disorders of Voluntary Muscle. Churchill Livingstone, Edinburgh, 1974, pp 1034–1072.

CHAPTER 4

Treatment Modalities

PHARMACOLOGY

Because pain is the presenting symptom in most patients with soft-tissue injuries, impairments, and disabilities, it must be dealt with early in therapy to permit initiation of more specific treatment modalities and to avoid further impairment, disability, or even chronic illness. Drugs have been the standard method of alleviating pain and will undoubtedly continue to play that role.

Medications aimed at relieving pain must be considered as intended to prevent disability and chronic illness by permitting and encouraging the patient to regain function and to resume normal activities. Medication must not create a need, a dependency, nor a manner of life.

The specific mechanisms of drug action have become a major aspect in the study of pain, as well as in other recent concerns of medical care.

Analgesics are pharmacologic agents which are considered to relieve pain by acting centrally. A possible mechanism has been postulated by the discovery of opiate receptors[1] in selected areas of the central nervous system (CNS) and of endogenous substances (enkephalins, also known as endorphins). The receptor sites have been termed mu, delta, and kappa.[2]

Opiate receptors are located in the medial thalamus—the area which processes deep, chronic, burning pain—as well as in areas of the cord gray matter, dorsal columns, and Rexed layers I and II. Opiate receptors are also greatly concentrated in the *amygdala*, a part of the limbic system.[3]

The presence of these receptors indicates that the body is capable of manufacturing its own narcotic-like substance. Two such substances have been discovered, both pentapeptides: tyrosine-glycine-glycine-phenyl-alanine-methionine and tyrosine-glycine-glycine-phenylalanine-leucine.[4]

Opium and morphine derivatives have been manufactured to be exogenous opioids.

One hypothesis is that opioids inserted at these sites activate the descending pathways to the midbrain periaqueductal gray (PAG) matter,[5] which inhibits ascension of nociception from the cord level.[6] Pain interruption has thus been asserted to occur at the cord level and at the dorsal root ganglia.

One study has postulated that opiates have an effect at the peripheral mechanism as well.[7] In this study, patients undergoing arthroscopic knee surgery followed by intra-articular morphine therapy had significantly diminished postoperative pain. The mechanism for this relief remains obscure.

The primary afferent nociceptor neuron is directed centrally to the spinal dorsal horn and its peripheral axons and proceeds distally to innervate the skin, muscle, and joint tissues. Opiate receptors are synthesized in the cell bodies of the receptors located in the dorsal root ganglia and are transported distally and centrally.

In pain it is considered that many agents sensitize primary afferent nociceptors directly by activating a G protein. The G protein activates adenylate cyclase which increases intracellular cyclic AMP (cAMP).[8] Opiates acting upon mu opiate receptors activate an inhibitory G protein which, in turn, inhibits adenylate cyclase with decreased production of cAMP.[9] The threshold of the nociceptor terminal is elevated and pain sensation is decreased. This action implies that pain mediation from opiates is essentially chemical intervention on the receptors of opiate action at various levels in the CNS: the median raphe of the midbrain, the dorsal root ganglia, and the peripheral nociceptor sites where initial trauma or irritation occurs.

Opioids, in addition to their direct action on the mu receptors, also act on the alpha and kappa receptors and on the postganglionic sympathetic terminals that block release of prostanoids.[10] Prostanoids are thought to be involved in sympathetic maintained-pain syndromes.

Opioids may also decrease the release of the pain-producing inflammatory mediator neuropeptide substance P. The lymphocyte-derived opioid peptide, considered to act upon peripheral opioid receptor, may be blocked by local opioid action.[11] How and if local opioids at the peripheral level influence other aspects of inflammation such as rubor, calor, and tumor remains a promising avenue for further research.

The local opioid liberated at the trauma site acting on the opioid receptor may not derive from the endogenous pituitary nor the adrenal medulla, but may actually be an opioid peptide derived from local lymphoid cells.

Therapies that aim to decrease influx of lymphoids at the trauma site may reduce endogenous peripheral pain–modulation opioids and increase the severity of local tissue damage.[12] This indicates the need to monitor the therapies carefully—both physical and medicinal modalities.

In treating pain resulting from acute peripheral inflammatory conditions, particularly the musculoskeletal aspects of the lumbosacral spine, it may be better to use local opioids at the periphery or at the dorsal root ganglia, rather than oral or intramuscular opioids acting at the central level with undesirable side effects.

Serotonin has been implicated in producing pain in cardiac conditions resulting from ischemic heart disease. Serotonin (5-hydroxytryptamine) is a vasoactive agent which acts by directly activating serotonergic and alpha-adrenergic receptors.[13] The role of serotonin in the treatment of pain has not been significantly explored but is a plausible factor.

During platelet aggregation from local tissue trauma, serotonin is released and this activity in turn furthers platelet aggregation. Serotonin binds 5-hydroxytryptamine receptors on epithelial cells and on smooth muscle cells, thus causing contraction (*spasm* of blood vessels). If the epithelial cells are normal, neutralizing chemicals are liberated that *wash out* these accumulating agents. If the tissue is damaged, however, these *neutralizers* are absent or diminished and vasoconstriction results.[14,15] This may well be the mechanisms of ischemic muscle pain.

Animal studies have strengthened the evidence for a serotonin pain-inhibitor mechanism in the CNS. Inhibition of serotonin (5-HT) synthesis by parachlorophenylalanine (pCPA) increases pain sensitivity. Administration of 5-hydroxytryptophan, a precursor of serotonin, restores depleted serotonin and returns the pain threshold to normal.[17] Lesions in the medial forebrain also reduce serotonin levels and lower the pain threshold, which can be restored to normal levels by administration of the serotonin precursor.[18] Injection of serotonin into the cerebral ventricles of rats and mice have raised their pain thresholds.[19]

Morphine depends on a serotonin mechanism for its effectiveness in moderating pain. Morphine decreases serotonin in the brain. This effect is modified by both pCPA and reserpine and can be reversed by administration of a serotonin precursor.

Because chronic pain is often associated with depression, a common mechanism regarding depletion or decrease in serotonin levels has been postulated.[20] Reserpine and 5-hydroxytryptophan cause depression and chlorimipramine (a selective serotonin reuptake blocking agent) is an antidepressant. This supports the theory that higher serotonin levels decrease pain tolerance and increase depression.

Pharmacologic intervention of pain, whether acute or chronic, can be administered orally, by numerous injection routes such as intramuscular, intradermal, epidural, dural, and intra-articular and even by mucosal routes. Many drugs are available that require extensive description,[21] and which cannot be fully discussed in this book. Each neuromusculoskeletal painful entity will have a pharmacologic intervention suggested, if the condition appears to be specific and not general.

PHYSICAL INTERVENTION

After the symptom of pain has been evaluated, the precise tissue site must be determined and its functional and psychologic significance established. The initial treatment of pain is a level sufficient to eliminate the nociceptor input and to allay the apprehension and impairment of the patient.

Haldeman[22] commented that the "proliferation of new technology and advanced skills for the investigation and treatment of spinal pain has not influenced the overall incidence, morbidity, cost or disability related to spinal pain disorders." This statement could well relate to other neuromusculoskeletal pains that are enumerated in this book. Statistics reflect an increasing incidence and higher expenses in the investigation and treatment of spinal and extremity disorders.

The term **nomogenic disorder** was proposed by Tyndel and Tyndel[23] as being analogous to iatrogenic: "any adverse mental or physical condition induced in a patient by effects of treatment by a physician or surgeon . . . such effects could have been avoided by proper and judicious care on the part of the physician, surgeon or dentist."[24] All modalities and techniques advocated in treatment protocols must be considered in light of this fact before physicians advocate and administer a specific treatment. The assessment of outcomes must also be guided by this factor.

Interruption of acute or recurrent pain is intended to ensure the prevention of ultimate chronic pain or to minimize its intensity, which, in itself, may become a disease rather than merely a symptom of one.

Interruption of the acute pathways of pain has been clearly discussed by Bonica in his classic two-volume text.[25] Acute pain consists of a complex constellation of unpleasant sensory, perceptual, and emotional experiences with certain associated autonomic, psychologic, emotional, and behavioral responses to a noxious stimulus produced by injury and disease.[25] All these factors must be addressed.

The quality of pain varies with the tissue responsible for the pain. Various adjectives such as sharp, pricking, burning, and stabbing are used to describe the more superficial tissue sites, such as skin and subcutaneous tissues. Other pains are described as aching or tightening, where deeper tissues are involved. Quality of pain is variously characterized as excruciating, frightening, or unbearable, implying the significance of the pain to the patient. Pain can be localized and localizing or it may be generalized and nonspecific as to site in the lumbosacral spine. Differentiations and interpretation of these symptoms depend upon the expertise and experience of the examiner. Because there are so few *objective* signs in many musculoskeletal soft tissue injuries, most symptoms are *subjective* in relation to pain.

Most soft tissue painful disorders can be considered as "benign"* posing a therapeutic challenge because although the cause may be considered innocuous by the examiner, it is not so acknowledged or accepted by the patient. Pain for which no cause or structural component can be determined understandably poses diagnostic and therapeutic problems.

Modalities

Sensitization of peripheral nociceptors by various types of trauma can also be enhanced by the application of modalities such as heat or ice.[27] This phenomenon within peripheral nociceptors causes pain from otherwise innocuous mechanical or thermal stimuli. There are many examples of this phenomenon of which sympathetic mediated pain (SMP) is a prime example.

Because of the possibility of the modality of thermal agents aggravating superficial pain, this must be considered in the application of such a modality for the purpose of pain relief.[28] Proper choice of a specific agent and appropriate application is therefore mandatory.

The noxious agents that accumulate at the peripheral trauma site including histamine, kinins, neuropeptides, and other algogens have a vasomotor effect: either vasodilatation or vasoconstriction. These nociceptive agents lower the threshold of the receptors of the A-delta and C-afferent fibers of the peripheral nervous system sending impulses cephalad. Intervention or elimination of these alogens at the trauma tissue site is the objective of the application of most modalities.

The local area becomes hypersensitive, creating pain known as *primary hyperalgesia. Secondary hyperalgesia* in the surrounding tissues results from antidromic activation of the C-primary afferents, which release substance P in the region.[29] This hypersensitivity may also be an after discharger from small primary afferents that release substance P. Electrical stimulation of the primary afferents has been shown to release substance P at their receptor ends. Reactive local skeletal muscle spasm then occurs, initiating a pain-spasm-pain cycle.[30]

The chemical and mechanical substances produced at the peripheral tissue site following injury are a mechanism of pain production that must be addressed in the treatment of *acute* and even some aspects of *chronic* pain.

---

*Benign: not recurrent or progressive and not malignant.[26]

Cryotherapy

Cryotherapy, the application of cold in the treatment of acute pain, has been an accepted modality for centuries. Three possible mechanisms for the effectiveness of local cold have been (1) a receptor adaptation;[31] (2) a counterirritant effect;[32] and (3) a neurogenic effect.[33] To date no evidence exists that cold thermal agents activate the endorphin system as has been postulated.

Cold lowers the temperature of the skin and underlying tissues by *removing* heat from them. Its local application as a treatment modality for a traumatized area is that (1) its being a vasoconstrictor decreases or inhibits bleeding; (2) it decreases local tissue metabolism that produces algogens; (3) it neutralizes the local histamine liberated by trauma; (4) it decreases local muscle spasm by lowering the sensitivity of the muscle spindle system;[34] and (5) it elevates the threshold of pain-transmitting nerves.

One local tissue reaction to trauma is the formation of edema. Edema occurs because of changes of hydrodynamics as vasoconstriction is followed by reflex vasodilatation. The afflicted vessels, the arterioles, the capillaries, the venules, and the lymphatics become distended. Endothelial cells separate and create gaps between the cells, thus allowing greater filtration of the serum with its contained constituents to enter the perivascular tissues.

This *edematous fluid* at first is merely a *transudate* containing water and dissolved electrolytes. It has a specific gravity of 1.012 and maintains osmotic balance. As permeability increases, the transudate becomes an *exudate* containing cells and protein, with a specific gravity of more than 1.012, which causes an imbalance of osmotic pressure causing further outward flow into perivascular tissues.

Both transudate and exudate create a mechanical impedance to further blood flow and result in ischemia. The protein contained in the exudate gradually causes chemical *thickening* of the fluid, which impairs physiologic movement between fascial planes.

Ice or cold applied to *inflamed* tissues intervenes in this transudate-exudate cycle by decreasing fluid transudate levels and lowering the metabolic rate. Cold also decreases tissue sensitivity, which permits active and passive exercises that mechanically express the exudate and transudate from the tissues.

Nerves differ in their reaction to cold[35] depending on their degree of myelination. The unmyelinated small diameter fibers are less responsive to cold than are A fibers with the large motor fibers (Alpha) the least affected.[36]

Exercise done after the application of cold generates more muscular tension.[37] The combined effects of ice, therefore, decreases pain, alters hydrodynamics, and permits greater strength of muscle contraction, decreasing edema and removing the accumulation of the nociceptive metabolites.

Therapeutic Heat.

The sequelae of the effects of heat on tissues depends on the level extent of increased temperature, the rate of application of heat energy, and the amount of tissue exposed to the heat application.[38] Elevation between 40° and 50°C increases blood flow, which is the therapeutic objective.

Temperature elevation increases blood flow which causes cooler blood to reach the site and displace the warmer blood. The rate of temperature increase influences its efficacy. A slow rise of tissue temperature may defeat the objective of heat application as it brings cooler blood into the inflamed tissue site. Too rapid an increase in temperature may also be deleterious, because the heat generated in the local tissues may stimulate pain receptors with adverse effect.

The effects of heat can be stated to be an alteration in metabolic activity, hemodynamic function, neural response, skeletal muscle activity, and modification of collagen tissue.[39] All these effects can be directly or indirectly related to the management of pain resulting from tissue trauma. The neural response more directly intervenes in transmission, but other effects of heat relate to the tissue dysfunction, which also enhances pain.

The neural effect of how heat provides analgesia and reduces muscle spasm, both functions of pain production, is not fully understood.[40,41] The latter, reduction of muscle spasm, is conceivably induced through the spindle system.[42] Heating the area over a peripheral nerve by high-intensity infrared radiation has induced[43] analgesia distal to the application. Much research remains to be performed relative to the precise neurophysiologic basis for relief from pain, but clinical experience seems to show validity.

Surface heating agents do not elevate muscle temperature needed to alter II or Ib afferent nerve activity, whereas skin temperature heating has decreased gamma (γ) efferent activity,[43] which may have an effect on diminished muscle spasm related to pain reduction.

Metabolic rate increases twofold to threefold with every 10°C rise. To increase the tissue temperature above 50°C burns the tissues, because their repair potential cannot cope with the protein denaturation of excessive heat. Chemical and metabolic activities are beneficially increased when therapy is kept below that temperature.

The hemodynamic effect of increasing blood flow occurs as superficial heat causes a reflex postganglionic sympathetic nerve activity to the smooth muscles of the blood vessels, supplying more blood flow to deeper organs such as muscle.[44]

The most effective heat modality proposed for therapeutic intervention has produced voluminous medical literature[45] and so will not be thoroughly evaluated here.

Moist heat transmitted using hot packs has many advocates.[46] Locally applied hot paraffin is effective in treating extremities as is hydrotherapy,[47] but it is not used in the low back, nor with ultrasound,[47] diathermy, pulsed electromagnetic fields, laser, and ultrasound. Whimsically, Licht[48] commented "the choice of source of heat will depend upon the training and experience of the physician, or empirically: the latter, a matter of local routine often based, regrettably on such considerations as cost, availability, convenience, hand-me-down habits, custom or publicity."

Modalities for Elongation

Connective tissue impaired by injury or disease benefits from heat application. Connective tissue, whether collagen, elastin, or fibrous, tends to shorten after injury.[49] The viscoelastic properties of connective tissues that permit elongation from physical stretch are known as *plastic deformation*.[50] Recoverable deformation is possible if the modalities of heat and passive-active stretch are applied to the deformed (i.e., shortened) tissues.[51]

The need to regain tissue flexibility in treating pain is apparent in that sensory nerves are enclosed within the soft tissues which often have become impaired after injury or during prolonged tension resulting from anxiety, anger, and emotional tension.

To return the physiologic elongation of damaged tissues to their normal length requires ensuring the appropriate temperature elevation as regards intensity, site, and duration. Consideration must also be given to the extent of intensity, duration, and velocity of physical stretch.[52] The techniques of stretch have been propounded varying from: (1) constant load to overcome impaired elasticity; (2) rapid stretch followed by holding the gained elongation; to (3) a slow progressive stretch.[52]

EXERCISE

For many years exercise has been the major conservative modality in the treatment of soft tissue pain. It is advocated in the management of acute and chronic pain, as well as prevention of recurrence.

Some controversy persists as to which form of exercise is appropriate in treating the various pain syndromes. Exercise is prescribed for flexibility, strength, endurance, aerobic fitness, stretching regimens, diminution of tension, or restoration of normal function. Controversy is exacerbated in respect to the virtues of active versus passive therapy.[53] Outcomes assessment of exercise regimens, long needed, has been undertaken recently with many articles appearing in medical journals[54–62] mostly concerned with low back disorders.

In a discussion of evaluation of the physical management of low back pain,[63] many modalities are discussed but exercise is not one of them. In a provocative 1988 article, Tollison and Kriegel[64] posed two questions: (1) what evidence supports the claim of the value of exercise; and (2) which exercises have proven most beneficial? Cady and associates[65] firmly established the role of physical exercise and general fitness in the *prevention* of back injuries and pain.

The literature on exercise in relation to soft tissue disorders and pain has had the following objectives: (1) decrease duration of the impairment and thus disability; (2) strengthen and increase endurance; (3) reduce mechanical stress (ergonomics); (4) correct posture; (5) restore general health; and (6) reduce pain.

In reduction of duration of pain and impairment, the exercise prescribed in the traditional model is "exercise according to pain severity . . . let pain be your guide." Fordyce and colleagues[66] initiated exercise at a fixed time but not at a fixed symptom, with a significant decrease in duration of disability.

DeVries,[67] through the use of EMG studies, concluded that muscular deficiency could be a causal factor in low back pain and that muscular fatigue was also significant.[68]

All these studies on back muscle strength and endurance indicate that susceptibility injuries are influenced by deficiency but fail to indicate the value of exercise after the patient has become symptomatic.

Reduction of mechanical stress (ergonomics) using exercise also remains controversial. *Body mechanics* involve eccentric muscle contraction (elongation/deceleration). Postural correction is considered to be a cause of low back, cervical, and shoulder disorders. Although supposedly improved by exercise, this remains unconfirmed.[69]

Pain reduction in the low back remains the predominant subject in treatment protocols. The statement that "exercise therapy is the cornerstone treatment for subacute and chronic pain"[70] is quoted in Bonica's classic volumes of the *Management of Pain.*[71] The statement continues "During acute pain exercise generally is contraindicated except for maintaining self administered passive range of motion (ROM) of all extremities and the trunk." Subacute pain, however, "is less intense . . . therefore therapeutic exercise is highly desirable and realistic 'for restoration of function to the affected area' . . . " This statement implies that exercise is mainly directed to the functional impairment of trauma or illness and only is indirectly applied to relief from pain.

In treating chronic pain, exercise is directed to the effects of decreased activity leading to atrophy, weakness, contracted joints, among others, with pain only indirectly addressed. In Basmajian's treatise on *Therapeutic Exercises,*[72] the use of exercise in treating syndromes involving pain is directed at specific areas or organ systems, such as low back or arthritis, without mention of exercise as a modality treating pain in a more general sense. DeVries[73] in his discussion of the physiology of exercise does not mention pain.

Fordyce,[74] whose *Operant Conditioning* has become an accepted effective treatment procedure in the treatment of chronic pain, uses exercise only to increase activity level. He states that "exercise is, with few exceptions, also a behavior that is incompatible with pain behavior."

No doubt remains that muscular weakness prevalent in many musculoskeletal pain syndromes,[75] as well as fatigue and debility such as occur in depression from chronic pain can be altered, in part, by exercise. In that respect exercise to regain strength and endurance, as well as flexibility and mobility, is a powerful adjunct in treatment of pain.

Exercise has been implied as increasing endorphin (endogenous opioid peptides) levels.[76] Endorphins are accepted neurotransmitters with a morphine-like action.[77] This modulation of pain perception and analgesia has been associated with the analgesia of electrical brain stimulation and acupuncture.[78]

Exercise results in elevation of adrenocorticotropic hormone, cortisol, and catecholamines, which are the precursors of beta endorphins. Many athletes have had decreased pain perception that has allowed them to make maximum effort "in spite of pain" and even claimed to reach an emotional high after extreme physical activity.[79]

Naloxone has altered pain perception experienced after running,[80] indicating that naloxone, as a narcotic antagonist which competes for endorphin-binding sites, substantiates the premise that endorphins are acting in the athlete. After 30 minutes of strenuous exercise, an elevation in the level of plasma endorphins has been noted. Further studies have, however, refuted these assertions,[81] when they found that mood changes attributed to endorphins after a 10-mile run were evident both with and without administration of naloxone.

Pitts[82] studied the effects of emotions and found an implied association of endorphins in stressful exercises postulated that the accumulated lactate from maximal exercising induced anxiety which has a mood-induced endorphin effect. This has been refuted[81] by the finding that elevated endorphin levels after stressful exercise may be noted without significant attendant elevation of lactates.

A recent paper[83] discussed an experiment wherein no analgesic effect from exercise was found, but that instead an analgesic effect resulted from the pain's *pretesting* itself. In this experiment subjects were exposed to pain pretesting, and that those who were tested exhibited analgesia from the test alone. Exercise following the test did not alter the analgesic effect.[84]

The conclusion of a relationship between endorphins and mood changes and analgesia related to strenuous exercise has not yet been ascertained but there is value in further studies. What seems, so far, apparent is that exercise must be strenuous in order to provide an analgesic effect and therefore its role in treatment of pain will depend on the physical and psychologic ability of the afflicted patient to implement this modality when confronted with persistent or chronic pain.

Exercise has a well-documented place in the physical treatment of most neuromusculoskeletal painfully disabling conditions. Its precise role in the treatment of acute low back pain, as an example of a soft tissue disorder, remains unclear as does its role in prevention of recurrence.

Further studies are needed to evaluate the efficacy of any exercise program and its objective. The provocative article of Headley[85] questioning the physiologic basis of treatment of *muscle spasm* is one indication because the muscles allegedly in *spasm* were electrically silent (see Chapter 3).

This should not be considered as refuting exercises in the therapy of patients with soft tissue disorders but rather be seen as a plea for a careful scientific outcomes assessment in evaluating the use of exercise in patients with these complaints.

Exercise is administered with a personal regard for the patient. Information and instruction given to the patient undoubtedly play a large role in either benefit or lack of it in the treatment program.

Discipline of the patient in performing the prescribed exercise also needs evaluation. Exercise requires effort, dedication, and a promise of value for the effort shown. The psychologic effect is evident. In today's incumbent economic consideration of any necessary prescribed medical care, it behooves professionals to evaluate their prescribed modalities carefully.

In this text exercise is discussed in relationship to the various neuromusculoskeletal disorders.

MANUAL THERAPY

Manual therapy encompasses techniques of passive movement such as massage, muscle stretching, traction-distraction, mobilization, and manipulation with guarded outcomes for long-term benefit.[86] The rationale for, indications for, and techniques of manipulation and mobilization are important and are discussed under the precise neuromusculoskeletal disorder in subsequent chapters.

The supposition that joints become *locked* and thus impaired has been a basis for manual therapy being used for their release. Soft tissues have a propensity to shorten when immobilized or restricted by injury; they require strengthening to regain their normal physiologic length.[87] To this end, several techniques of stretch have been proposed: (1) constant load to overcome impaired elasticity; (2) more rapid stretch followed by holding the gained elongation; and (3) slower, more progressive stretch.[88]

Manipulation may possibly also have an effect upon modification of the gamma-alpha neuronal interaction, but this remains without scientific verification.

In regards to manipulative (chiropractic) treatment of low back pain, which is one of the major indications for this type of manipulative intervention, the following conclusions were reached:[89]

"Manipulation, the abrupt passive movement of a vertebra beyond its physiological range, whether by chiropractors, osteopaths, orthopedists or physical therapists, has enjoyed broad acceptance by acute and chronic back sufferers in spite of the fact that few scientific studies have demonstrated that it affords anything more than temporary relief."[89-93]

"There is absolutely no scientific basis for it but if the patient feels more secure it would not seem to be unreasonable to taper off the treatments for up to two months."[89]

Chiropractors furnish 94% of manipulative care in this country.[94] "The fact that chiropractic manipulation, which may or may not differ materially from similar care administered by osteopaths, physical therapists, trainers or orthopedic surgeons, can take only part of the credit for favorable outcome. One cannot overestimate the positive impact of the dietary advice, nutritional supplement and professional counseling given the patient and there is nothing in the literature to prove that the manual component of the care, in isolation from these modalities, can affect visceral disorders."[94]

The aim of manipulation is to restore full range and quality of motion to affected and dysfunctional muscles, ligaments, and joints. It begins with the patient's joint being positioned so that muscles or joints are placed at maximum stretch and that the stretched muscle cannot effectively resist the thrust of manipulation.

The additional abrupt thrust (stretch) on the maximally extended muscle is thought to stimulate the muscle spindles and connective tissue's proprioceptive organs resulting in relaxation of the muscles, as well as effect the pain mechanism.[94-96]

Because manual therapy is so widely advocated in soft tissue injuries, it has been given greater emphasis, while admitting that the scientific basis for it remains obscure.

ANALGESIC NERVE BLOCKS

The original text of Bonica's *The Management of Pain* stated in its title "with Special Emphasis on the Use of Analgesic Block in Diagnosis, Prognosis, and Therapy."[98] This laid the groundwork for interrupting all peripheral tissue sites of nociception by analgesic nerve blocks. This concept is still valid for use in acute and recurrent pain for its diagnostic localization, treatment, and even prognosis.

Diagnostic nerve blocks, although less sensitive and accurate than diagnostic imaging and electrodiagnosis,[99] are valuable in locating and identifying a structural abnormality. After *the structure* or *the tissue* has been ascertained, interruption of its sensory nerve supply can be therapeutic as well as diagnostic.

The purpose of analgesic nerve blocks is to interrupt transmission of nociceptive impulses of the afferents to the gray matter of the cord from the damaged or traumatized tissues. Interruption of the nerve of the afflicted organ or tissue becomes a diagnostic tool. Interruption of the acute pain is therapeutic and allows other modalities to be initiated to assure healing and functional recovery. It, at the very least, allows the patient comfort during the healing process.

Knowing that repeated or continuous afferent impulses from the terminal of the afflicted organ increases the sensitivity of the dorsal root ganglion, the dorsal column neurons, and even the thalamic pathway's interruption of the acute initial barrage of afferent impulses diminishes enhancement of subsequent peripheral and central nervous system sensitivity. Avoidance of subsequent chronic pain is achieved, or the pain is, at least, minimized.

Bonica states that "Analgesic blocking, skillfully performed, can play a significant role in the management (of acute low back) pain, regardless of its etiology." He continues with the statement "it is . . . an important adjunct to other treatments . . . even though it may produce complete and permanent relief of pain." He also stressed that analgesic blocks are effective in relieving muscle spasm "as known." As has been stated and will be stated again, the mechanism of *spasm* remains conjectural, yet nerve blocks do relieve the pain and limitation is considered to result from this *spasm.*

Analgesic blocks are also administered into tender muscles, ligaments, tendons, and joint cavities. Caudal and peridural blocks are also effective, albeit as interrupting precise nerves, and so are to be considered only when pain persists in spite of administration of other modalities.

The techniques of performing nerve blocks have been extensively described in medical, surgical, and anesthesia textbooks.[98–101] The precise nerve supply of every tissue is well known, but, technically, interrupting this nerve supply is not necessarily within the range of skill of the average clinician and such activity may not be indicated as an initial procedure.

Analgesia occurring after nerve block, which continues after the expected duration of the injected chemical, remains effective for reasons currently unknown.

The value of nerve blocks in treating soft tissue injuries is accepted as a primary modality as well as an adjunctive therapy. It has played and continues to play a major role in pain, impairment, and disability and should be included in the armamentarium of every clinician.

REFERENCES

1. Pert, CB and Snyder, SH: Opiate receptors: Demonstration in nervous tissue. Science 179:1011–1014, 1973.
2. Hughes, J: Isolation of an endogenous compound from the brain with pharmacological properties similar to morphine. Brain Res 88:295–308, 1975.
3. Cailliet R: Pharmacological intervention in pain. In Cailliet, R: Pain: Mechanism and Management. FA Davis, Philadelphia, 1993, pp 91–99.
4. Hughes, J: Search for the endogenous ligand of the opiate receptor. Neurosci Res 13:55–58, 1975.
5. Basbaum, AI and Fields, HL: Endogenous pain control system: brain stem spinal pathways and endorphin circuitry. Annu Rev Neurosci 7:309–338, 1984.
6. Yaksh, TI and Rudy, TA: Analgesia mediated by direct spinal action of narcotics. Science 192:1357–1358, 1976.

7. Stein, C, Comisel, K, Haimeri, E, et al: Analgesic Effect of Intracarticular Morphine After Arthroscopic Knee Surgery. New Engl J Med 325:1123–1126, 1991.

8. Taiwo, YO, Bjerknes, LK, Goetzl, EJ, and Levine, JD: Mediation of primary afferent peripheral hyperalgesia by the cAMP second messenger system. Neuroscience 32:577–580, 1989.

9. Levine, JD and Taiwo, YO: Involvement of the mu-opiate receptor in peripheral analgesia. Neuroscience 32:571–575, 1989.

10. Taiwo, YO and Levine, JD: k- and alpha-opioids block sympathetically dependent hyperalgesia. J Neurosci 11:928–932, 1991.

11. Basbaum, AI and Levine, JD: Opiate analgesia. How central is a peripheral target. N Engl J Med 325:1168–1169, 1991.

12. Jessell, TM and Iversen, LL: Opiate analgesics inhibit substance P release from rat trigeminal nucleus. Nature 268:54–61, 1977.

13. Coderre, TJ, Chan, AK, Helms, C, et al: Increasing sympathetic nerve terminal-dependent plasma extravasation correlates with decreased arthritic joint injury in rats. Neuroscience 40:185–189, 1991.

14. Stein, C, Hassan, AHS, Przewlocki, R, et al: Opiodes from immunocytes interact with receptors on sensory nerves to inhibit nociception in inflammation. Proc Natl Acad Sci, U S A, 87:5935–5939, 1990.

15. Lam, JY, Chesebro, JH, Steele, PM, et al: Is vasospasm related to platelet deposition? Relationship in a porcine preparation of arterial injury in vivo, Circulation 75:243–248, 1987.

16. Vanhouttee, PM and Shimokawa, H: Endothelium-derived relaxing factor and coronary vasospasm. Circulation 80:1–9, 1989.

17. Harvey, JA and Lints, C: Pharmacologist 20:211, 1968.

18. Akil, H, Mayer, DJ, and Liebeskind, JC: Antagonism of stimulation-produced analgesia by p-CPA, a serotonin synthesis inhibitor. Brain Res 44:692–697, 1972.

19. Calcutt, CR, Handley, SL, Sparkes, CG, and Spencer, PSJ: In Kosterlitz, HW, Collier, HOJ, and Villareal, JA (eds): Agonist and Antagonist Actions of Narcotic Analgesic Drugs. University Park Press, Baltimore, 1973.

20. Sternbach, RA, Janowsky, DS, Leighton, YH, and Segal, DS: Effects of Altering Brain Serotonin Activity on Human Chronic Pain. In Bonica, JJ and Albe-Fessard, D (eds): Advances in Pain Research and Therapy, vol 1. Raven Press, New York, 1976.

21. Gennaro, AR (ed): Remington's Pharmaceutical Sciences, ed 18. Mack Publishing, Easton, Penna., 1990.

22. Haldeman, S: Failure of the pathology model to predict back pain. Spine 15:718–724, 1990.

23. Tyndel, M and Tyndel, FJ: Post-traumatic stress disorders: A nomogenic disease. Emotional First Aid 1:5–10, 1984.

24. Thomas, CL (ed): Taber's Cyclopedic Medical Dictionary, ed 16. FA Davis, Philadelphia, 1989, p 885.

25. Bonica, JJ: The Management of Pain, ed 2. Lea & Febiger, Philadelphia, 1990, pp 651–1621.

26. Thomas CL (ed): Taber's Cyclopedic Medical Dictionary, ed. 15. FA Davis, Philadelphia, 1989.

27. Sherrington, CS: The Integrative Action of the Nervous System. Yale University Press, New Haven, 1947.

28. Michlovitz, SL: Thermal Agents in Rehabilitation, ed. 2, FA Davis, Philadelphia, 1990.

29. Dubner, R and Bennett, GJ: Spinal and trigeminal mechanisms of nociception. Annu Rev Neurosi 6:381, 1983.

30. Lynn, B: The detection of injury and tissue damage. In: Wall, PD and Melzack, R (eds): Textbook of Pain. Churchill-Livingstone, New York, 1984, pp 19–33.

31. Travell, J: Myofascial trigger points: Clinical view. In Bonica JJ and Able-Fessard, DG (eds): Advances in Pain Research and Therapy, vol 1. Raven Press, New York, 1976, pp 919–926.

32. Goldscheider, A: Ueber den Schmertz in Physiologischer und Klinischer Hensicht. Hirschwald, Berlin, 1894.

33. Gammon, GD and Starr, I: Studies on the relief of pain by counter-irritation. J Physiol 72:392, 1931.
34. Michlovitz, SL: Cryotherapy: The use of cold as a therapeutic agent. In Michlovitz, SL (ed): Thermal Agents in Rehabilitation, ed. 2. FA Davis, Philadelphia, 1990, pp 63–87.
35. Douglas, WW and Malcolm, JL: The effect of localized cooling on conduction in cat nerves. J Physiol 130:53, 1955.
36. Li, C-L: Effect of cooling on neuromuscular transmission in the rat. Am J Physiol 194:200, 1958.
37. McGown, HL: Effects of cold application on maximal isometric contraction. Phys Ther 47:185, 1967.
38. Lehmann, JF and deLateur, BJ: Therapeutic Heat. In Lehmann, JF (ed): Therapeutic Heat and Cold, ed 4. Williams & Wilkins, Baltimore, 1990.
39. Michlovitz, SL: Biophysical principles of heating and superficial heat agents. In Michlovitz, SL (ed): Thermal Agents in Rehabilitation. FA Davis, Philadelphia, 1990 pp 88–108.
40. Lehmann, JD, Brunner, GD, and Stow, RW: Pain threshold measurements after therapeutic application of ultrasound microwaves and infrared. Arch Phys Med Rehabil 39:560, 1958.
41. Currier, DP and Kramer, JF: Sensory nerve conduction: Heating effects of ultrasound and infrared. Physiotherap Can. 34:241, 1982.
42. Mense, S: Effects of temperature on the discharges of muscle spindles and tendon organs. Pflugers Arch 374:159, 1978.
43. Fischer, E and Solomon, S: Physiological response to heat and cold. In: Licht, S (ed): Therapeutic Heat and Cold, ed 2. Waverly Press, Baltimore, 1965.
44. Guyton, AC: Textbook of Medical Physiology, ed. 7. WB Saunders, Philadelphia, 1986.
45. Wright, V and Johns, RJ: Physical factors concerned with the stiffness of normal or diseased joints. Bull Johns Hopkins Hosp 106:215, 1960.
46. Lehmann, JF and DeLateur, BJ: Diathermy and Superficial Heat, Laser and Cold Therapy. In Kotke, FJ and Lehmann, JF (eds): Krusen's Handbook of Physical Medicine and Rehabilitation, ed 4. WB Saunders, Philadelphia, 1990, pp 283–367.
47. Michlovitz, SL: Thermal Agents in Rehabilitation, ed 2. FA Davis, Philadelphia, 1990, pp 258–273.
48. Licht, S: Physical Therapy. In Licht S (ed): Rehabilitation and Medicine. Physical Medicine Library, Waverly Press, Baltimore, 1968, pp 16–17.
49. Cailliet, R: Soft Tissue Concepts. In Cailliet R: Soft Tissue Pain and Disability, ed. 2. FA Davis, Philadelphia, 1988, pp 3–17.
50. LeBan, MM: Collagen tissue: Implications of its response to stress in vitro. Arch Phys Med Rehabil 43:461, 1962.
51. Kottke, FJ, Pauley, DI, and Ptak, RA: The rationale for prolonged stretching for correction of shortening of connective tissue. Arch Phys Med Rehabil 47:345, 1966.
52. Warren, GC, Lehmann, JF, and Koblanski, JN: Heat and stretch procedures: An evaluation using rat tail tendon. Arch Phys Med Rehabil 57:122, 1976.
53. Waddell, G: A new clinical model for the treatment of low back pain. Spine 12:632–644, 1987.
54. Nutter P: Aerobic exercise in the treatment and prevention of low back pain. Spine: State-of-the-Art Reviews 2(1):137–145, 1987.
55. Kraus, H: Backache, stress, and tension: causes, prevention, and treatment. Simon & Schuster, New York, 1965.
56. Kraus, H, Nagler, W, and Melleby, A: Evaluation of an exercise program for back pain. Am Fam Physician 28:153–158, 1983.
57. Deyo, RA: Historic perspective on conservative treatments for acute back problems. In Mayer, TG, Mooney, V, and Gatchel, RJ (eds): Contemporary Conservative Care for Painful Spinal Disorders. Lea & Febiger, Philadelphia, 1991, pp 169–180.
58. Faas, A, Chavannes, AW, van Eijk, JThM, and Gubbels, JW: A randomized, placebo-con-

trolled trial of exercise therapy in patients with acute low back pain. Spine 18:1388–1395, 1993.

59. Farrell, JP and Twomey, LT: Acute low-back pain: Comparison of two conservative treatment approaches. Med J Aust 1:160–164, 1982.

60. Davies, JR, Gibson, T, and Tester, L: The value of exercises in the treatment of low back pain. Rheumatoid Rehabil 18:243–247, 1979.

61. Lindequist, S, Lundberg, B, Wildmark, R, et al: Information and regime of low back pain. Scand J Rehabil Med 16:113–116, 1984.

62. Berwick, D, Budman, S and Feldstein, M: No clinical effect of back school in an HMO, a randomized prospective trial. Spine 14:338–344, 1989.

63. Rose, MJ: Evaluation of the physical management of low back pain. Int Rehab Med 1:83–86, 1979.

64. Tollison, CD and Kriegel, ML: Physical exercise in the treatment of low back pain: Part 1: A review. Orthop Rev 17:724–729, 1988.

65. Cady, LD, Bischoff, DP, O'Connell, ER, et al: Strength and fitness and subsequent back injuries in fire fighters. J Occup Med 21:269, 1989.

66. Fordyce, WE, Brockway, JA, Bergman, JA, and Spengler, D: Acute back pain: A control-group comparison of behavioral vs. traditional management methods. J Behav Med 9:127, 1986.

67. DeVries, H: EMG fatigue curve in postural muscles. A possible etiology for idiopathic low back pain. J Phys Med 47:175, 1968.

68. Jackson, CP and Brown, MD: Is there a role for exercise in the treatment of patients with low back pain? Clin Orthop Rel Res Ther 179:39, 1983.

69. Nachemson, AL: The load on lumbar disks in different positions of the body. Clin Orthop 45:107, 1966.

70. Grabois, M: Treatment of pain syndromes through exercise. In Lowenthal, DT, Bharadwaja, K, and Oaks, WW (eds.): Therapeutics Through Exercise. Grune & Stratton, New York, 1979, pp 181–187.

71. Lee, MHM, Itoh, M, Yang, G-F W, and Eason, AL: Physical therapy and rehabilitation medicine. In Bonica JJ: The Management of Pain, ed. 2, vol II. Lea & Febiger, Philadelphia, 1990, pp 1778–1781.

72. Basmajian, JV (ed): Therapeutic Exercise, ed. 4. Williams & Wilkins, Baltimore, 1984.

73. DeVries, HA: Physiology of Exercise for Physical Education and Athletics, ed. 3, William C. Brown, Pub, Dubuque, 1966.

74. Fordyce, WE: Exercise and the increased inactivity level. In: Fordyce, WE (ed): Behavioral Methods for Chronic Pain and Illness. CV Mosby, St. Louis, 1976, pp 168–183.

75. Haberg, M and Kvarnstrom, S: Muscular endurance and electromyographic fatigue in myofascial shoulder pain. Arch Phys Med Rehabil 65:522–525, 1984.

76. Francis, KT: The role of endorphins in exercise: A review of current knowledge. J. Orthop Sports Phys Ther 4:169–173, 1983.

77. Markoff, RA, Ryan, P, and Young, T: Endorphins and mood changes in long distance running. Med Sci Sports Exerc 14:11–15, 1982.

78. Mayer, D and Watkins, L: Role of endorphins in endogenous pain control systems. Mod Probl Pharmacopsychiatry 17:68–96, 1981.

79. Appenzeller, O: What makes us run? N Engl J Med 305:578–579, 1981.

80. Haier, R, Quaid, B, and Mills, J: Naloxone alters pain perception after jogging. Psych Res 5:231–132, 1981.

81. Farrell, PA, Gates, W, Maksud, M, and Morgan, W: Increases in plasma β-endorphin/β-lipotropin immonoreactivity after treadmill running in humans. J Appl Physiol 52:1245–1249, 1982.

82. Pitts, F: Biochemical factors in anxiety neurosis. Behav Sci 16:82–91, 1971.

83. Padawer, WJ and Levine, FM: Exercise-induced analgesia: fact or artifact? Pain 48:131–135, 1992.

84. Mayer, DL, Wolfle, H, Akil, B, and Carder, J, Liebeskind Science, 164:444, 1969.
85. Headley, BJ: Muscle inhibition. Phys Therap Forum 224–226, 1993.
86. Ottenbacher, K and DiFabio, RP: Efficacy of spinal manipulation/mobilization therapy—a meta-analysis. Spine 10:833–837, 1985.
87. Kottke, FJ, Pauley, DI, and Ptak, RA: The rationale for prolonged stretching for correction of shortening of connective tissue. Arch Phys Med Rehabil 47:345, 1966.
88. Warren, GC, Lehmann, JF, and Koblanski, JN: Heat and stretch procedures: An evaluation using rat tail tendon. Arch Phys Med Rehabil 57:122, 1976.
89. Feffer, HL and Nachemson, AL: Standards for Assessment and Management of Low Back-Pain in Health Care Containment. In Greenwood, J and Taricco, H (eds): LRP Publications, Horsham, 1992, pp 155–200.
90. McAndrews, BG, Phillips, RB, and Feffer, HL: Chiropractic Cost Containment. NCCI Digest. 7:1–16, 1993.
91. Deyo, RA: Conservative therapy for low back pain: distinguishing useful from useless therapy. JAMA 250:1057–1062, 1983.
92. Hadler, NM, Curtis, P, Gillings, DB, and Stinnett, S: A benefit of spinal manipulation as adjunctive therapy for low back pain: a stratified controlled trial. Spine 12:703–706, 1987.
93. Kane, RL, Olsen, D, Leymaster, C, et al: Manipulating the patient—a comparison of the effectiveness of physician and chiropractic care. Lancet 1:1333–1336, 1974.
94. Meade, TW, Dyer, S, Browne, W, et al: Low back pain of mechanical origin: randomized comparison of Chiropractic and hospital outpatient treatment. Br Med J 300:1431–1437, 1990.
95. Sandoz, R: Some reflex phenomena associated with spinal derangements and adjustments. Ann Swiss Chirop Assoc 15:45, 1981.
96. Vervest, ACM and Stolker, RJ: The treatment of cervical pain syndromes with radiofrequency procedures. Pain Clin 4:103–112, 1991.
97. Greenman PE: Manual and manipulative therapy in whiplash injuries. In Teasell, RW and Shapiro, AP (eds): Cervical Flexion-Extension Whiplash Injuries, Spine. Hanley & Belfus, Philadelphia, pp 517–530.
98. Bonica, JJ: Management of Pain. Lea & Febiger, Philadelphia, 1953.
99. White, AH: Structural diagnostic tests. In Mayer, TG, Mooney, V, and Gautschel, RJ (eds): Contemporary Conservative Care for Painful Spinal Disorders. Lea & Febiger, Philadelphia, 1991, pp 364–379.
100. Pecina, MM, Krmpotic-Nemanic, J, and Markiewitz, AD: Tunnel Syndromes. CRC Press, Boca Raton, 1991.
101. Travell, JG and Simon, DG: Myofascial Pain and Dysfunction. The Trigger Point Manual. Williams & Wilkins, Baltimore, 1983.

CHAPTER 5

Low Back Pain

Predominant among activity-related spinal disorders, 70% of low back pain is related to symptoms in the lumbar region and consumes 75% of all compensation claims.[1] An estimated 7000 publications discussing low back pain were available in the literature in 1993.[2] The mechanisms, evaluation, and management of low back pain and disability remains an enigma with many diagnostic procedures remaining unconfirmed.

Treatment of chronic pain originating from soft tissue and back injuries has undergone significant change in recent years. Current emphasis is being placed on functional restoration rather than on mere reduction or elimination of pain.[3]

Numerous treatises exist on the mechanics of the low back with analysis of faulty function leading to pain and impairment.[4] Faulty neuromusculoskeletal function has been determined to be the major cause of low back pain and its resulting impairment, but the resulting *disability*, on being further examined, was found to be disproportionate to impairment.

Fear of reinjury from any or all motion has been considered a significant factor in persistent, recurrent, and chronic pain and dysfunction. Objective findings regarding the injured low back pain patient remain sparse because most symptoms are subjective and difficult to equate.[5] Pain has been defined as ". . . an unpleasant sensory and emotional experience associated with tissue damage or potential tissue damage, or described in terms of such damage."[6] Most treatment protocols of low back pain (as an example) have been in search of relief of this pain and to assist the patient to cope with the pain. This approach has largely either completely failed or been inadequate, thus the current emphasis is on restoration of function. Objectivity of findings is attempting to replace subjectivity.

Most low back disorders (LBD) occurring in the workplace involve muscular overexertion injuries with the patient's bending and twisting in asymmetric manner being the predominant causes of injury. Inappropriate and repetitive dynamic activities currently termed cumulative trauma disorders (CTD) are foremost in the list of causes.[7-9]

Because muscular activity is predominant in causing symptomatic pathology, it is becoming a major focus of research. The resulting structural diagnosis remains the basis of classification of LBD. Investigation based solely on anatomic structures fails to determine an accurate diagnosis in 80% to 90% of patients with LBD.[10] A pathoanatomic diagnosis is available in fewer than 15% of patients with LBD.

To correct this faulty basis for diagnosis, the Quebec Study[12] was developed. This report recognized that many patients do not have a clearly identifiable structural abnormality and most have only limited disability. Functional assessment becomes the basis of diagnosis using this scheme; ignorance of a pathoanatomic diagnosis remains one of its weaknesses, however.

Functional assessment of LBD is based on the premise that the trunk musculature both supports and loads the spine in home or workplace activities.

With a neuromusculoskeletal cause of LBD, exercise has become the major modality in this approach. Providing significant benefit not only in restoration of function but also in diminution of pain,[13] this newer concept implies that restoration of normal physiologic function is as necessary as is relief of the concomittant psychologic aspect of pain.

The benefits of exercise have also been under scrutiny, however. Restoration of flexibility (i.e., range of motion) has been strongly advocated without setting clear norms.[14] Range of motion is also a much misused term that needs clarification if the phrase is to be used as a basis for assessment during examination and treatment.

Muscle pain, which has largely been relegated to describe myofascial pain, is also a function of the soft tissue component of the low back pain syndrome. Unlike cutaneous pain, muscle pain is poorly localized; it thus has a referral pain pattern, as well as localized pain. The exact mechanism of this referral pattern remains obscure and is probably a conversion-projection connection within the central nervous system (CNS).[15,16]

The psychologic aspects of muscular pain have been proposed in some reports, refuted in others,[17] and considered prevalent in another group.[18] Pain has been found to be both acute and chronic: the latter is more prevalent. Chronic pain syndromes include somatoform disorders, depression, anxiety, substance abuse, and personality disorders. This has been related in reference to the current edition of the Diagnostic and Statistical Disease Manual of the American Psychiatric Association.[19]

To understand the nature of low back pain, and its etiology, mechanism, diagnosis, and appropriate management, it is mandatory that the term **functional anatomy** be understood. It is becoming increasingly more important, however, to determine all these aspects and give them a proportionate value within the gathering of a meaningful history and providing a careful physical examination. Functional anatomy implies an understanding of the neuromuscular forces normally imposed upon the spine—when these are abnormal in any aspect, tissue pathology may result.

FUNCTIONAL ANATOMY

The basis of function and malfunction of the lumbosacral spine occurs within the involved anatomic unit. It is within this unit that the nociceptors that present pain when irritated or inflamed exist. It is also within this unit that normal function occurs when it is viewed as a small, but pertinent, component to range of motion within the vertebral column as a whole. Total motion is a precisely controlled musculoskeletal activity both neurologically and psychologically. Deviation from normal function results in pain, impairment, and disability. Internal musculoskeletal structures within the functional unit are exposed to structural changes through their movement's being so close to the axis of motion as they counteract external forces. The internal forces generated far exceed the external forces. Before discussing these forces, the pathoanatomic structures of the functional unit are described.

Functional Unit

The functional unit is composed of two adjacent vertebrae with an interposed intervertebral disk (Fig. 5–1). The disk is a hydrodynamic structure that permits weight bearing and mobility of the unit itself and of the entire vertebral column. The study of all aspects of the disk consumes volumes of medical literature;[20] only major aspects can be discussed in this text.

The intervertebral disk is a fibrocartilaginous structure containing an envelope of annular fibers with a central nucleus. Its major substance is a mucopolysaccharide gel that consumes fluid for its sustenance.[21] The enclosed collagen fibers whose structure and function have been described in Chapter 1 provide stability and flexibility.

These collagen fibers (Fig. 5–2) are arranged in sheets with each fiber attached from the adjacent end plates of the vertebrae and crossing at approximately a 30° angulation. The angulation of the fibers changes diametrically within each sheet (Fig. 5–3).

The deterioration and destruction of the collagen fibers provide the basis of many symptomatic injuries to the spine. The physiologic effects on the collagen fibers from forces imposed upon the spine are illustrated in Figure 5–4. Each collagen fiber elongates to its physiologic limit and resumes its rest-

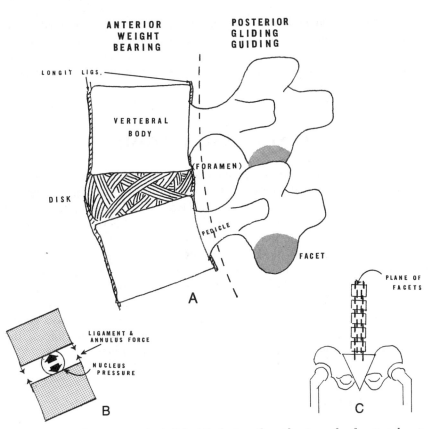

Figure 5–1. The intervertebral disk. (A) depicts the side view of a functional unit showing the crisscrossing of annular fiber in the disk in the anterior weight-bearing position of the unit. (B) is a schematic version of the nucleus with small arrows indicating the force within the nucleus that separates the vertebrae. The annular and ligament forces (*smaller arrows*) contains the nuclear force. (C) shows a sagittal view of the facets illustrated in the posterior gliding guiding portion of the function unit (A).

ing length upon cessation of the deforming force. It is only when the force exceeds physiologic limits that the fiber undergoes damage and loses its elasticity and structural integrity.

The nucleus is a major component of the hydrodynamic function of the disk. It is a contained mucopolysaccharide gel in which few annular fibers are present. The nucleus acts hydrodynamically because of its intrinsic pressure as a fluid enveloped within a flexible container. It has the ability to deform, permitting changes in the alignment of the functional unit (Fig. 5–5).

The intervertebral disk is a mechanical structure devoid of vascular and nerve supply, thus it acts in a purely mechanical manner. Its action is pertinent

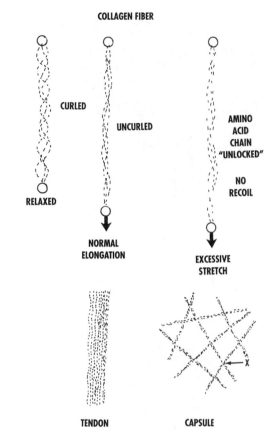

Figure 5–2. Collagen fibers of the nucleus pulposus. The nucleus of the disk is a mucopolysaccharide gel containing irregularly directed collagen fibers shown in the upper three illustrations. In tendons, these fibers are parallel, whereas in capsules, they are irregular as in the disk nucleus.

to proper mechanical function of the vertebral column and can become a source of impairment and disability when it is damaged and unable to perform its physiologic function with attendant irritation and inflammation, of the nociceptive tissues. No nociceptive nerve endings are present within the intervertebral disk except possibly in the very outer annular layers.

The disk ceases to operate properly when hydrodynamic function is impaired, thus denying adequate separation of the vertebral end plates with resulting loss of movement and weight bearing.

Zygapophyseal Joints

Posteriorly the zygapophyseal joints (facets) are incorporated within the laminae. These joints are lined with cartilage (Fig. 5–6). These joints, by virtue of their alignment, direct the motion of the functional unit and either

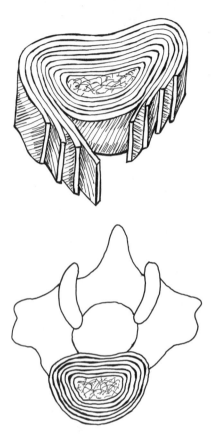

Figure 5–3. Annulus fibrosus. The annulus is a series of concentric annular fibers that run in opposite directions in an oblique manner in each layer. The fibers originate from one vertebral end plate into the opposite end plate. The annulus contains a pulpy nucleus (nucleus pulposus).

prevent or significantly restrict contrary motion. The zygapophyseal joints' sagittal placement allows flexion and extension and restricts lateral flexion and rotation of the functional unit, thus minimizing rotatory stress upon the intervertebral disk's annular fibers.

The zygapophyseal joints have an articular capsule sufficiently fibrous to allow flexibility yet also rigid enough to afford stability to the joint. The joints contain fat pads (menisci) that give congruity to the joints. The capsule and the enclosed pads are innervated with nerve fiber endings that offer proprioception, as well as nociception.

Ligaments. Numerous ligaments afford stability to the functional unit and restrict motion, thus further protecting the intervertebral disk and the facets. The major ligaments are the anterior longitudinal and posterior longitudinal. They line the entire vertebral column and reinforce the outer layers of the intervertebral disks. They are innervated with proprioceptive and nociceptive nerve endings. Intervertebral ligaments also attach laterally to the trans-

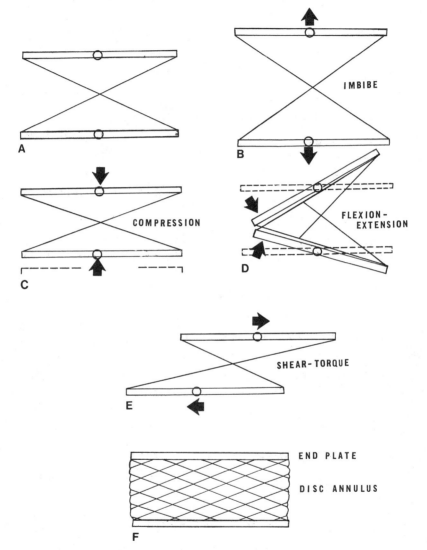

Figure 5–4. Annular fiber angulation under various forces. (*A*) shows the angulation of the annular fibers with the intervertebral disk under no external pressure. They angle at approximately 30°. (*B*) as the disk expands during imbibition, the angle becomes less acute. (*C*) under external compression, the angle becomes more acute. (*D*) during flexion and extension of the functional unit, the fibers angle according to their anterior or posterior positions. (*E*) shows the angulation and the length of annular fibers during shear or torque force. (*F*) shows the attachments of the angled fibers to the endplates of adjacent vertebrae.

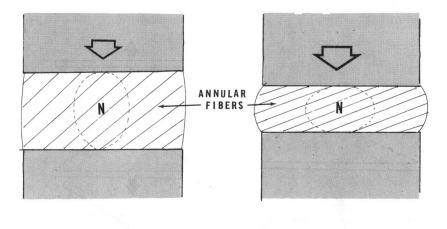

A   **B**

Figure 5–5. Change in shape of nucleus and angulation of annular fibers from compression. (A) with a limited external pressure (*arrow*) the nucleus (N) retains it physiologic form and annular fibers angulate at approximately 30°. (B) with greater external force (*large arrow*) the nucleus deforms and the fibers assume a more acute angulation and length. The disk physiologically *bulges* circumferentially.

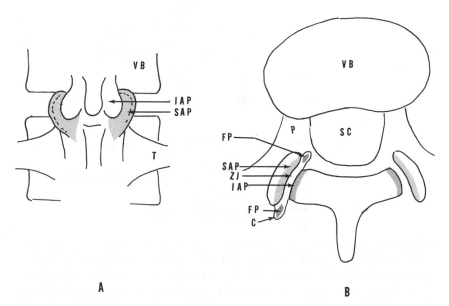

A   **B**

Figure 5–6. The zygapophyseal joints (facets). (A) is a posterior view of two vertebrae (a functional unit). IAP = inferior articular processes; SAP = superior articular process of the inferior vertebra (VP). T = transverse processes. (B) superior view of a vertebra. ZJ = zygapophyseal joint; C = a facet capsule; FP = the fat pads; P = pedicles; SC = spinal canal.

verse processes and posteriorly to the posterior superior spines. The function of those latter ligaments is essentially to limit motion.

Dynamic motion influences the viscoelastic properties of osteoligamentous tissues. With the spine fully flexed, osteoligamentous limitation of the spine has been determined to be 10° short of its elastic limit,[22] indicating little chance of damage from extreme trunk flexion.

Viscoelasticity is reduced and even overcome by rapid elongation. Rapid elongation also increases immediate *stiffness* of a ligament that progressively decreases with repetition unless there is a recovery period[23] before the next elongation. This viscoelasticity exists in the ligamentous structures, as well as in the annular fibers of the disk.

Interspinous Muscles. The interspinous muscles are the erector spinae and the smaller intrinsic muscles that motor the vertebral column. They are controlled by intrinsic muscle fibers—the spindle system—that determines their precise contraction. In the erect static posture, the erector spinae muscles sustain isometric contraction. In forward flexion they act *eccentrically** by decelerating forward flexion. In resuming the erect posture, they act *concentrically*.†

The smaller intrinsic muscles play a role in rotation of the vertebral spine. Because only very limited rotational motions are permitted, these muscles are short in form and act through a small lever arm.

Whereas external forces generated by similarly external activities create movement about the spine that is counterbalanced by the smaller intrinsic muscles acting through a smaller movement arm, these muscles are exposed to injury. Their failure has been considered responsible for LBD.[24]

Neural Tissues Within the Functional Unit

Only innervated structures can be a source of pain. The ligamentum flavum and internal venous plexus are known to have no innervation. Free nerve endings have been found in the following structures:

(1) Facet joint capsules[25-27]
(2) Anterior longitudinal ligaments, posterior longitudinal ligaments, and annulus fibrosus[28-30]

The functional unit has been divided into ventral and dorsal compartments[31-33] with their sensory and motor supply occurring through the nerve roots that emerge through the intervertebral foramena (Fig. 5–7). These roots are contained within a dural sheath (Fig. 5–8).

---

*Eccentric involves force exerted while the muscle is lengthening.
†Concentric involves force exerted while the muscle is shortening.

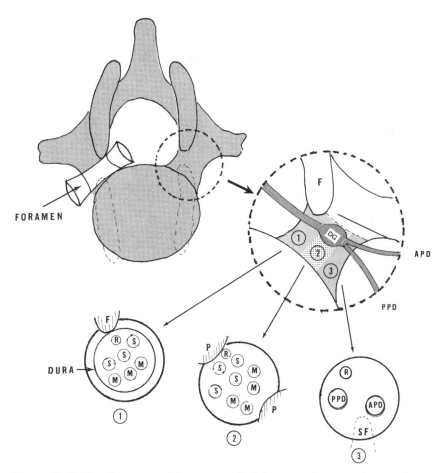

Figure 5–7. Neural contents of the intervertebral foramen. The upper drawing shows the foramen (*dotted circle on the right*) as a funnel-shaped tubular opening (*left*). The figure within the dotted circle shows the contents: F = facet; SF = superior facet of the inferior vertebra; P = pars portion of the lamina; DG = dorsal root. The contents of the foramen are (*1*), (*2*), and (*3*) revealing the contents of the root in those foramenal segments. S = sensory roots; R = recurrent nerve of Luschka, M = motor; PPD = posterior primary division; APD = anterior primary division.

The tissues of the functional unit are innervated by the recurrent nerve of Luschka (Fig. 5–9). The ventral compartment (vertebra, longitudinal ligaments, disk, and anterior aspect of the nerve root) is not supplied by a single nerve root but instead by interconnected neural pathways in the anterior and posterior longitudinal ligaments and the ventral dura (Fig. 5–10).[34,35]

Nerves of the anterior longitudinal plexus are branches of communicating

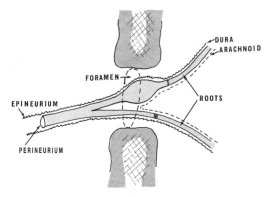

Figure 5–8. Dural and arachnoid sheaths of the nerve root. The sensory nerve roots (S) and the motor nerve roots (M) merge at the intervertebral foramen. The arachnoid terminates at the foramen, whereas the dura continues and becomes epineurium and perineurium.

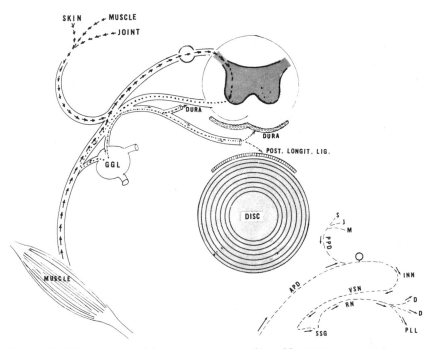

Figure 5–9. Innervation of the recurrent nerve of Luschka. PPD = posterior primary division; APD = anterior primary division; GGL = sympathetic ganglion; INN = internuncial neuron; VSN = ventral sensory nerve; SSG = sensory sympathetic ganglion; RN = recurrent nerve of Luschka; D = dura; PLL = posterior longitudinal ligament.

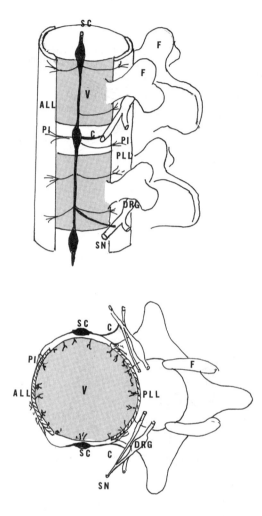

Figure 5–10. Innervation of a vertebral functional unit. Upper figure shows a functional unit of two adjacent lumbar vertebrae (V) and their innervation. ALL is the anterior longitudinal ligament and PLL is the posterior longitudinal ligament on which is a nerve plexus (P1), which ascends and descends several units. The spinal nerve (SN) with the sensory dorsal root ganglion emerges through the foramen inferior to the facets (F), sends the somatic nerve to the vertebral structures, and is joined by branches of the autonomic nervous system (SC) through communicating branches (C). The lower drawing depicts a superior view of the functional unit and depicts the plexi sending branches into the outer layers of the intervertebral disk.

rami, sympathetic chains, and perivascular nerves innervating the vertebral body and annulus fibrosus for three to five levels. The posterior longitudinal plexus consists of branches of the communicating rami which reenter the vertebral canal as the recurrent nerve of Luschka. This plexus supplies two to four levels bilaterally and multisegmentally.

The dorsal compartment (lamina, facets, ligaments, and muscles) is supplied by medial and lateral branches of the dorsal rami, which span two to three segments. Only the dorsal dura is not innervated multisegmentally; it receives monosegmental innervation. This multisegmental innervation explains why the nerve root blockade procedure so often fails to relieve pain resulting from LBD.[36]

The finding of innervation, especially in the ventral compartment sharing common pathways with areas of autonomic and rami communication,[37] indicates clearly that the autonomic nervous system plays a role in maintaining spinal pain.[38,39]

NORMAL BODY MECHANICS

The basis for both normal function and impairment and disability is found in neuromusculoskeletal patterns. In the erect static posture, muscles are in a state of tonus with minimal contraction. The support is essentially provided by intervertebral disk pressure, the tonus of the ligaments, the muscular fascia, and the zygapophysial capsular tonus. The physiologic curves are informed by genetic, cultural, sexual, and occupational factors. The range of *normal* postural curves have not been confirmed by degree of flexion. The provision of physiologically minimal energy requirements, being pain free and having a cosmetically acceptable appearance have been the criteria to determine a *normal* person.

In initiating any activity, the center of gravity changes. Bending forward or accelerating are similar in this respect. The static forces are changed. The muscles change from kinetic to static energy and contract eccentrically to decelerate flexion or concentrically to ambulate.

These units change in form as well as function. The disks deform as required by pressure changes altering the relationship of the various vertebral end plates. In flexion the anterior end plates approximate and the posterior separate. The nucleus migrates and the annular fibers elongate accordingly. The facets glide, either separating or approximating with the cartilages' compressing lubricant. The capsules and ligaments elongate to their physiologic limits. Muscles contract or elongate within fascial limits.

The muscular action that initiates this activity is precisely coordinated by feedback from the Golgi and spindle systems. The *exact* action is determined by its appropriateness following the intended motion.

Proper function requires well-conditioned tissues and that all activities remain within physiologic limits. Proper conditioning indicates adequate flexibility, precise activity by similarly well-conditioned muscle, and a neuromusculoskeletal sequence unbroken by perturbers.

By far the most prevalent cause of low back pain and disk disruption is violation of normal *kinetic function.* Normally as a person bends forward and then resumes an erect posture, the spine must conform to correct motion of all its segments.

The pelvis is fixed initially because it is the supporting structure of the spinal column. The erect lordosis assumes a gradual kyphosis, that is, the erector spinae muscles elongate to decelerate trunk flexion (Fig. 5–11). The facets separate and the intervertebral disks alter their contour by compressing anteri-

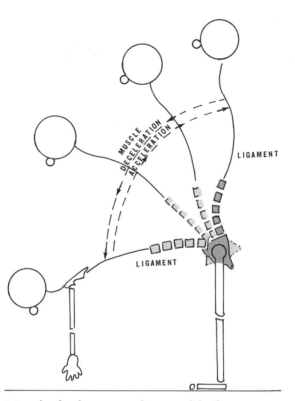

Figure 5–11. Muscular deceleration-acceleration of the flexing spine. From an erect stance, the flexing spine flexes as the erector spinae muscles decelerate descent. On reaching full flexion, the muscles relax and support now relies exclusively on ligamentous and fascial support.

orly and expanding posteriorly. The disk nucleus migrates posteriorly and the posterior ligaments elongate to their gradual physiologic lengths. The muscle fascia also elongates to its limits of physiologic elasticity.

Once fully flexed, supporting tissues are the ligaments (longitudinal and paraspinous), the muscles' fascia, and the facet capsules. As the spine has rotated (flexed), the pelvis gradually also undergoes rotation until its posterior musculature (hamstrings and glutei) has fully elongated in its decelerating action.

During this flexion action, the tissues are all kinetic and depend on their elasticity and neuromuscular coordination to provide the necessary strength and endurance.

Resumption of an erect posture requires the exactly opposite activity: return from total kyphosis to erect lordosis and then gradual return of pelvic rotation to the erect position. This is a muscular activity coordinated by precise neurologic pattern engrams, which are subconscious and result from habit and training.

Proper resumption of the erect position is termed **lumbar pelvic rhythm**, indicating correlated lumbar motion with a simultaneous pelvic rotation (Fig. 5–12). This undoubtedly derives from cortical patterns that are genetic, moderated by training, and influenced by *perturbers*.

Perturbers are external factors that impair normal neurologic patterns. Among the most common are fatigue, distraction, anger, impatience, depression, and various other emotional or mental states. Examples of physical perturbers include trauma, impact, obstacles, or improper motions (Fig. 5–13).

Return to the erect posture depends not only on muscular activity but also on facet alignment, which essentially permits movement only in the sagittal plane. Because many bending and return motions also invoke rotation, this activity requires an asymmetric relationship among the facets, as well as the action of torque on the disk fibers. In flexion, the facets separate on the convex side and approximate on the concave side. Annular fiber permits elongation of only approximately 5° rotation. Excessive rotation can tear the annular fibers,

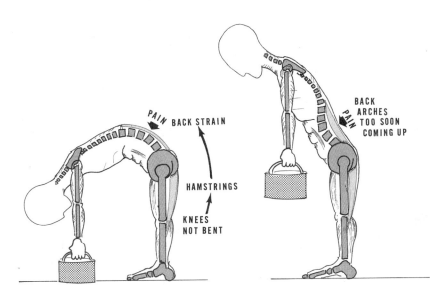

Figure 5–12. Faulty lifting technique. (*Left*) shows improper lifting of an object far from the center of gravity with the legs unbent and the lift being accomplished exclusively with the low back. (*Right*) shows the low back being re-extended prematurely in the lift effort causing the erector muscles to do most of the extension in the lift. This is a violation of the lumbar-pelvic rhythm.

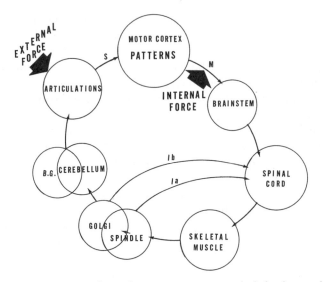

Figure 5–13. Perturber influence on neuromusculoskeletal control.

the capsules of the facets, the parasinous ligaments and the fascia of the muscle, if not the bellies of the muscles themselves.

Reextension must *derotate* in the direction opposite to which it rotated during flexion. Failure to do so in a coordinated manner can impinge the facets on the concave side, thus changing the axis of rotation and concurrently damaging the intervertebral disk. Any or all the soft tissues involved in these maneuvers can be traumatized. These factors are learned during taking a pertinent patient history. Any resultant tissue injury can be ascertained by physical examination.

HISTORY

In eliciting a history of low back pain, the physician must learn how the patient's low back was injured, as well as where the pain is felt and which movements or positions will aggravate the pain. Clearly, pain occurring only in the low back must be differentiated from pain in both the low back *and* the leg.

Ascertaining the mechanism of a low back injury is necessary to determine which tissues, as well as which motion(s), are implicated. The ergonomics required of the patient's work must also be determined to assure avoidance or recurrence. The majority of LBD incidents in the workplace involve muscular overexertion injuries. An acute problem will become chronic when such actions are repeated.

Manual materials handling and lifting are the most frequent causes of LBD—such motion has been determined to be tridimensional[38] and to involve eccentric, as well as concentric, forces (Fig. 5–14).

In assessing asymmetric (tridimensional) lifting strength, studies have shown that there is a loss of 6% to 9% in lifting limits with every 30° of asymmetry with losses of 12%, 21%, and 31% at 30°, 60°, and 90° of asymmetry, respectively.[39]

Velocity of motion also affects strength of action. Velocity within a saggital plane affects strength at various degrees of motion (both flexion and extension) and torque decreases force by as much as 78% of maximum as velocity increases from zero to maximum.[40,41]

It is apparent from these factors above that trunk angle, asymmetric movement, and velocity affect trunk efficiency and strength. In dynamic motion, all degrees of rotation, flexion–re-extension velocity, and degrees of trunk angle must be analyzed in studying activities in the workplace. Because eccentric trunk strength exceeds concentric strength,[42] this may explain the

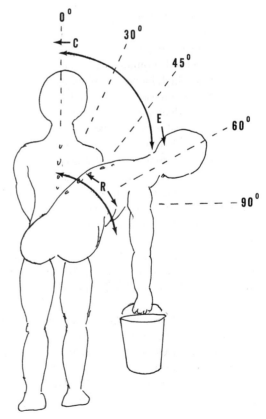

Figure 5–14. Tridimensional forces in trunk flexion and lifting. Zero degrees indicates the fully extended position. As the person flexes and rotates (R), strength diminishes with every 30° of rotation. Muscular efforts are concentric (C) in extending and eccentric (E) in lowering. Velocity affects the strength expended.

high incidence of low back injuries in nursing practitioners, who often lower an inert patient onto a bed at a slow velocity.

Muscular activity directly affects the pressure and movement of disk annular fibers. Because disk tolerance to compression is greatly reduced when it is loaded under symmetric motion,[43] disk failure occurs from these forces,[44] and even more frequently from asymmetric loading.[45]

Coactivation occurs at various levels of acceleration of contraction.[46] Coactivation indicates *simultaneous* contraction of agonist and antagonist muscles, rather than antagonist relaxation during agonist contraction. In the trunk, the abdominal muscles must be the antagonists while the agonists, or erector spinae, contract. The flexors, oblique abdominal, and latissimus dorsi muscles are farthest from the center of movement and thus are at an advantage during the process of acceleration. In asymmetric motion, the small spinal muscles, which counterbalance the larger external muscles, are at a disadvantage and may fail. Such small muscle failures have been identified as a cause of some LBDs.[24]

Certain limitations of range of motion so frequently analyzed and noted in the examination of the LBD patient must be noted:[47]

1. Limitation because of increasing discomfort when approaching the end point.
2. A decrease caused by bending forward alters the center of gravity with increased moment. This action is counterbalanced by the back muscles, which increases spinal loading.
3. With decrease in trunk motion, there is also a decrease in acceleration, which decreases trunk forces. There is a 50% decrease in flexion velocity in patients with LBD regardless of their having legs extended or flexed. Extension velocity is also decreased, possibly because the extensor muscles are irritated.

For the trunk to accelerate coactivation (stiffness) must be reduced—the antagonist must relax to allow contraction of the agonists, yet there is an attendant increase in coactivation during acceleration, thus creating a delicate balance.

As there is greater change in the oblique muscles in tridimensional motion with diminished force from the erector spine, there is also a greater degree of shear that results and damages the disks.

Recent review of trunk-strength and lifting-strength measurement has summarized very well the current acceptance of these measures,[48] but current traditional measures used for *objective* evaluation of LBDs have been unable to provide meaningful, reproducible quantitative parameters to classify or monitor LBDs accurately.

Physicians attempt to classify LBDs according to pathoanatomic sources of LBD, but these measures afford a precise diagnosis in fewer than 15% of patients with LBD.[48] It has been estimated that over 25% of healthy asymptomatic individuals can provide image-based evidence of abnormal disk herniation.

The Quebec Study[1] revealed that structural abnormalities are not always identifiable in LBDs and that LBDs were time dependent. Objective functional assessment systems have been explored in which measurements of the amount of force or strength the patient is willing to generate under isometric, isokinetic, and isodynamic conditions can be compared with those generated by normal, or asymptomatic, people. These measures usually require maximum voluntary force to be exerted against a set resistance, usually in one plane of motion. Results are influenced by the patients' pain tolerance, which is a highly variable factor.

Most of these tests give mixed results and are not precisely repeatedly reproducible in similar tests. These strength-testing measures externally load the trunk in a manner that does not reflect learned patterns or coordinated neuromuscular control systems, nor do they replicate actual work situations. Most studies were computed to equate the activity with compressive forces upon the spine and so largely ignored shear and rotational forces or acceleration during complex lifting tasks.[49]

Epidemiologic evidence emphasizes that twisting and symmetric trunk motion that involve shear and rotation are related to the increase in LBDs.[50,51] In vitro studies have shown that spinal segments have a lower capacity to withstand compressive forces imposed simultaneously with torsional and shearing forces.[52,53] Cyclic rotation of torsional loads also increases compressive and shearing forces.[54]

Most systems analyses to date have studied linear forces but not the actual complex spinal motions—simultaneous flexion, extension, lateral flexion, and rotation—which oversimplifies the action of the neuromuscular system.

In the normal neuromuscular system, there is a constant instantaneous interplay between the agonist and antagonist muscle systems that conforms to a pattern of tridimensional forces with controlled acceleration. In a simple linear motion, fewer muscles are activated than are activated in complex tridimensional motion. In a tridimensional system the numerous muscles involved are in a constant state of flux at various points in the motion, when many muscles are cocontracting rather than undergoing reciprocal action-relaxation. For this reason, electromyographic (EMG) evaluations are confusing. Linear studies misrepresent shear and torsional forces because not all muscles are constantly being represented.

Marras and Wongsam[47] developed a system to measure trunk unloaded free dynamic motion patterns in home and workplace situations. These studies measured velocity in tridimensional measures of motion found to occur in everyday activities. Single motor units studied by EMG have been enhanced by introducing the concept of recruitment and coactivation of muscle units,

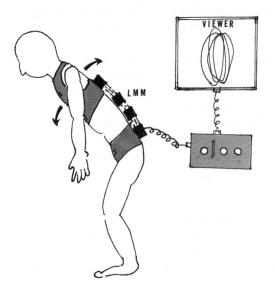

Figure 5–15. Lumbar motion monitor (LMM). This externally applied equipment with a chest portion and a pelvic portion is connected with a triaxial electrogoniometer, and the paths of trunk motion are viewed on a monitor that can be recorded on computer disk. The person can flex and extend, laterally flex, rotate, and do any combination and the range of motion as well as the velocity and acceleration are recorded over time. (Equipment was developed by Biodynamics Laboratory and Statistics and the Division of Orthopedic Surgery, Ohio State University, Columbus, Ohio.)

such as occurs during a complex action such as the tridimensional activities of the spine.

The biomechanical studies of Marras and associates[51] used equipment they developed called a *lumbar motion monitor* (LMM) (Fig. 5–15), which is an externally applied triaxial electrogoniometer which assesses the changing instantaneous positions of the lumbar spine in a tridimensional space.[53] It tracks position, velocity, and acceleration by recording with an analogue-to-digital converter and a microcomputer. The repeated dots are lined forming a reportable curve upon a computer disk.

The relationship between the correlation of faulty motion to specific tissue sites of pain and impairment have as yet not been confirmed, but the study of faulty motion indicates that motion is a learned or cognitive process and resultant pathology (e.g., LBDs) may reflect changes in coordinated recruitment of the neuromuscular system with resultant tissue injury (Fig. 5–16). Faulty body mechanics that have been impugned as causative for many decades are becoming clarified during study. The functional impairment becomes the basis for *diagnosis*, rather than being seen as a strict pathoanatomic base.

Free dynamic measurement, rather than strength-base loaded studies, is more subtle and informative because it simulates actual daily activities which stress-loaded studies do not do.

Cognitive processes affect biomechanical processes and thus explain how

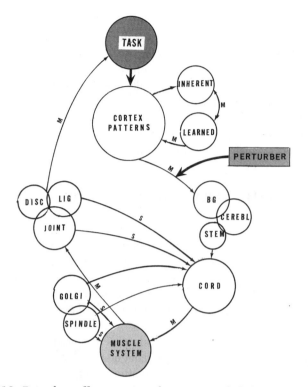

Figure 5–16. Perturber effect on normal neuromusculoskeletal function. Normal neuromusculoskeletal function occurs when the desired TASK is initiated. The cerebral cortex, which contains basic (inherent) neuromuscular patterns, are affected by training into learned actions and then pass to the spinal cord through the basal ganglia (BG), the cerebellum (CEREBL), and the brain stem (STEM) for central coordination. Within the cord, the motor neurones are activated, monitored, and modified by the Golgi and spindle systems as to force, rapidity, and duration. The muscle system determines the recruitment and reciprocal action to initiate movement. This movement demands participation of the joints, ligaments, and, in the low back, the disks. Ultimately, the **task** is performed. Should there be perturbers (i.e., fatigue, anger, anxiety, impatience, monotony, depression) the neuromuscular sequence described is impaired and the resultant dysfunction occurs at the disk, ligament, and joint levels with resultant pain and impairment. S depicts the sensory pathways and M depicts the motor.

learned behaviors are influenced by pain sensitivities.[55,56] The deviations caused by pain-inhibition fear avoidance,[57] psychologic distress,[58] and illness behavior[59] are revealed in unloaded acceleration tridimensional studies. These modifiers of normal neurophysiologic mechanisms have been termed **perturbers** (see Fig. 5–13).

This model (LMM) may ultimately reveal patterns for specific LBDs as well as an understanding of the ergonomics of the workplace. Once standardized, it may set a basis of neuromuscular function in the patient with LBD and also provide a basis for monitoring progress from a therapeutic approach.

If the action of faulty neuromuscular activity is understood, the resultant pathoanatomic sequelae will become more comprehensible and therapeutic approaches will be monitored physiologically in a recordable manner.

Many of these studies have been implemented in chronic low back pain patients with fairly well-established patterns. It remains to be seen if similar studies will be effective in evaluating acute LBDs when the developing neuromuscular patterns remain in developmental stages.

EXAMINATION OF THE LOW BACK PAIN PATIENT

A patient presenting with symptoms of pain in the low back must be evaluated to determine the presence of low back pain alone or combined with leg pain. "The history is more pertinent than is the examination." An adequately performed examination should inform the examiner as to the *structural* basis of the impairment, the tissue site, and thus the *mechanical* basis of the complaints.

A rational diagnosis of low back syndromes is handicapped by the lack of reliable objective tests.[60] Pain is the fundamental basis of low back symptoms; thus, a nociceptive site must be identified after taking a careful history has determined the mechanism of the factors irritating these tissues. The tissue sites of potential nociception within a functional unit can be summarized as:

1. External fibers of the intervertebral disk annulus
2. Posterior longitudinal ligament
3. Nerve root dura
4. Synovial capsular tissue of the facets
5. Ligaments, both interspinous or supraspinous
6. Erector spinae muscles (and their fascia)

Mechanical pain can be simplistically classified as being either discogenic or myogenic.[61] Additionally, there are other tissues such as the facets, ligaments, and the dura of the nerve roots, the function of which need consideration.

The examination begins by observing the patient's facial expression, attitude, posture, and manner of mobility. The emotional tone used by the patient during the eliciting of the history is also to be observed. Because pain is subjective, it is manifested to the observer by the facial expression of the patient, as well as by the tone of the verbal complaint.

Determining the degree of impairment is the objective of the physical examination, but the determination of the resultant disability must also be established from the history, that is, the subjective component of impairment. Impairment has been defined by the World Health Organization as "any loss or abnormality of psychologic, physiologic, or anatomic structure or function."[62] This can be amplified to include "leading to loss of normal bodily function."[63-65] Social Security guidelines[66] have defined impairment as "being demonstrable by medically acceptable clinical and laboratory diagnostic techniques."

Clinical assessment of impairment should therefore be based solely on reliable *objective* clinical signs that are clearly separable from cognitive, psychologic, or behavioral features of the illness. The impairment identified must specifically relate to the disability claimed or demonstrated by the patient. Therein lies the dilemma of disability evaluation.

Techniques of Examination

The examination begins with the first observation as the patient enters the examining room, and as the patient arises from a seated position, undresses, and responds to requested motions and positions. All these motions or actions depict the *disability*, which indicates to the examiner "how the patient hurts," and to what extent and what movements he or she finds it "painful" and "how it impairs their function."

The term **disability** essentially describes what the patient cannot do at all or do only with pain. The *objective* reasons for that disability should be found in the *impairments* that the examination reveals.

The gait reveals any impaired motor function of the legs and the trunk. A *limp* must be analyzed regarding its mechanism and limiting basis. Complaints of pain during gait focus the specific time and therefore the basis of the limp as described by the patient. The observer can only analyze the gait and judge from the evinced grimace and verbal complaint that pain is elicited.

Gait abnormalities reveal motor weakness of involved muscle groups,[67] such as a drop foot, steppage gait, trunk asymmetry, or even pain on weight bearing. Abnormal gaits that are created by fear of pain or that depict the *disability* experienced must be carefully evaluated as being expected from the ultimate findings, exaggerated, or nonphysiologic. Appropriate neurologic and orthopedic examination of the foot, ankle, and lower leg will reveal the basis for the limp.

Sitting or arising from the seated position must be observed as to assess trunk physiologic movements and leg weakness. Pain must be evaluated as occurring during sitting, after being seated, and upon arising. The physiologic movements of the lumbosacral spine that occur during these activities must be analyzed. Physiologic sitting requires some reversal of the lordosis and central sitting position without functional scoliosis (Fig. 5–17).

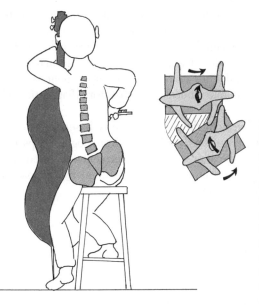

Figure 5–17. Pelvic angulation in a musician. Being seated obliquely, as required by functional position, here causes a pelvis obliquity with superincumbent scoliosis. The laterally curved lumbar spine (*arrows*) functional unit causes an oblique deformity of the disk and approximates the facets of the concave side (*small side of drawing*).

TISSUE SITES OF PAIN AND THEIR MANIFESTATIONS

The history has revealed which actions, movements, and positions result in pain and limitation. The examination attempts to ascertain which tissue is the source and causation of the pain. During the examination, the purpose should be to reproduce the precise pain complained of by the patient, depicting the mechanism of the pain and indicating the tissue responsible.

Tissue Sources of Pain

The principal sources of pain are: (1) injury to the supporting *soft tissues* especially ligaments, muscles, and tendons; (2) injury or inflammation of the posterior joints (facets); and (3) injury to the disk structures.

Injury to soft tissues such as ligament are rarely as massive as those that occur in knees, shoulders, and other extremity injuries. Ligamentous injuries in the spine are usually secondary to overload, inappropriate movements, or external forces.

Muscles tear more readily than tendons or ligaments. Muscles also tear more readily in eccentric contracture (lengthening while under tension), which is a frequent muscular function of the spine during bending and lifting. Muscular tears, when they occur, do not occur within their midsubstance but rather at their myotendinous junction.[68] Residual pain results from the area of the tendon to the bony attachments of these injured tissues.

Inflamed muscles may undergo **compartment syndrome**, in which there is swelling within an inflexible compartment (fascia) with resultant ishemia. Little or no evidence exists that compartment syndrome occurs in the erector spinae muscle groups.[69,70]

Fibromyalgia or fibrositis has been associated with low back injuries.[71] The diagnosis of myofascial pain as a cause of low back pain must meet the criteria discussed in Chapter 3.

Examination of Muscles and Tendons

Muscle pain is accompanied by muscle tenderness, which is palpable by the examiner, but the response by the patient is *subjective* as to its presence and its severity. Pain can also be elicited by passive stretching, but this motion also involves other periarticular soft tissues. Pain can be reproduced by actively contracting the involved muscle, but such active contraction increases pressure within the disk as well, so this does not represent an isolated tissue response. No laboratory or imaging studies confirm myogenic pain, so in such a finding, subjectivity predominates.

Facet Pathology and Examination

Badgley[72] first confirmed that abnormalities within the facet joints could be a source of persistent (i.e., chronic) pain. He postulated the innervation of the capsule and periosteum of the facets as deriving from the medial branch of the posterior primary ramus. Inman and Saunders[73] in 1940 revealed numerous overlapping neurologic innervations occur to these spinal structures, as well as an overlapping of somatic nerves with autonomic nerves.[74,75]

There is no question that lumbar zygapophyseal joints can be a source of low back and referred leg pain, but a question does arise as to whether facet pain can be diagnosed clinically without resorting to invasive diagnostic blocks.[76]

The **facet arthrosis syndrome** is characterized by morning stiffness and pain aggravated by rest. It is reproduced by lumbar extension and relieved by gentle flexion movement.[77] Fairbanks and colleagues[81] identified certain features which they related as being *specific* for the diagnosis of facet pain:

1. Acute onset of LBP from bending and twisting motions (these twisting motions should preferably be done upon reextension).
2. Increase in pain from sitting and forward flexion. (I prefer using extension.)

3. Relief during walking.
4. Pain occurring more proximally in the leg and aggravated by straight leg raising (SLR). Fairbanks[78] stated that "these are admittedly non-precise".
5. Relief after facet anesthetic injection.

In a retrospective study,[79] the following criteria were postulated:

1. LBP is associated with groin or thigh pain.
2. Localized paraspinal tenderness is present.
3. Pain is reproduced by lumbar extension and rotation toward the symptomatic side.

The last criteria in both of these postulations merely suggest that the facets are the cause of low back and leg pain. Three-level nerve blocks are the most confirmatory tests implicating the facets.[76]

Percutaneous injection of a local anesthetic to relieve pain was originally assumed as resulting from anesthetizing the facet joints,[80] but because the facets have multiple innervations, the facets were invalidated as the primary site of pain.

Injection of a hypertonic saline solution into the joint created low back pain, but as these findings were not radiographically confirmed,[81] the study was invalidated. Repetition of this study under radiologic localization confirmed the facet joints to be sites of nociception.[82]

The amount of hypertonic saline injected increased the area of pain. A small amount caused pain into the buttock. With increased amounts, the pain was referred down the posterior thigh and the calf.

Local tenderness over a facet has been described as has lateral manipulation through the posterior spinous process.[83] Hyperextension of the lumbosacral spine, combined with lateral flexion, is thought to impinge on the unilateral facets on the concave side, but this test is purely subjective. Only intra-articular injections are reasonably confirmatory.

LUMBAR DISK PAIN: ITS EXAMINATION

In patients with low back pain *and* leg pain, objective signs are more meaningful and diagnostic even though they do not always clearly relate to the subjective disability claimed by the patient.

The standard tests performed to measure and substantiate impairment can be listed as follows:

1. Excessive (abnormal and symptomatic) lordosis
2. Lumbar kyphosis

3. Lumbosacral (functional) scoliosis
4. Sacral angle
5. Lumbar flexion: range of motion (ROM)
6. Lumbar extension (sagittal and with lateral flexion)
7. Lateral flexion
8. SLR or Lasegue's test
9. Contralateral SLR
10. Tenderness
    interspinous
    paraspinous
    buttocks or lower extremity
11. Strength testing
    trunk flexors
    trunk extensors
    lower extremities
12. Precise pain reproduction

These *standard tests* will be discussed to consider which are subjective or objective in order to make a precise pathoanatomic diagnosis.

STANDARD PHYSICAL EXAMINATION TESTS

Lordosis

Excessive lordosis, or abnormal lumbosacral angle, has been advocated as the major cause of postural pain, whether it is discogenic, facetal, or radicular. The sacral angle implies the concept of *pelvic tilt*, because the sacrum is firmly attached to the pelvis, which rotates about the hip joints (Fig. 5–18). The manner of determining pelvic tilting is merely a visual observation and varies with the individual examiner and also when and how the patient is examined. It is an inaccurate and *subjective* measurement not dependent on instrumentation. Pain elicited by passively or actively accentuating the lordosis is subjective, but does implicate the movement as causative of the patient's symptoms.[84,85]

Because posture influences lumbar lordodsis, there are predominant influences upon the posture that must be recognized:[86-88]

1. Familial or hereditary factors.
2. Structural anomalies either congenital, acquired, neurological, muscular, or skeletal.
3. Postures of habit or training during the developmental years and those acquired from prolonged occupational stresses.

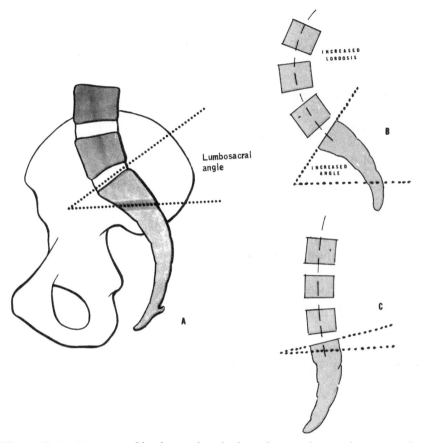

Figure 5–18. Variations of lumbosacral angle dependent on the sacral rotation. The physiologic lumbosacral angle is shown on the left (A). With an increased angle (B), the superincumbent lordosis increases whereas (C) a decreased angle decreases the lordosis.

That abnormal posture involving the lumbosacral spine causes pain remains unconfirmed,[89] yet reproducible symptomatic hyperlordosis during the examination may well be a factor in low back pain (Fig. 5–19), and may be elicited in the history and then reproduced during the examination (Fig. 5–20).

Lumbar Flexion

Forward flexion reverses the lumbar lordosis and its range of motion is *documented* in all reports. It is reduced in acute low back disorders possibly as a protective mechanism because it is *not* reduced in patients with chronic low

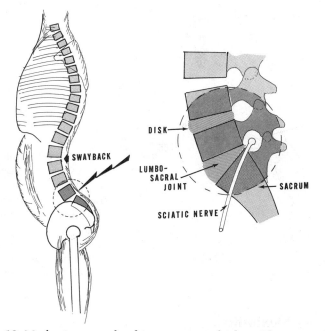

Figure 5–19. Mechanisms postulated in symptomatic lordosis. The increased lordosis, termed "swayback," increases the lumbosacral angle, which causes closure of the foramen between L5-S1 and compresses the sciatic nerve. The lumbosacral joint is between fifth lumbar vertebra and the sacrum with the intervertebral disk shown.

back pain.[90–92] Only when there are concurrent leg symptoms is this deduction valid.

Lumbar flexion limitation is often influenced by hamstring elongation limitation (Fig. 5–21). The influence of the hamstrings can be avoided if lumbar flexion is observed with the patient in the seated position (Fig. 5–22).

Physical therapists have long known that warm up exercises done before measurement of flexibility increases the range of motion tested,[93] thus recording ROM without preceding flexibility exercises is inaccurate.

Lateral and Rotational Flexibility

Lateral and rotational flexibility are tested (Figs. 5–23, 5–24, 5–25) as if they were *objective signs*, yet they are subjective and influenced by pain and fear.[94–98]

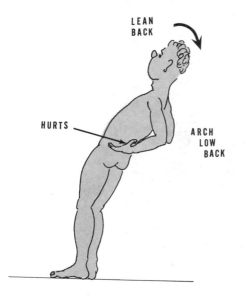

Figure 5–20. Confirmation of lordosis causing backache. In the clinical setting, the complaint of low backache is considered as being caused by excessive lordosis and can be reproduced by causing the patient to lean back excessively (*arrow*) at the low back region.

Hamstring Flexibility

When trunk flexion is considered to be impaired by inflexible hamstring muscles (Fig. 5–26), this hypothesis must be tested and evaluated accurately. If limited SLR is considered as being exclusively muscular and fas-

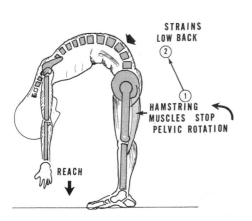

Figure 5–21. Standing test for degree of lumbar flexion and hamstring tightness. To evaluate the degree of lumbar flexion and where a loss of flexion occurs, as well as to determine the degree of hamstring tightness, the patient is viewed from the side. The patient with legs extended flexes fully in an attempt to touch the floor ahead of his feet. The patient is asked to flex fully, but slowly, to avoid low back strain. Pain may be produced in doing the test, which indicates structural problems. In case of a sciatic neuritis, this test causes pain radiation down the posterior aspect of the afflicted nerve root.

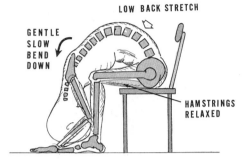

Figure 5–22. Testing low back flexibility without hamstring involvement. Having the patient seated, the hamstring muscles are totally relaxed. Having the patient flex forward demonstrates the flexibility of the lumbosacral spine.

cial and not resulting from nerve root tension, pain will be considered as *muscular* and there will be attendant negative *dural signs*. What this means is that the pain will be unilateral and will not be significantly aggravated by ankle dorsiflexion and simultaneous nuchal flexion such as occurs in a nerve root entrapment.

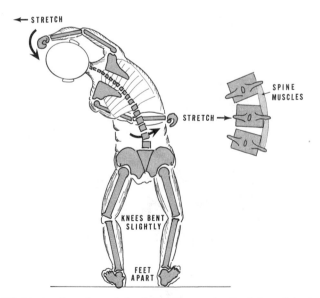

Figure 5–23. Testing lateral trunk flexibility. To test the flexibility of the lateral trunk soft tissues, the patient, standing with feet slightly apart and the knees slightly bent, is asked to bend as far as possible to one side and then to the other side. The small drawing depicts the tissues being tested. Bringing the arms overhead to either side also tests the flexibility of the latissimus dorsi muscle groups.

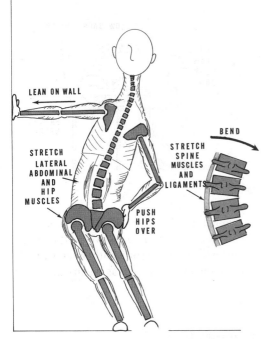

SIDE BENDING 2

LEAN ON WALL

STRETCH
LATERAL
ABDOMINAL
AND
HIP
MUSCLES

PUSH
HIPS
OVER

BEND

STRETCH
SPINE
MUSCLES
AND
LIGAMENTS

Figure 5–24. Another test of lateral trunk flexibility. To test the flexibility of the lateral trunk soft tissues, the patient, with feet together, is asked to lean against a wall. With the contralateral hand, the pelvis is pushed toward the wall. This maneuver tests the flexibility of the lateral abdominal and hip muscles as well as the paraspinous muscle and ligaments (*small side figure*).

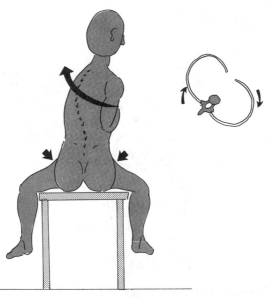

Figure 5–25. Testing trunk rotational flexibility in the seated position. To test the rotational flexibility of the trunk, the patient sits straddled over the examining table, which fixes the trunk. The patient actively turns the upper trunk to the right and then to the left. The degree of rotation is estimated and compared, left to right.

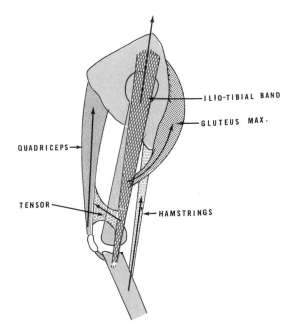

Figure 5–26. Muscles acting on the pelvis. In evaluating truncal flexibility, the muscles acting on the pelvis are also involved. Their flexibility should also be individually evaluated. These tissues are the iliotibial band, the gluteus maximus, the quadriceps muscles group, the tensors, and the hamstrings.

STRENGTH TESTING

Strength testing of the trunk muscles as an objective test for the cause of low back pain symptoms has also been advocated. It has led to development of instrumentation for documenting this weakness.

The exercises used for testing abdominal strength is the sit-up which, because it can be done properly or improperly, thus casts question on the validity of the test. Done with the knees and hips flexed and in stages (Fig. 5–27), the test can be performed without causing pain and remain valid.[99] Abdominal strength can also be tested from the shortened (fully flexed) position and gradual backward descent (Fig. 5–28).

In a physically unfit person, a sit-up done with legs extended can cause painful lordotic extension (Fig. 5–29). Because of the resultant low back pain, it cannot be considered a valid test of strength.

Testing abdominal strength by bilateral SLR (Fig. 5–30) is also feasible *if* the person has strong abdominal muscles but in a poorly conditioned person, resultant low back pain can make the test invalid.

Extensor muscle strength testing can be done by manual resistance of lift-

SITUP:STAGES

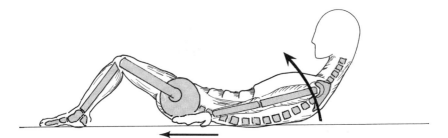

Figure 5–27. Trunk flexor strength testing: stages. The trunk flexors, the abdominal muscles, are best tested in stages of sitting up from the supine position. These stages are also used in exercises for trunk strengthening (to be discussed). The first stage is the elevation (flexing) of the head and neck, which causes a coordinated contraction of the abdominal muscles.

ing variable weights. In this test the proper way the patient lifts can also be evaluated (Fig. 5–31). Most strength tests are invalidated by pain, pain fear and avoidance, deconditioning, and patient failure to make maximum effort. An objective test is therefore not gained. Muscle strength tested in the usual manner does not indicate this as the mechanism of chronic low back pain.

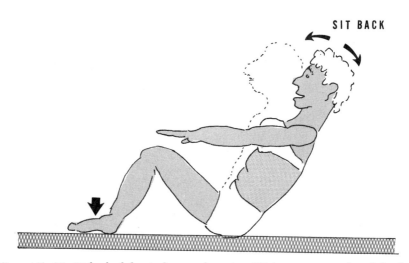

SIT BACK

Figure 5–28. Sit-back abdominal strength testing. With patient seated and the feet possibly held down, the patient slowly sits back and "holds" at various degrees. This test can be done with arms extended forward if the patient is poorly conditioned or with arms behind the head if reasonably strong.

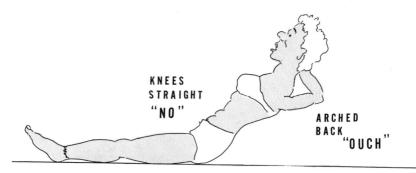

Figure 5-29. Poorly conditioned patient doing a painful situp. From the supine position with legs extended and feet possibly held down, the patient sits up or sits back, which causes low back pain from hyperextension if the abdominal muscles are extremely weak.

Lumbar Extension

Lumbar extension has also been used to elicit low back pain. Reproducing the low back symptoms by having the patient hyperextend the low back and maintain that posture for several seconds is considered diagnostic. This, however, demands exclamation of pain by the patient and thus is not wholly *objective*. McKenzie[100] implies that *passive* hyperextension can cause anterior migration of an internally herniated disk (Fig. 5-32) and can thus relieve a symptomatic bulge.

For these tests to be considered as *objective* will require patient effort, compliance, and performance often despite pain. They therefore remain *subjective* and need careful evaluation.

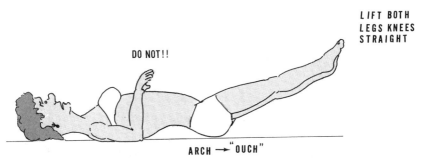

Figure 5-30. Abdominal strength testing with bilateral leg raising. If patient has extremely weak abdominal muscles, this test usually causes a painful low back extension. Otherwise, it can be used to test rectus abdominal muscle strength and endurance.

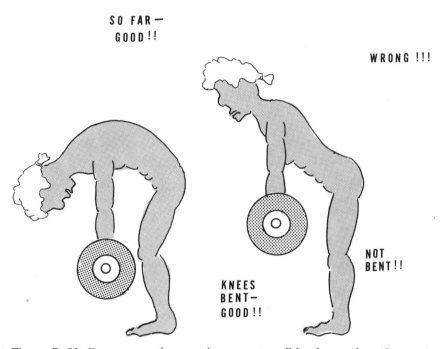

SO FAR—
GOOD!!

WRONG!!!

KNEES
BENT—
GOOD!!

NOT
BENT!!

Figure 5–31. Extensor muscle strength testing. As will be discussed in Chapter 7, there are many machines designed to test trunk extensor strength. A simple test is to have the patient lift a measured weight. This test should conform to a proper physiologic mechanism, and thus is done with legs and back slightly flexed. Avoid extension during the lift.

OBJECTIVE NEUROLOGIC EXAMINATION

The SLR test, otherwise termed **the Lasegue test**, if performed accurately, is objective.[101,102] The purpose of the SLR test is to determine whether the resultant pain elicited behind the thigh is derived from muscular or nerve irritation. Essentially the SLR test merely extends the hip with the lower leg extended to elicit pain and determine at which angle of flexion the pain occurs.

The hamstring muscles elongate to their physiologic flexibility as the extended leg is flexed. Resultant pain is the myofascial component of the hamstring muscle group that is shortened. Muscular pain in the SLR test is usually identical in both legs and occurs at the same level of straight leg raising.

Pain resulting from performing the straight leg procedure must be defined as either from a muscular source or from sciatic nerve stretch. Confusion in terminology was carefully analyzed by van Akkerveeken[103] who differentiated **radicular pain** from that termed **sciatica**. The former term should be

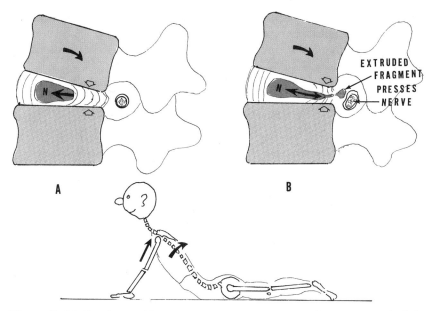

EXTRUDED
FRAGMENT
PRESSES
NERVE

A

B

Figure 5–32. Lumbosacral hyperextension causing root pain from intervertebral disc protrusion. As the lumbosacral spine is extended (*lower drawing*), the nucleus (N) of the disk migrates anteriorly (*A*). If the disk is extruded, this position (*B*) encroaches on the nerve root and forces the fragment to compress the root.

used to describe the condition in patients suffering from pain resulting from pathology of the spinal nerve *root*, whereas the latter is a neuralgia of the sciatic nerve *trunk*.

Verbiest[104,105] postulated that pain from compression of a nerve root resulted from irritation of the nervi nervorum of the root sheath when he eliminated the pain from an inflamed nerve root by placing a drop of cocaine upon the sheath. The basis for a *dural* straight leg raising being seen as a nervous rather than a muscle stretch phenomenon is thus clarified.

The SLR test may be performed in two ways:

1. With the leg fully extended at the knee, the leg is passively flexed at the hip joint.
2. With the person seated and thus with the hip flexed to 90°, the lower leg can be passively extended.

Both of these tests measure only the muscular flexibility of the posterior thigh muscles. The sciatic nerve is also extended but if not inflamed or under tension, the test produces no pain. If inflamed or under tension, however, SLR testing is limited with pain occurring early and usually in one leg.

The dural sign can be confirmed by flexing the neck or dorsiflexing the foot and ankle after accomplishing full passive straight leg raising (Figs. 5–33 and 5–34). A confirmatory dural test is the Fajersztain test,[106] also known as the *well leg-raising test* or *crossed* nerve stretch. Sciatic pain radiation occurs down the afflicted leg from raising the opposite *normal* leg.

Straight leg raising only tests the lower root segments (L-4, L-5, S-1) be-

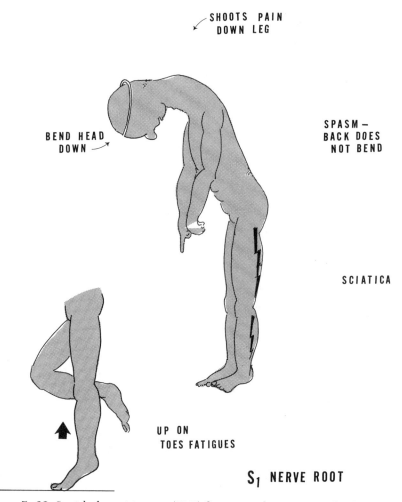

Figure 5–33. Straight leg raising test (SLR) from a standing position: the dural sign. In the presence of a herniated lumbar disk, as the patient flexes forward with legs extended, the low back does not flex and the straight leg is essentially flexed (SLR). This alone may cause sciatic neuritic pain. The *dural sign* is then elicited by flexing the neck and head. Suspecting an S-1 root involvement, the strength of the gastroc-soleus muscle (*lower drawing*) is tested by having the patient arise repeatedly on the toes. Fatigue or weakness confirms S-1 involvement.

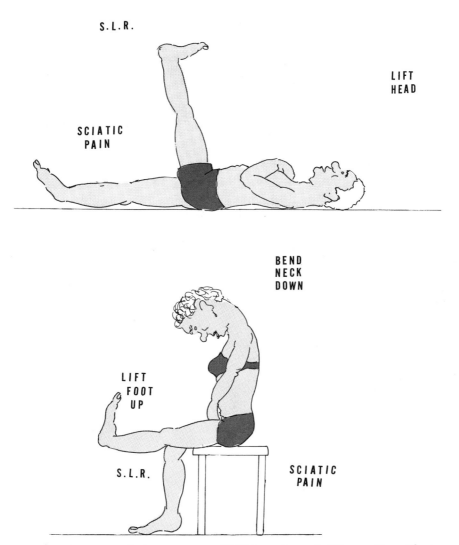

Figure 5–34. Straight leg raising test (SLR) in supine and sitting positions. The top drawing shows the method of eliciting nerve root pain from straight leg raising. The extended leg is slowly flexed at the hip and compared with the other leg. Flexing the head-neck elicits the "dural sign" as would dorsiflexing the foot after raising the leg (not illustrated). The bottom picture demonstrates the same test in the seated position. Here, the dural test includes the ankle dorsiflexion, as well as nuchal flexion.

cause only these roots extend into the lower leg. If neuritis, from whatever cause, involves upper lumbar segments, such as L-2 or L-3, which form the femoral nerve, the root segments are not stretched during the SLR test.

Nerve root involvement of the upper lumbar plexus is tested using the femoral stretch test (Fig. 5–35). This test is performed with the patient prone and with the hip extended flexing the knee (i.e., the foot approaching the buttocks). This test stretches the quadriceps as well as the femoral nerve. No dural component is known.

Neurologic Determination of Nerve Root Involvement

All lower extremity muscles and sensory nerves emerge from the lumbosacral spine. Each must be individually tested to determine which is entrapped, inflamed, or under tension and at which spinal level.

Clinical dermatome and myotome levels are depicted (Table 5–1). All muscles are innervated by peripheral nerves that contain more than one nerve root (Table 5–2).

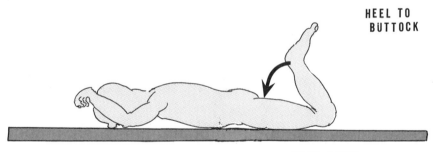

HEEL TO BUTTOCK

PAIN DOWN FRONT OF THIGH

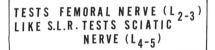

TESTS FEMORAL NERVE (L_{2-3}) LIKE S.L.R. TESTS SCIATIC NERVE (L_{4-5})

Figure 5–35. Femoral Nerve Stretch Test. When the upper nerve roots (L-2, L-3, and possibly L-4), which form the femoral nerve, are entrapped they cause a positive test termed the "prone femoral nerve test." With the patient prone, the lower leg is flexed to approach the foot to the buttocks. In a positive test, pain is felt down the front of the thigh. This pain must be differentiated from muscle (quadriceps) stretch pain by being compared with the other leg.

Table 5–1. SCHEMATIC DERMATOME AND MYOTOME LEVEL OF NERVE ROOT IMPINGEMENT

Nerve Root	Intervertebral Space	Subjective Pain Radiation	Sensory Area	Bladder and Bowel Dysfunction*	SLR†	Ankle Jerk‡	Knee Jerk‡	Motor Dysfunction (Myotome)§
L-3	L2-L3	Back to buttocks to posterior thigh to anterior knee region	Hypalgesia in knee region	+/-	Usually -	+	+	Quadriceps weakness
L-4	L3-L4	Back to buttocks to posterior thigh to inner calf region	Hypalgesia inner aspect of lower leg	+/-	Usually - Maybe +	+	-	Quadriceps and possible anticus weakness
L-5	L4-L5	Back to buttocks to dorsum of foot and big toe	Hypalgesia in dorsum foot and big toe	+/-	++	+	+	Weakness of anterior tibialis, big toe extensor, gluteus medius
S-1	L5-S1	Back to buttocks to sole of foot and heel	Hypalgesia in heel or lateral foot	+/-	+++	-	+	Weakness of gastrocnemius, hamstring, gluteus maximus

*Bladder and bowel dysfunction can occur at any level. †Related to extent of nerve root movement of each level. ‡Ankle jerk is absent only at L5-S1; knee jerk at L3-L4. §Only the more obvious and functional muscles are listed.

**Table 5-2. RELATIONSHIP OF SPECIFIC ROOTS,
MUSCLES, AND PERIPHERAL NERVES**

Root	Muscle	Peripheral Nerve
L-2	Sartorius (L2-3)	Femoral
	Pectineus (L2-3)	Obturator
	Adductor longus (L2-3)	Obturator
L-3	Quadriceps femoris (L2-3-4)	Femoral
L-4	Quadriceps femoris (L2-3-4)	Femoral
	Tensor fascia lata (L4-5)	Superior gluteal
	Tibialis anterior (L4-5)	Peroneal
L-5	Gluteus medius (L4-5 S1)	Superior gluteal
	Semimembranosus (L4-5 S1)	Sciatic
	Semitendinosus (L4-5 S1)	Sciatic
	Extensor hallucis longis (L4-5 S1)	Deep peroneal
S-1	Gluteus maximus (L4-5 S1-2)	Inferior gluteal
	Biceps femoris—short head (L-5 S1-2)	Sciatic
	Semitendinosus (L4-5 S1)	Sciatic
	Medial gastrocnemius (S1-2)	Tibial
	Soleus (S1-2)	Tibial
S-2	Biceps femoris—long head (S1-2)	Sciatic
	Lateral gastrocnemius (S1-2)	Tibial
	Soleus (S1-2)	Tibial

Each dermatomal area of the lower extremity is subserved by specific nerve roots. Dermatome areas can be mapped out by the examiner by rubbing the skin with a piece of cotton, the end of a pin, or a wheel. The patient literally draws the map by indicating where the test object is felt. Dermatomal mappings are present in every neurologic text (Fig. 5-36); the most usual are those of Keegan and Garret,[10] Bolk,[108] or Hansen.[109]

The dermatomal area has already been designated by the subjective claim of the patient during the history taking and is confirmed by "where the pain is felt" during the SLR test.

The myotome designation is performed by the patient actively initiating the precise muscle group upon demand of the examiner. The nerve supply to that muscle group is deducted by the response. The objectivity of this test is colored by the willingness of the patient to cooperate fully.

The S-1 nerve root innervates the gluteus maximus and the gastrocnemius-soleus group. The former is tested by placing the patient in the prone position and elevating (extending) the flexed leg. This tests the hip extensors, primarily the glutei (S1-2 & L4-5) and is compared to the other side. Preferably endurance is tested by repeating the effort several times on both legs.

The gastrocnemius-soleus muscle (S1-2) is tested by asking the patient to

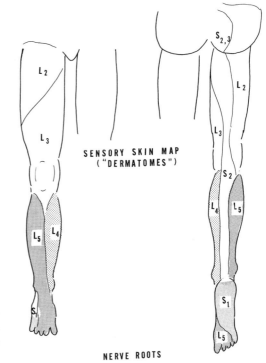

SENSORY SKIN MAP
("DERMATOMES")

NERVE ROOTS

Figure 5–36. Dermatomal areas of the lower extremity. This is the classic dermatomal mapping of Keegan (see text).

rise up on the toes of each leg and comparing the two. Endurance is tested here by having the patient arise several times. Merely walking up on one's toes to test strength in gastrocnemius muscle is not satisfactory (Fig. 5–37).

Tenderness of the myoneural junctions has been postulated[110] as having localizing characteristics (Fig. 5–38), but this demands a careful search by the examiner's probing finger, and findings remain highly subjective.

Tests to Increase Intrathecal Pressure

Admittedly *objective* and reproducible, these tests depend on verbal reports by the patient which brings in an element of subjectivity. These tests are based on the fact that increased intrathecal pressure also increases the pressure upon the involved and obstructed nerve root. The tests are more objective when used to confirm leg pain as emanating from a source in the low back.

Milgram Test. Lying supine on the examining table, the patient attempts to hold both legs approximately 2" above the table for 30 seconds (Fig.

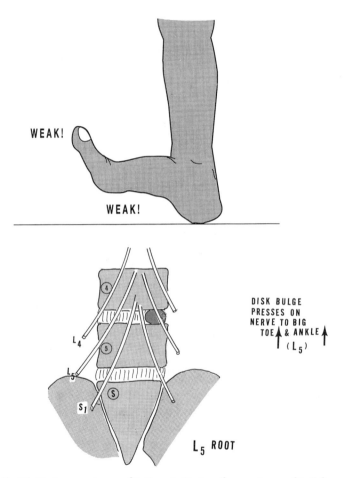

Figure 5–37. Testing myotome of L-5 root. Testing the myotome of L-5 for weakness or fatigue of the extensor hallucis longus (big toe extensor). This usually indicates an L-5 lesion although some clinicians also implicate the S-1 root (see text). Fatigue of one leg should be compared with the other leg to be diagnostic.

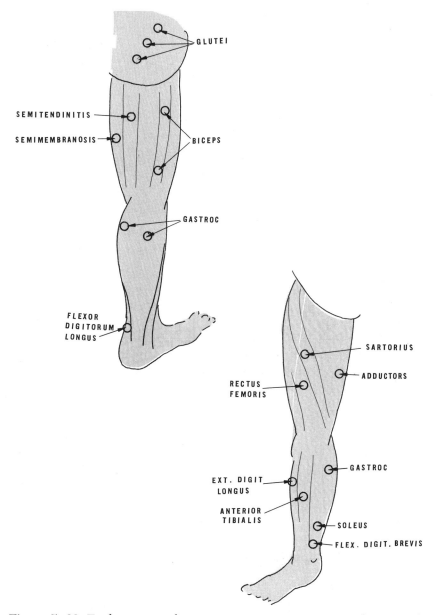

Figure 5–38. Tender myoneural junction points. Deep pressure tenderness at the sites of myoneural junctions have been postulated as localizing nerve root lesions. The innervation of the muscles being palpated must be known and it must be remembered that most muscles have multiple innervations and not merely one root.

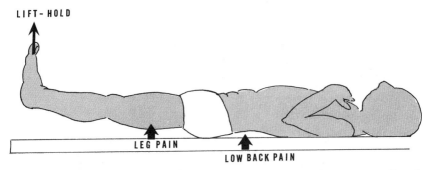

LIFT-HOLD

LEG PAIN

LOW BACK PAIN

Figure 5–39. The Milgram test. When considered "positive," this test originally indicated increased intrathecal pressure. It requires the patient to hold both legs some inches from the table for 30 seconds. This test also causes low back pain from lumbosacral hyperextension in patients with subnormal abdominal musculature, but this is not a positive response.

5–39).[110] If no pain occurs, no intrathecal pathology is present, whereas with pain, pathology can be considered to occur. What pathology must then be determined. This maneuver also causes a stressful hyperextension in the presence of weak abdominal muscles; and thus is a mechanical test not involving intrathecal pressure.

Naffziger Test. The Naffziger test increases the intrathecal pressure, during which the jugular veins are compressed gently for approximately 10 seconds until the patient's face flushes (Fig. 5–40). The physician's request for the patient to cough should produce pain if there is increased pressure. In the

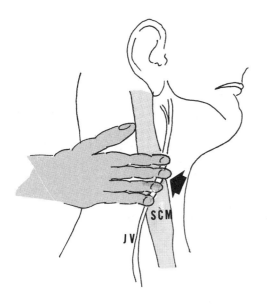

SCM

JV

Figure 5–40. The Naffziger test. Compression of the jugular vein until the patient's face begins to flush causes an increase in intrathecal pressure if accompanied by a cough. JV = jugular vein; SCM = sternocleidomastoid muscle.

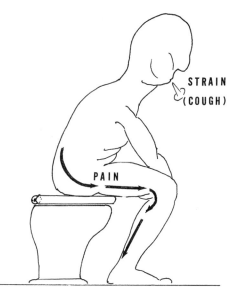

STRAIN
(COUGH)

PAIN

Figure 5–41. The Valsalva maneuver. When the patient bears down, as in moving the bowels or coughing, there is an increase in intrathecal pressure. If any of these maneuvers causes posterior leg pain, it indicates pressure upon the theca somewhere in the cord.

presence of discogenic nerve compression, this test can be considered *objective*; however, the same result can also present in other cord and nerve compressive syndromes.

Valsalva Maneuver. The patient is asked to *bear down* as if to move the bowels or to strain while not breathing. This maneuver increases intrathecal pressure (Fig. 5–41). It is *positive*, if this maneuver produces pain in the low back or down the leg and thus becomes *objective*. It does not, however, signify only disk pathology, because any other space-consuming thecal pathology also causes a positive test.

Kernig Test. The supine patient's head is forcefully flexed (Fig. 5–42) upon the chest which is thought to stretch the spinal cord dura including that covering the nerve root distally. It is a modification of the "well leg straight-leg raising test" previously described. Because it may be positive as a result of pathology or cord compression at any point along the cord, it is, thus, not specific for lumbosacral pathology.

Confirmatory Tests for Sciatic Radiculitis

An EMG examination will document objective evidence of nerve root compression, demyelinization, or inflammation. Radiographs, computed tomographic (CT) scans, and magnetic resonance imaging (MRI) will also confirm compression on nerve roots and indicate the pathologic lesion.

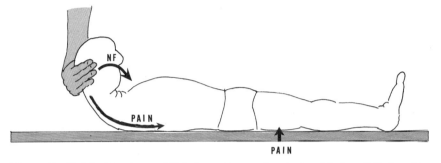

Figure 5–42. The Kernig test. With the patient supine the head is forcefully flexed to bring the chin on the chest. If pain radiates down the spine and into the leg, it indicates dural irritation or compression somewhere along the cord or pathologic abnormality within the cord. The clinical examination confirms the site of cord (dural) compression. NF=nuchal flexion.

Test for Malingering

Certain tests are designated to determine whether the patient is malingering, even though there is disagreement as to whether malingering indicates a psychologic aberration.

The problem relates to whether the patient is providing inaccurate information *consciously and intentionally*. The definition of malingering is "deliberately faking symptoms for the sole purpose of obtaining an extrinsic goal."[111]

There is no good marker that correlates the objectivity of findings with the subjectivity of the incurred disability.[112]

Psychologic disorders are most often diagnosed in patients with chronic low back pain and disability who have symptoms out of proportion to the structural pathology. These include depression, secondary gain, and learned pain patterns.

In many patients with chronic low back pain disease, there is a preponderance of abandonment, as well as a history of emotional, physical, and sexual abuse in their childhoods.[113] These must be considered before alleging the patient is malingering. Such possibilities should also be evaluated before undertaking surgical intervention for chronic pain.

In summarizing the necessity for accurately diagnosing low back disorder and implementing prolonged therapy and surgical intervention, the true basis of disability must be ascertained using meaningful diagnostic procedures. With essentially limited results from surgical intervention, the rates of hospitalization for cervical surgery increased more than 45% and for lumbar spine surgery more than 33% in the years between 1979 and 1990. Lumbar spine fusions have increased more than 60%.[114]

Most low back problems are self limited with approximately 75% to 90% of patients recovering within 6 weeks, regardless of the applied treatment, yet *care* for the patient with low back problems continues to exert a tremendous cost in treating such an injured patient. Of all claims for worker's compensation[115-117] 16% are from low back pain with 32.4% being for medical costs, compared with 65.8% for indemnity.

In appreciating the subjectivity as compared with objectivity of the low back soft tissue injury, a full review of this disease entity certainly is indicated.

TREATMENT PROTOCOL FOR LOW BACK PAIN

Low back pain must be differentiated into acute, chronic, or recurrent forms.

Patients with benign low back pain get well regardless of the treatment in 80% of cases. Consequently, treatment is aimed at hastening recovery, returning to daily activities, and preventing chronicity.

Pain has been discussed in Chapter 2. Only those modalities specifically pertaining to low back will be addressed here. The noxious agents that accumulate at the peripheral trauma site from trauma—intrinsic or extrinsic, comprising histamine, kinins, neuropeptides, and numerous other algogens, have a vasomotor effect—either vasodilatation or vasoconstriction. These nociceptive agents lower the threshold of the receptors of the A-delta and C-afferent fibers of the peripheral nervous system sending impulses cephalad. Intervention or elimination of these algogens at the trauma tissue site is the objective of the application of most modalities.

The local area becomes hypersensitive creating pain known as **primary hyperalgesia**. A **secondary hyperalgesia** occurs in the surrounding tissues from antidromic activation of the C primary afferents which releases substance P in the region.[118] This hypersensitivity may also be an after discharge from small primary afferents that release substance P. Electrical stimulation of the primary afferents has been shown to release substance P at their receptor ends. Reactive local skeletal muscle spasm occurs, thus initiating a pain-spasm-pain cycle.[119]

The chemical and mechanical substances produced at the peripheral tissue site following injury are a mechanism of pain production that must be addressed in the treatment of acute, and even some aspects of chronic, pain.

Following ice application, the application of heat is therapeutic in that it increases blood flow, which causes cooler blood to reach the site and remove the warm blood. The process by which heat provides analgesia and reduces muscle spasm is not fully understood.[120,121]

The hemodynamic effect of increasing blood flow occurs as superficial heat causes reflex postganglionic sympathetic nerve activity to the smooth muscles of the blood vessels to supply greater flow of blood to deeper organs, such as muscle.[122]

Modalities to increase flexibility are divided into active and passive procedures. Connective tissue, whether collagen, elastin, or fibrous tends to shorten after injury.[123] The viscoelastic properties of connective tissues that permit elongation from physical stretch are collectively known as **plastic deformation**.[124] Recoverable deformation is possible if the modalities of heat and passive-active stretch are applied to the deformed (i.e., shortened) tissues.[125]

Techniques for stretch have been propounded varying from constant load to overcome impaired elasticity, rapid stretch followed by holding the gained elongation, or a slow progressive stretch.[126]

ANALGESIC NERVE BLOCK IN TREATING PAIN

In treating acute low back pain, with or without radiation of pain to the leg, the site of nerve block is not precise. Bonica initially[127] stated that "analgesic blocking, skillfully performed, can play a significant role in the management of acute low back pain, regardless of the etiology." He continues "it is . . . an important adjunct to other treatment . . . even though it may produce complete and permanent relief of pain." He stresses that analgesic blocks are effective in relieving muscles spasm "as known."

The analgesic blocks are administered into the tender muscle(s), into the ligaments of the apophyseal, sacroiliac, and sacrococcygeal joints (Fig. 5–43), which do not interrupt the nerve supply to the affected tissues.

Of neural blocks the caudal and peridural are effective but are usually considered only when pain persists and does not respond to other modalities. Perivertebral blocks also fall into this category of therapy.[128]

The techniques of performing nerve blocks have been extensively described in textbooks of anesthesia and acute pain.

Epidural injections are rarely used for acute low back pain unless the pain persists, in which case it becomes chronic pain.[129]

The technique of epidural injection is well documented (Fig. 5–44). In itself, the benefit is limited and its value is only subjectively palliative, while remaining of temporary value.

EXERCISE TREATMENT OF ACUTE LOW BACK PAIN

The literature is replete in proclaiming exercises as *the* major modality in treating low back pain, whether acute or chronic, but which exercise remains as unclear as the basis for the intended benefit of exercise. The outcomes assessment of exercise regimes is gradually receiving attention.[130–134] Tollison and Kriegel 1988,[135] posed two questions: what evidence is there to support the claim of the value of exercise; and which exercises have proven beneficial?

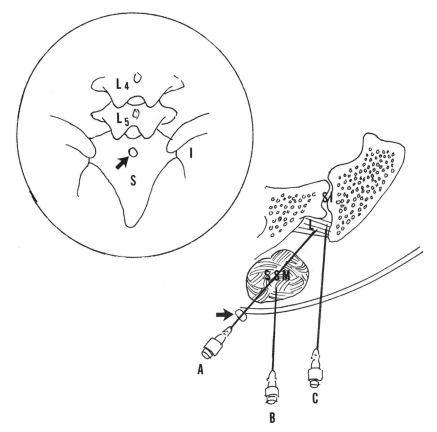

Figure 5–43. Injection sites of paraspinous muscles, sacroiliac ligaments, and the sacroiliac joint. The drawing in the circle is a posterior view of the sacrum (S), the fifth lumbar vertebra (L-5), the fourth lumbar vertebra (L-4), and the ilium (I). The site of injection (*circle indicated by arrow*) is in the center between both posterior superior spines. The needle *A* is inserted at a 45° angle toward the sacroiliac ligaments (L) further into the sacroiliac joint (SI). Needle *B* inserts into sacrospinalis muscle (SSM). Needle *C* in a direct injection into the SI joint and its ligaments.

For centuries the traditional exercises for the low back were the Williams' type[136] which were essentially flexion exercises to attempt to decrease lordosis. MacKenzie[100] refuted the flexion aspect. His concept was that the extension of the lumbosacral spine returned the disk nucleus anteriorly away from the sensitive tissues posteriorly. Both of these exercises invoked movement within the functional units, not the external muscles themselves.

More recently[137] the concept that muscle spasm occurs after an injury has been refuted because the muscle that prevented motion were electrically *silent*. Any motion resistance present was attributed to "functional contrac-

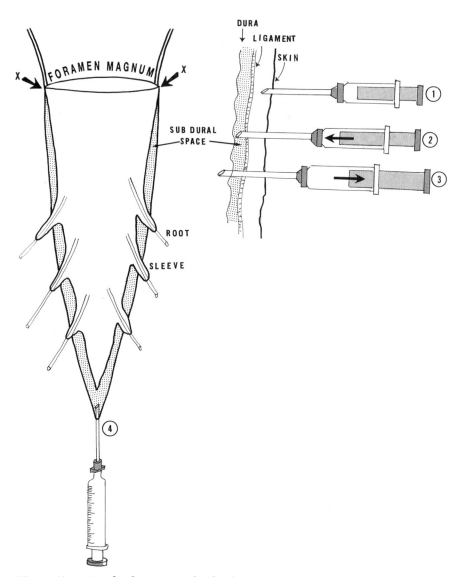

Figure 5–44. Epidural injection. The dural sac is closed at the foramen magnum (*X*) then descends distally enclosing the nerve roots as they emerge through the foramena. The technique of injection includes (*1*) spinal needle penetration of the skin into the subcutaneous tissues toward the dura. At this stage there is no pressure change in the syringe. (*2*) Penetration through the ligament into the subdural space where pressure is less and the plunger enters the syringe. If the needle penetrates the dura (*3*) it becomes an intradural (spinal) tap and the spinal fluid pressure is higher and forces the plunger out of the syringe. (*4*) Another epidural route is at the caudal tip through the sacral notch.

ture" from impairment of the gamma-alpha neuronal cycle (see Chapter 3 for more detailed discussion).

"Exercise therapy is the cornerstone treatment for subacute and chronic."[138] Bonica continues "During acute pain exercise generally is contraindicated except for maintaining self administered passive range of motion of all extremities and the trunk."

Neurophysiologic and clinical studies have verified that there is no doubt that muscular weakness and fatigue are prevalent in many musculoskeletal pain syndromes.

Rest, so frequently prescribed without definition and duration, has proven to be detrimental both physiologically and psychologically, therefore exercise is a good antidote of these sequelae. After 24 to 48 hours of bed rest, self-administered exercise to gradually increase flexibility and isometric exercises for maintainance of muscle tone should be initiated along with other modalities. Self-applied stretching exercises in all planes of motion and combined tridimensional planes done slowly, progressively, and frequently ensure regaining flexibility of all soft tissues of the back and lower extremities.

Exercise for the treatment of chronic and recurrent low back disorders has more complete documentation.[139] Walking remains the best form of exercise (Figs. 5–45 and 5–46). Walking addresses every aspect of the body including all the trunk muscles, upper and lower extremity muscles, all fascial sheaths, and even the annular fibers of the intervertebral disks (Fig. 5–47). Walking properly with good stride and pace actually has cardiovascular value, psychologic benefit, and even postural training.

Improving the static low back pain as determined from taking the history and making a physical examination requires attention to the patient's posture. This may require a corset if pain is acute and persistent but that modality should be brief and only be applied while exercises for posture are implemented. Daily ergonomics, such as standing and sitting in physical activities or in routine daily life should be evaluated and modified.

Strengthening exercises have become the current model. Strength testing has been illustrated as sufficient to determine the precise weakness, and so the precise exercise. Numerous machines have been devised to measure strength and endurance, which have failed to analyze daily requirement of activities, because most are done unphysiologically, in a single plane, against isometric resistance and using only limited muscles of the trunk and total body. Recently,[140] a lumbar motion monitor (see Fig. 5–15) has been devised that measures tridimensional trunk activity determining acceleration, coordination, and range of motion. The monitor can be implemented in the workplace and determines the functional deficiency. It also establishes a base line and monitors the outcomes of therapeutic exercises. Extensive clinical application remains untested at this moment, but the prospect is encouraging.

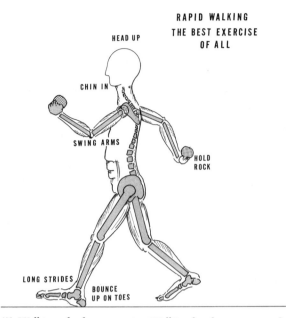

Figure 5–45. Walking: the best exercise. Walking has been accepted as the best comprehensive exercise. With swinging of the arms the trunk undergoes active flexion gentle rotation and lateral flexibility at each step. With attention, good posture is also enhanced. Holding a weight in each hand is optional. Besides trunk benefit there is no stress on the lower extremities and there is psychologic and cardiovascular benefit.

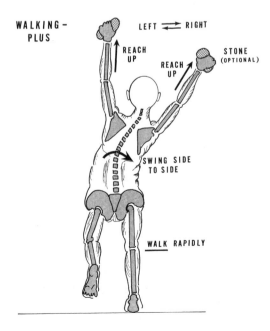

Figure 5–46. Walking plus. An addition to walking (Fig. 5–45), the walking depicted here increases active stretching of the lateral trunk muscles and also stretches and strengthens the latissimus dorsi muscles, which are the muscles involved in proper back function.

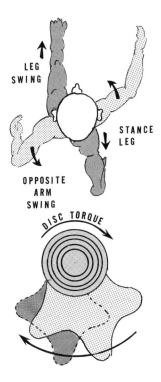

Figure 5–47. Physiologic effect of walking on the intervertebral disk. The determinants of gait specify that as the forward leg swings the hind leg remains the stance leg and the arms swing in the opposite direction. This imposes a rotational torque on the spine at an estimated 8° of rotation. The vertebral disk undergoes this torque albeit with a slight degree of compressive force from the body weight and the contraction of the trunk muscles. The torque is impressed on the annular fibers of the disk enhancing their "rigidity," hence walking is physiologically beneficial.

Exercises to correct any weakness ascertained by a meaningful clinical examination should be instituted. Flexors as well as extensors must be addressed especially the abdominal obliques. The protocols for each exercise are well documented in the literature.[139]

Teaching proper body "mechanics" is probably of the most significance in treating the chronic and recurrent low back disorder. Physiologic bending, rearising, and lifting must be taught and practiced until they become automatic for the patient.

The psychologic aspects of the patient who suffers low back disorders have become prominent in recent concepts,[141] both in continuance of pain, fear of recurrence,[142] and the psychologic aspects of perturbers in normal neuromuscular mechanisms (see Fig. 5–13). These psychologic factors of disability must be suspected and recognized and therapy invoked early so that psychologic testing is not implemented "later when patient is not improving" implying that the pain is "all in the mind."

There are other modalities of treatment advocated such as traction,[142] epidural analgesic agents, biofeedback, and transcutaneous electrical stimulation, which have been discussed in Chapter 4 and in other medical literature.

MANIPULATION

Manipulation of the spine has been practiced since antiquity with both Eastern and Western medical history sources replete with antecdotal evidence of *cures*.

Late in the 19th century, two philosophies of spinal manipulation evolved. In 1874, Andrew Taylor Still proposed the modality of osteopathy in which manipulation was the predominant modality. In 1885, D. D. Palmer proposed what is currently called chiropractic. Palmer's concept was that spinal joint dysfunction affected contiguous nerve function with resultant pathology occurring in the organs related to these nerves.

The influence of nerve function on these organs was considered the "law of the nerve," whereas initially osteopathy attributed pathology to impaired vascularity improved by manipulation: hence the "law of the artery."

Osteopathy has been modified so that in most states, osteopaths have become allied to the American Medical Association, although still advocating manipulation as a precise modality. The practice of chiropractic has been modified tremendously in recent decades and its practitioners are now represented by the American Chiropractic Association (ACA). A typical graduate of a Council on Chiropractic Education–accredited college takes premedical courses and 4 to 5 years of graduate medical education. The graduates are considered specialists in the function of joints of the spine and extremities.

Chiropractors furnish 94% of manipulative care in the United States. In addition to manipulation, however, they also administer dietary advice, nutritional input, changes in life style and general exercise programs so any benefit from their ministrations cannot be attributed exclusively to manipulation.

Of the patients seeking chiropractic care, low back pain involves 42%. Of others, 10.3% refer to the face and neck, 9.6% to headache, and 9.6% consult for "back adjustments."[143–149]

That literature research fails to reveal scientific bases for chiropractic does not refute that spinal manipulation therapy, as practiced by qualified licensed chiropractors, provides effective relief for musculoskeletal disorders, both acute and chronic.

Manipulation has enjoyed advocacy in the treatment of low back pain problems so that it must be considered in the realm of treatment protocol.[150–152] Many practitioners claim that manipulation of the spine *unlocks*, mobilizes a *jammed facet*, reflexively releases muscle spasm, elongates the facet capsule, or realigns a *subluxed joint*.

Therapy varies from gentle stretching to forceful application of manual force. The former is termed mobilization and the latter is manipulation. In many geographic regions, the latter can be administered only by a physician and the former remains the domain of the physical therapist.

The concepts of benefit from manipulation as postulated include:

1. A facet becomes immobilized by an acute synovial reaction and adherence of the adjacent facet joint surfaces from an inappropriate motion or an abnormal external force. Manipulation separates these surfaces.
2. A meniscus that normally exists within the facet joint becomes entrapped from an nonphysiological motion.
3. The redundant facet capsule becomes lodged between the adjacent articular surfaces.
4. The mechanoreceptors of the joint capsule are desensitized by an abrupt nonphysiologic motion of the joint, preventing further motion.
5. The spindle system of the involved muscles are impaired by a nonphysiologic motion. Manipulation allegedly reflexively stimulates and reciprocally relaxes the extrafusal muscles.
6. The involved spinal segments become malaligned by a nonphysiologic movement and are realigned into physiologic position by manipulation. This explains the term **adjustment**.
7. Manipulation is a placebo which benefits the patient by the *laying on of hands*.

The physiologic movements of joints are limited in their range by the elasticity of the capsules, the periarticular ligaments, and the fascial limits of the contiguous muscles. Joints have an active and a passive range (Fig. 5–48).

Exactly what occurs during manipulation remains conjectural. It affords benefit in many patients but the basis for the improvement gained is obscure. Lasting benefits have also not been confirmed.

Manipulation is usually a force applied in the direction of restriction to regain that lost motion. Manipulation in the opposite direction, away from the locked position, has been advocated by Maigne.[153] A critical evaluation of manipulation is that it is often applied in a *total* manner without specifically designating which precise functional unit that allegedly needs to be *unlocked*. The long-arm technique is gross rotary motion of the entire lumbosacral spine and

Figure 5–48. Concept of manipulation. A joint has an active range of motion that can passively be physiologically exceeded. When that range is reached, a firm but gentle thrust achieves the desired *joint play* that restores motion that frequently is lost.

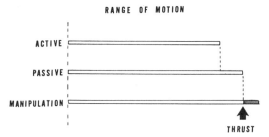

the short-arm technique is aimed at a precise segment but how this locale is to be determined remains moot.

The stated goal of manipulation is to regain mobility but it has also been advocated as improving the "stability" of a joint by realignment to its physiologic position. **Clinical instability** is defined as the "loss of the ability of the spine under physiologic loads to maintain relationships between vertebrae in such a way that there is either damage or subsequent irritation to the spinal cord or nerve roots . . . and development of incapacitating deformity or pain from structural changes."[154]

How the instability of a spinal segment is to be clinically determined has neither a clear nor a valid definition. Even radiologic studies fail to ascertain this instability. The role of muscles in clinical stability also remains obscure.

Hesitations about the modality of manipulation derive from its unproven basis and that it is a passive therapy with no patient assistance. Long-range benefits (outcomes assessment) need confirmation. Its immediate benefit has been claimed and this cannot be disproved, albeit by subjective findings. The prolonged repeated application of adjustments with recurrence of the pain and disability is to be deplored and avoided.

The Rand group[149] agreed that review of the literature specified uneven quality of assessment of spinal manipulation with the following statement:

> "While many studies are randomized controlled trials, there is a great diversity in the initial selection and evaluation of patients for study, assignment of these patients to spinal manipulation or control treatment, the type of manipulation given, and the method of assessing a response. Given that caveat, support is consistent for the use of spinal manipulation as a treatment for patients with acute low-back pain and absence of other signs or symptoms of lower limb nerve root involvement. Support is less clear for other indications, with the evidence for some insufficient, while the evidence for others is conflicting."

Consensus standards of quality chiropractic care, and thus including the validity of manipulations as a specific modality, including treatment frequency, treatment duration, maintainance care, relevance of radiologic studies invoked by the chiropractic profession, and outcomes assessment remain unconfirmed, but currently are being studied.

SPINAL STENOSIS

Lumbar spine stenosis has been defined as a condition involving any type of narrowing of the spinal canal, nerve root canals, or tunnels of intervertebral foramina.[155] The narrowing not only reduces the anteroposterior and lateral diameters but also alters the cross-sectional configuration of the spinal canal. The precise determination of what constitutes stenosis relies exclusively on radiologic measurement, cadaver dissections, or observations during surgery.

The condition termed **spinal stenosis** was initially described by Verbiest in 1954,[156] and was divided into absolute stenosis of the lumbar spine (ASLC) and relative stenosis of the lumbar spine (RSLC). The definition of narrow canals varied with the examiner with the predominent rating being canal to body: anteroposterior diameter (A-PD).[157] An A-PD narrower than 10 mm was considered pathologic,[161] although numerous other authors have given varying numbers with 12 mm being the most consistent among them.

The normal lumbosacral canal is narrowest in its A-PD at the third and fourth lumbar vertebra and its size increases caudally. At L5-S1 the shape of the canal is trefoil. The measurement of the canal is purely an indication of potential for the development of symptoms and does not reveal the site of the stenotic symptoms.[159]

The dorsolateral wall of the spinal canal is formed by the L-5 lamina and superior facet of the sacrum, whereas the ventrolateral wall is the superior facet of the sacrum and the inferior facet of the fifth lumbar vertebra that forms the entrance of the root canal (foramen) (Fig. 5–49).

Spinal stenosis can be considered as either congenital or developmental; the latter is further subdivided as idiopathic or achondroplastic. Acquired stenosis is further subdivided into degenerative (central, peripheral, or spondylolisthesis), iatrogenic (postlaminectomy, postfusion, postchemonucle-

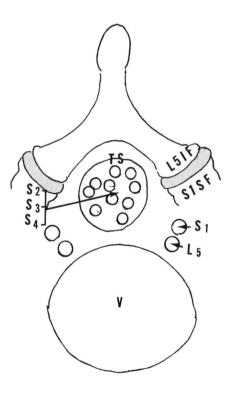

Figure 5–49. Spinal canal contents. The posterior wall of the canal comprises the lamina, which form the facets. At the L5-S1 joints the L-5 inferior facet (L5IF) articulates with the superior facets of the sacrum (S1SF). The thecal septum (TS) encloses the S-2, S-3, and S-4 nerve roots and the L-5 and S-1 roots pass within the foramen between the facets and the vertebral body (V).

olysis), post-traumatic or secondary to systemic disease such as Paget's disease.[160] Narrowing is also considered as secondary to disk herniation.

Narrowing can occur in one or several locations of the same vertebral segment or can affect several segments with similar changes. The size of the canal can be decreased by soft tissue changes or bony changes such as hypertrophy of the facets by posterior bulging of the disk, or by hypertrophic degenerative spurs of the vertebrae such as occur secondary to structural scoliosis.

Reduced space of the lumbosacral canal or dural space does not necessarily produce neurogenic syndrome. Only if the nerve roots are excessively stretched by the stenosing material is the neurogenic syndrome present.

Symptoms of spinal stenosis have been attributed to postural problems with aggravation occurring from extension and relief from flexion. A catheter transducer connected to an amplifier and a recorder has been inserted into[161] the epidural space and patients were placed into hyperextension for a time then moved into a flexed posture.[164] Those in extension showed significant elevation of epidural pressure compared with those in flexion. This did not explain the mechanism by which radiculopathy occurs.

The vascular arrangements of the nerve roots are highly vulnerable to compression or traction. The veins consist of complicated sinusoidal channels.[162] Exercise of a limb has been shown to dilate the blood vessels of the emergent nerve roots within the foramenal canals.[163]

Apparently, then, it is not only the mechanical stenosis that produces symptoms, but also the spinal movement. The clinical condition considered as a sequelae of spinal stenosis (ASLC or RSLC) was termed **neurogenic claudication** because of compression of the nerves of the cauda equina.[159,160] The symptoms of neurogenic claudication given included pain, paresthesias, or impairment of sensory or motor power noted in the leg(s) on walking or standing. Back pain often exists with leg pains occurring later. Back symptoms are stiffness upon awakening, lessening with activity but aggravated by prolonged standing and walking. Sleeping postures are impugned with discomfort in the prone position and relief being gotten in assuming the fetal position.

What classically designates the condition is the syndrome termed **pseudoclaudication**. Walking or leg exercises give symptoms of vascular claudication in that the symptoms occur and increase with exercise and intensify during prolonged exercise. Unlike in a truly vascular condition, hence the prefix "pseudo," is that the pain does not cease from merely stopping exercise as occurs in vascular claudication but ceases or diminishes in stopping *AND* assuming a flexed posture of the lumbosacral spine. Lower extremity pulses are also not diminished as in vascular condition.

Neurologic findings are sparse so pseudoclaudication remains a subjective diagnosis alluded to as being spinal stenosis *IF* radiologic findings demonstrate measurable stenosis.

Conservative treatment seeks to achieve a flexed lumbosacral spine, that is, to decrease the lumbar lordosis including trunk flexion exercises and to avoid extension exercises. A corset or brace may be of value. Surgical decompression is indicated when conservative measures fail and neurologic deficit increases.

SPONDYLOLYSIS
AND SPONDYLOLISTHESIS

The terms **spondylo** relates to spine and **lysis** means dissolution and **listhesis** from the Greek *olisthesis*, means slipping or falling. This lesion is often found incidentally in radiologic studies without clinical significance.

Spondylolisthesis indicates a forward or backward translation of the body of a superior vertebra upon its immediate adjacent inferior vertebra (Fig. 5–50).

There are five types of spondylolisthesis:

- *Type I (isthmic):* There is an anatomic defect in the pars interarticularis. It is seen usually in adolescents and considered to be the result of trauma causing a fatigue fracture. The fracture usually heals with fibrous tissue and becomes stable.[164]
- *Type II (congenital):* The posterior elements are structurally inadequate because of developmental causes.
- *Type III (degenerative):* The facets and their ligamentous supporting structures have become deficient from various causes.

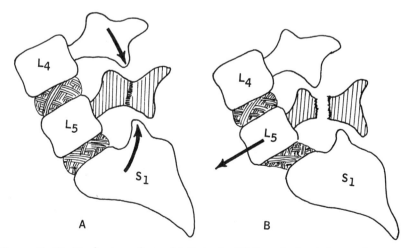

Figure 5–50. Mechanism of spondylolisthesis. (A) Reveals the defect in the pars interarticularis (*shaded area*) but no listhesis. (B) A fracture occurs with separation of the pars and (*straight arrow*) forward listhesis of L-5. The curved arrows in (A) are considered to be the basis of fracture from severe extension (*curved arrows*).

- *Type IV (elongated pedicles):* The neural arch is elongated placing the facets more posteriorly. This is essentially a variant of the isthmic type.
- *Type V (destructive disease):* This is a secondary manifestation of a metabolic, metastatic, or infectious disease. Any systemic bone pathology can be involved.

Spondylolisthesis type I at L5-S1 spinal space usually does not progress between age 20 and age 70 but listheses above it have a higher incidence of neurologic signs, tend to progress, and may often lead to spinal stenosis.

Symptoms

The major symptom of spondylolisthesis is low back pain. Examination reveals signs of limited flexibility and a "ledge" may be palpated at the upper aspect of the listhesis. There may be a segmental lordosis which when aggravated by the examiner causes or increases the pain. On rectal examination the prominent sacrum may be palpated as a "mass." Limited hamstring extensibility is often associated with spondylolisthesis. Radiologic signs are well documented.

Treatment

Treatment depends upon the severity of symptoms and the resultant impairment, disability, and confirmation that the spondylolisthesis is the major cause of the symptoms. Lordosis must be decreased using a brace, corset, or cast if indicated (Fig. 5–51). Exercises to decrease the lordosis and strengthen the muscles involved must be instituted. Ergonomics at home or in the workplace must be modified.

Surgical intervention is indicated usually by presence and progression of neurologic symptoms and conceivably, when a cast benefits the patient subjectively enough to relieve the pain.

PIRIFORMIS SYNDROME

Low back pain with sciatic radiation may be caused by entrapment of the sciatic nerve as it emerges from under the piriformis muscle (Fig. 5–52).

Symptoms include those of a sciatic radiculopathy with the exception that on examination, the SLR test reproduces the referred pain by simultaneous external rotation of the leg which when performed actively by the patient tenses the piriformis muscle. Deep palpation throughout the gluteus maximus or during a pelvic or rectal examination reveals a tender piriformis and nerve.

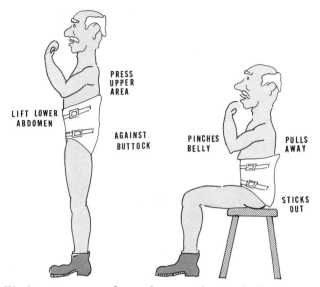

Figure 5–51. Corsetting in standing and sitting. The upright bracing presses against the buttocks and the lower thorax with uplift of the abdomen. This ensures a decrease of the lordosis. The brace in the seated position often fails as the contact points are lost and the anterior portion wrinkles and pinches the abdomen.

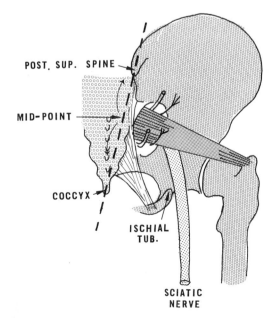

Figure 5–52. Piriformis muscle. The piriformis muscle and its anatomic relationship to the sciatic nerve is shown.

Treatment requires a direct local injection into the piriformis muscle through the vagina or through the gluteus maximus. The nerve must be kept from direct injection which requires that the injection be done with the patient awake. Surgical resection of the piriformis muscle insertion may be required after an injection fails to afford permanent relief.

REFERENCES

1. Spitzer, WO, LeBlanc, FE, Dupuis, M, et al: Scientific approach to the assessment and management of activity related spinal disorders: A monograph for clinicians. Report of the Quebec Task Force on Spinal Disorders. Spine 12:51–59, 1987.
2. Cutler, RB, Fishbain, DA, Rosomoff, HL, et al: Does nonsurgical pain center treatment of chronic pain return patients to work. Spine 19:643–652, 1994.
3. Mitchell, RI and Carmen, GM: The functional restoration approach to the treatment of chronic pain in patients with soft tissue and back injuries. Spine 19:633–642, 1994.
4. Cailliet, R: Low Back Pain Syndromes, ed 4. FA Davis, Philadelphia, 1988.
5. Waddell, G: A new clinical model for the treatment of low-back pain. Spine 12:632–644, 1987.
6. IASP Subcommittee on Toxonomy. Pain terms: A list with definitions and notes on usage. Pain 6:249–252, 1979.
7. Kelsey, KL, Githens, PB, and White, AA, III: An epidemiological study of lifting and twisting on the job and risk for acute prolapsed lumbar intervertebral disc. J Orthop Res 2:61–66, 1984.
8. Andersson, GB: Epidemiologic aspects of low back pain in industry. Spine 6:53–60, 1981.
9. Putz-Anderson, V: Cumulative Trauma Disorders: A Manual for Musculoskeletal Diseases of the Upper Limbs. Taylor & Francis, New York, 1988.
10. Spratt, KF, Lehmann, TR, Weinstein, JW, et al: A new approach to low-back examination: Behavioral assessment of mechanical signs. Spine 15:96–102, 1990.
11. Nachemson, A: Advances in low-back pain. Clin Orthop 200:266–278, 1985.
12. Spitzer, WO, LeBlanc, FE, Dupuis, M, et al: Scientific approach to the assessment and management of activity-related spinal disorders. A monographs for clinicians. Report of the Quebec Task Force on Spinal Disorders. Spine 12:S1–S59, 1987.
13. Tollison, CD and Kriegel, ML: Physical exercise in the treatment of low back pain. Parts I, II, and III. Orthop Rev 17:724,913,1002, 1988.
14. Sullivan, MS, Dickinson, CE and Troup, JDG: The influence of age and gender on lumbar spine sagittal plane range of motion. A study of 1126 healthy subjects. Spine 19:682–686, 1994.
15. Mense, S: Referral of Muscle Pain: New aspects. American Pain Society Journal 3:1–9, 1994.
16. Ruch, TC: Visceral sensation and referred pain. In Howell, WH, Fulton, JF (eds) with collaboration of Barron, DH: Howell's Textbook of Physiology, ed 16. WB Saunders, Philadelphia, 1949, pp 385–401.
17. Yunus, MB: Psychological factors in fibromyalgia syndrome: An overview. J Musculoskeletal Pain 2:87–91, 1994.
18. Kinney, RK, Gatchel, RJ, Polatin, PB, et al: Prevalence of psychopathology in acute and chronic low back pain patients. J Occupational Rehabil 3:95–103, 1993.
19. American Psychiatric Association. Diagnostic and Statistical Manual of Mental Disorders, ed 3, rev. American Psychiatric Association, Washington, 1987.
20. Cailliet, R: Low Back Pain Syndromes, ed 5., FA Davis, Philadelphia, 1995.

21. McDevitt, C: Proteoglycans of the intervertebral disc. In Ghosh, P (ed): The Biology of the Intervertebral Disc, vol I. CRC Press, Boca Raton, 1988, pp 151–170.

22. Adams, MA, Hutton, WC: Has the lumbar spine a margin of safety in forward bending? Clin Biomech, 1:3–6, 1986.

23. Adams, MA, Dolan, P: A technique for quantifying the bending moment acting on the lumbar spine in vivo. J Biomech 24:117–126, 1991.

24. Nachemson, A: The future of low back pain research. In New Perspectives on Low Back Pain. American Academy of Orthopedic Surgeons, Park Ridge, Ill, 1989, p 383.

25. Pederson, HE, Blunck, CFJ, and Gardner, E: The anatomy of lumbosacral posterior rami and meningeal branches of spinal nerves (sinu-vertebral nerves) J Bone Joint Surg 38A:377–391, 1956.

26. El-Bohy, A, Cavanaugh, JM, Getchell, ML, et al: Localization of substance P and neurofilament immunoreactive fibers in the lumbar facet joint capsule and supraspinous ligament of the rabbit. Brain Res 460:379–382, 1988.

27. Gronblad, M, Korkala, O, Konttinen, YT, et al: Silver impregnation and immunohistochemical study of nerves in lumbar facet joint plical tissue. Spine 16:34–38, 1991.

28. Groen, GJ, Baljet, B, and Drukker, J: Nerves and nerve plexuses of the human vertebral column. Am J Anat 188:282–296, 1990.

29. Korkala, O, Gronblad, M, Liesi, P, and Karaharju, E: Immunohistochemical demonstration of nociceptors in the ligamentous structures of the lumbar spine. Spine 10:156–157, 1985.

30. Coppes, MH, Marani, E, Thomeer, RTWM, et al: Innervation of annulus fibrosis in low back pain. Lancet 336:189–190, 1990.

31. Bogduk, N, Tynan, W, and Wilson, AS: The nerve supply to the human intervertebral discs. J Anat 132:39–56, 132.

32. Bogduk, N, Wilson, AS, and Tynan, W: The human dorsal rami. J Anat 134:383–397, 1982.

33. Auteroche, P: Innervation of the zygapophyseal joints of the lumbar spine. Anat Clin 5:17–28, 1983.

34. Groen, GJ: Contributions to the Anatomy of the Peripheral Nervous System. Unpublished Thesis, University of Amsterdam, 1986.

35. Groen, GJ, Baljet, B, Boekelaar, AB, and Drukker, J: Branches of thoracic sympathetic trunk in the human fetus. Anat Embryol 176:401–411, 1987.

36. Jackson, RP, Jacobs, RR, and Montesano, PX: Facet joint injection in low back pain. Pain 13:966–971, 1988.

37. Stolker, RJ, Vervest, ACM, and Groen, GJ: The management of chronic spinal pain by blockades: a review. Pain 58:1–20, 1994.

38. Marras, WS, Sudhaker, LR, and Lavander, SA: Three-dimensional measures of trunk motion components during manual materials handling in industry. In Proceedings of the Human Factor's Society 33rd Annual Meeting. Human Factors Society, Santa Monica, 1989, pp 662–666.

39. Garg, A and Badger, D: Maximum acceptable weights and maximal volunteer isometric strengths for asymmetrical lifting. Ergonomics 29:879–892, 1986.

40. Marras, WS, King, RA and Joynt, RL: Measurements of loads on the lumbar spine under isometric and isokinetic conditions. Spine 9:176–188, 1984.

41. Marras, WS, Joynt, RL, and King, AI: The force-velocity relation and intra-abdominal pressure during lifting activities. Ergonomics 28:603–613, 1984.

42. Reid, JG and Costigan, PA: Trunk muscle balance and muscular force. Spine 12:783–786, 1987.

43. Troup, JDG and Edwards, FC: Manual handling and lifting. Her Majesty's Stationery Office, London, 1985.

44. Chaffin, DB and Baker, WH: A biomechanical model for analysis of symmetrical sagittal plane lifting. AIIE Transact 2:16–27, 1970.

45. Marras, WS and Mirka, GA: Muscle activities during asymmetric trunk angulation accelerations. J Ortho Res 8:824–832, 1990.

46. Marras, WS: Toward an Understanding of Dynamic Variables. In (ed): Ergonomics. Occupational Medicine: State of the Art Reviews. Hanley & Belfus, Philadelphia, 1992, p 4.
47. Marras, WS and Wongsam, PE: Flexibility and velocity of the normal and impaired lumbar spine. Arch Phys Med Rehabil 67:213–217, 1986.
48. Nachemson, AL: Advances in low back pain. Clin Orthop 200:266–278, 1985.
49. Mirka, GA and Marras, WS: A stochastic model of trunk muscle coactivation during trunk bending. Spine 18:1396–1409, 1993.
50. Keyserling, W, Punnett, L, and Fine, L: Trunk posture and back pain: Identification and control of occupational risk factors. Appl Ind Hyg 3:87–92, 1988.
51. Marras, WS, Lavender, S, Leurgans, S, et al: The role of dynamic three dimensional trunk motion in occupationally related low back disorders: The effects of workplace factors, trunk position and trunk motion characteristics on risk of injury. Spine 18:617–628, 1993.
52. Gunzburg, R, Hutton, W, and Fraser, R: Axial rotation of the lumbar spine and the effects of flexion: An in vitro and in vivo biomechanical study. Spine 16:22–28, 1991.
53. Pearcy, M and Tibrewal, S: Axial rotation and lateral bending in the normal lumbar spine measured by three dimensional radiography. Spine 9:582–587, 1984.
54. Lui, Y, Goel, V, Dejong, A, et al: Torsional fatigue of the lumbar intervertebral joints. Spine 10:894–900, 1985.
55. Wolf, SL, Basmajian, JV, Russe, CT, and Kutner, M: Normative data on low back mobility and activity levels. Am J Phys Med 58:217–229, 1979.
56. Wolf, SL, Nacht, M, and Kelly, JL: EMG biofeedback training during dynamic movement for low back pain patients. Behav Ther 13:395–406, 1982.
57. Waddell, G, Sommerville, D, Henderson, I, and Newton, M: Objective clinical evaluation of physical impairment in chronic low back pain. Spine 17:617–628, 1992.
58. Waddell, G, Main, CJ, Morris, EW, et al: Chronic low-back pain, psychologic distress, and illness behavior. Spine 9:209–213, 1984.
59. Cooke C, Menard MR, Beach GN, et al: Serial lumbar dynamometry in low back pain. Spine 17:653–662, 1992.
60. Laros, GS: Differential Diagnosis of Low Back Pain. In Mayer, TG, Mooney, V, and Gatchel, RJ (eds): Contemporary Conservative Care of Painful Spinal Disorders. Lea & Febiger, Philadelphia, 1991, pp 122–130.
61. Laros, GS, Ozanne, S, and McCarron, RF: Six categories of low back pain: a prospective study. Submitted [to Spine] 1993.
62. WHO: International classification of impairments, disabilities and handicaps. World Health Organization, Geneva, 1980.
63. AMA: Guides to the evaluation of permanent impairment of the extremities and back. JAMA 166(suppl): 1–122, 1958.
64. Garrad, J and Bennett, AE: A validated interview schedule for use in population surveys of chronic disease and disability. Br J Prev Soc Md 25:97–104, 1971.
65. Waddell, G, Bircher, M, Findlayson, D, and Main, CJ: Symptons and signs: Physical disease or illness behaviour? BMJ 289:739–741, 1984.
66. U.S. Bureau of Disability Insurance: Disability evaluation under social security. A handbook for physicians. U.S. Government Printing Office, Washington, DC, 1970.
67. Inman, VT, Ralston, HJ, and Todd, F: Human Walking. Williams & Wilkins, Baltimore, 1981.
68. Woo, SL and Buckwalter, JA: Injury and Repair of the Musculoskeletal Soft Tissue. American Academy of Orthop Surg, Chicago, 1988, pp 171–207.
69. Jones, DA, Newham, KJ, Obletter, G, and Giamberaridino, MA: Nature of exercise-induced muscle pain. Adv Pain Res Ther 10:207–218, 1987.
70. Bobbert, MF, Hollander, AD, and Huijing, PA: Factors in delayed onset of muscle soreness of man. Med Sci Sports Exercise 18:75–81, 1986.
71. Moldofsky, H, Scaribrick, P, England, R, and Smythe, H: Musculoskeletal symptoms and

non-REM sleep disturbance in patients with "fibrositis syndrome" and healthy patients. Psychosomatic Med 37:341–351, 1975.

72. Badgley, CE: The articular facets in relationship to low back pain and sciatic radiation. J Bone Joint Surg 23A:481–496, 1941.

73. Inman, VT and Saunders, JB: Referred pain from skeletal structures. J Nerv Ment Dis 99:660–667, 1944.

74. Paris, SB: Functional Anatomy of the Lumbar Spine. Doctoral thesis. Union Graduate School, Atlanta, 1983.

75. Cailliet, R: Pain mediated through the sympathetic nervous system. In Cailliet, R: Pain: Mechanisms and Management, ed 1. FA Davis, Philadelphia, 1993.

76. Schwartzer, AC, Derby, R, Aprill, CN, et al: Pain from the lumbar zygapophyseal joints: A test of two models. J Spinal Disord 7:331–336, 1994.

77. Eisenstein, SM and Parry, CR: The lumbar facet arthrosis syndrome—clinical presentation and articular surface changes. J Bone Joint Surg (Br) 69:3–7, 1987.

78. Fairbanks, JCT, Park, WM, McCall, IW, and O'Brien, JP: Apophyseal injection of local anesthetic as a diagnostic aid in primary low-back pain syndromes. Spine 6:598–605, 1981.

79. Helbig, T and Lee, CK: The lumbar facet syndrome. Spine 13:61–64, 1988.

80. Steindler, A and Luck, JV: Differential diagnosis of pain in the low back: Allocation of the source of pain by procaine hydrochloride method. JAMA 110:106–113, 1938.

81. Hirsch, D, Inglemark, B, and Miller, M: The anatomical basis for low back pain. Acta Orthop Scand 33:1–17, 1963.

82. Mooney, V and Robertson, J: The facet syndrome. Clin Orthop 115:149–156, 1976.

83. Maigne, R: Diagnostic et Traitment des Douleurs Communes d'Origine Rachidienne. Expansion Scientifique Francaise, Paris, 1989.

84. Nelson, RM and Nestor, DE: Standardized assessment of industrial low-back injuries: Development of the NIOSH low back atlas. Topics in Acute Care and Trauma Rehabilitation 2:16–30, 1988.

85. NIOSH: National Institute for Occupational Safety and Health Low Back Atlas. U.S. Department of Health and Human Services, Morgantown, West Virginia, 1988.

86. Feldenkrais, M: Body and Mature Behavior: A Study of Anxiety, Gravitation and Learning. International Universities Press, New York, 1949.

87. Lowman, CL: Postural Fitness: Significance and Variances. Lea & Febiger, Philadelphia, 1960.

88. Roaf, R: Posture. Academic Press, New York, 1977.

89. Hansson, T, Bigos, S, Beecher, P, et al: The lumbar lordosis in acute and chronic low-back pain. Spine 10:154–155, 1985.

90. Mayer, TG, Tencer, AT, Kristoferson, S, and Mooney, V: Use of noninvasive techniques for quantification of spinal range of motion in normal subjects and chronic low back dysfunction patients. Spine 9:588–595, 1984.

91. Rae, P, Venner, RM, and Waddell, G: A simple clinical technique of measuring lumbar flexion. J Roy Coll Surg 29:281–284, 1981.

92. Burton, AK: Patterns of lumbar sagittal mobility and their predictive value in natural history of back and sciatic pain. Ph D thesis. The Polytechnic, Huddersfield, England, 1988.

93. Biering-Sorensen, F: Physical measurements as risk indicators for low back trouble over a one-year period. Spine 9:106–119, 1984.

94. Guccione, AA: Physical therapy diagnosis and relationship between impairments and function. Phys Therapy 71:36–41, 1991.

95. Nagi, SZ: Some conceptual issues in disability and rehabilitation. In Sussman, MB (eds): Sociology and Rehabilitation. American Sociology Association, Washington, DC, 1965, pp 100–113.

96. Nagi, SZ: Disability and Rehabilitation. Ohio State University Press, Columbus, 1969.

97. Waddell, G, Sommerville, D, Henderson, I, et al: Pain, disability and fear avoidance beliefs. Pain (submitted for publication).

98. Waddell, G, Main, CJ, Morris, EW, et al: Chronic low back pain, psychological distress and illness behavior. Spine 9:209–213, 1984.

99. Cassell, EJ: The evaluation of disability due primarily to pain. In Fordyce, WE (ed): IASP Task Force on Pain in the Workplace. International Association for the Study of Pain, (in press).

100. McKenzie, R: A Physical Therapy Perspective on Acute Spinal Disorders. In Mayer, TG, Moony, V, and Gatchel, RJ (eds): Contemporary Conservative Care for Painful Spinal Disorders, Lea & Febiger, Philadelphia, 1991, pp 211–220.

101. Forst, JJ: Contribution sur l'etude dexique de la sciatique. Paris, These, no. 33, 1881.

102. DePalma, A and Rothman, RH: The Intervertebral Disc. WB Saunders, Philadelphia, 1970, p 227.

103. van Akkerveeken, RF: On pain patterns of patients with lumbar nerve root entrapment. Neuro-Orthopedics 14:81–102, 1993.

104. Verbiest, H: Chronischer lumbaler vertebragener Schmerz, Pathomechanismus und Diagnose. In Benini, A (ed): Komplikationen und Misserfolge des lumbalen Diskuschirurgie. Huber, Bern, 1989.

105. Verbiest, H: The management of cervical spondylosis. Clin Neurosurg 20:262–294, 1973.

106. Fajersztajn J: Ueber das gekreuzte Ischiasphanomen. Weiner Klin Wochenschr 14:41–47, quoted In Woodhall, B and Hayes, GJ: The Well-Leg Raising Test of Fajersztajn in the Diagnosis of Ruptured Lumbar Intervertebral Disc. J Bone Joint Surg 32A: 786–792, 1950.

107. Keegan, JJ and Garret, FD: The segmental distribution of the cutaneous nerves in the limbs of man. Anat Rec 102:409–437, 1948.

108. Bolk, L: De segmentale innervatie van romp en ledematen bij de mens. Bohn, Haarlem, 1910.

109. Hansen, K and Schliack, H: Segmentale Innervation, ihre Bedeutung in Klinik und Praxis. Thieme, Stuttgart, 1962.

110. Hoppenfeld, S: Physical Examination of the Spine and Extremities. Appleton-Century-Crofts, New York, 1976, pp 258–263.

111. Leavitt, F and Sweet, JJ: Characteristics and frequency of malingering among patients with low back pain. Pain, 25:357–364, 1986.

112. Department of Health and Human Services. Report of the Commission on the Evaluation of Pain and Disability. US Government Printing Office, Washington, DC, 1987.

113. Blair, JA, Blair, RS, and Rueckert, P: Pre-injury emotional trauma and chronic back pain. Spine 19:1144–1147, 1994.

114. Davis, H: Increasing rates of cervical and lumbar spine surgery in the United States 1979–1990. Spine 19:1117–1124, 1994.

115. Webster, BS and Snook, SH: The cost of 1989 Workers' Compensation low back pain claims. Spine 19:1111–1116, 1994.

116. Snook, SH and Webster, BS: The effectiveness of a standardized treatment protocol in reducing disability from low back pain. Arbete och Halsa 17:270–272, 1992.

117. Waddell, G: A new clinical model for the treatment of low back pain. Spine 12:632–644, 1987.

118. Dubner, R and Bennett, GJ: Spinal and trigeminal mechanisms of nociception. Annu Rev Neurosci 6:381, 1983.

119. Lynn, B: The detection of injury and tissue damage. In Wall, PD and Melzack, R (eds): Textbook of Pain. Churchill-Livingstone, New York, 1984, pp 19–33.

120. Lehmann, JD, Brunner, GD, and Stow, RW: Pain threshold measurements after therapeutic application of ultrasound microwaves and infrared. Arch Phys Med Rehabil 39:560, 1958.

121. Currier, DP and Kramer, JF: Sensory nerve conduction: Heating effects of ultrasound and infrared. Physiotherap Can, 34:241, 1982.

122. Guyton, AC: Textbook of Medical Physiology, ed 7. WB Saunders, Philadelphia, 1986.

123. Cailliet, R: Soft Tissue Concepts. In Cailliet, R: Soft Tissue Pain and Disability, ed 2. FA Davis, Philadelphia, pp 3–17.

124. LeBan, MM: Collagen tissue: Implications of its response to stress in vitro. Arch Phys Med Rehabil 43:461, 1962.
125. Kottke, FJ, Pauley, DI, and Ptak, RA: The rationale for prolonged stretching for correction of shortening of connective tissue. Arch Phys Med Rehabil 47:345, 1966.
126. Warren, GC, Lehmann, JF, and Koblanski, JN: Heat and stretch procedures: An evaluation using rat tail tendon. Arch Phys Med Rehabil 57:122, 1976.
127. Bonica, JJ: Management of Pain. Lea & Febiger, Philadelphia, 1953.
128. White, AH: Structural Diagnostic Tests. In Mayer, TG, Mooney, V, and Gatchel, RJ (eds): Contemporary Conservative Care for Painful Spinal Disorders. Lea & Febiger, Philadelphia, 1991, pp 364–379.
129. Goldie, J and Peterhoff, K: Epidural anaesthesia in low back pain and sciatica. Acta Orthop Scand 39:261–269, 1968.
130. Waddell, G: A new clinical model for the treatment of low back pain. Spine 12:632–644, 1987.
131. Nutter, P: Aerobic exercise in the treatment and prevention of low back pain. Spine: State-of-the-Art Reviews 2(1). Hanley & Belfus, Philadelphia, 1987, pp 137–145.
132. Kraus, H, Nagler, W, and Melleby, A: Evaluation of an exercise program for low back pain. Am Fam Physician 28:153–158, 1983.
133. Faas, A, Chavannes, AW, van Eijk, JThM, and Gubbels, JW: A randomized, placebo-controlled trial of exercise therapy in patients with acute low back pain. Spine 18:1388–1395, 1993.
134. Davies, JR, Gibson, T, and Tester, L: The value of exercises in the treatment of low back pain. Rheumatoid Rehabil 18:243–247, 1979.
135. Tollison, CD and Kriegel, ML: Physical exercise in the treatment of low back pain. Part 1: A review. Orthop Rev, pp 18:724–729, 1988.
136. Williams, PC: Lesions of the lumbosacral spine. Part 1. J Bone Joint Surg (Am) 19:343, 1937, and Part II, 19:690, 1937.
137. Headley, BJ: Muscle Inhibition. Physical Therapy Forum, Nov 1993, 24–26, 1993.
138. Grabois, M: Treatment of pain syndromes through exercise. In Lowenthal, DF, Bharadwaja, K, and Oaks, WW (eds) Grune & Stratton, New York, 1979, pp 1281–1287.
139. Cailliet, R: Treatment protocols for low back pain syndrome. In Cailliet, R: Low Back Pain Syndrome, ed 5, FA Davis, Philadelphia, 1995.
140. Marras, WS and Fattalah, F: Accuracy of the three dimensional lumbar motion monitor for recording trunk motion characteristics. International Journal of Industrial Ergonomics 9:75–87, 1992.
141. Waddell, G: Biopsychosocial analysis of low back pain. Baillieres Clin Rheumatol 6:523–557, 1992.
142. Waddell, G, Newton, M, Henderson, I, et al: A fear-avoidance beliefs questionnaire (FABQ) and the role of fear avoidance beliefs in chronic low-back pain and disability. Pain 52:157–168, 1993.
143. Deyo, RA and Voh-Jane, TW: Descriptive epidemiology of low back pain and its related medical care in the USA. Spine 12:264–268, 1987.
144. Coyer, AB and Curwin, I: Low back pain treated by manipulation. Br Med J pp 1:707–709, 1955.
145. Hoehler, FK and Tobis, J: Appropriate statistical methods for clinical trials of spinal manipulation. Spine 12:409–411, 1987.
146. Macdonald, RS, Bell, CM, and Janine, JM: An open controlled assessment of osteopathic manipulation in non-specific low back pain. Spine 44:851–854, 1957.
147. Meade, TW, et al: Comparison of chiropractic and hospital outpatient management of low back pain: A feasibility study. J Epidemiol & Community Health 40:12–17, 1986.
148. Twomey, L and Taylor, J: Spine update: Exercise and spinal manipulation in the treatment of low back pain. Spine 20:615–619, 1995.
149. Haldeman, S: Spinal manipulative therapy: a status report. Clin Orthop 179:62–70, 1983.

150. Stoddard, A: Manipulative procedures in the treatment of intervertebral disc lesions. Br J Phys Med May, 101–106, 1951.
151. Ray, MB: Manipulative treatment. Br J Phys Med 13:241–254, 1950.
152. Parsons, WB and Roake, HK: Manipulation for backache and sciatica. Applied Therapeutics 8:954–961, 1966.
153. Maigne, R: The concept of painless and opposite motion in spinal manipulations. Am J Phys Med 44:55, 1978.
154. Murray, DG (ed): Instructional Course Lectures, Volume XXX, 1981. The American Academy of Orthopedic Surgeons. C.V. Mosby, St Louis, 1981, pp 457–483.
155. Arnoldi, CC, Brodsky, AE, Cauchoix, J, et al: Lumbar spinal stenosis and nerve root entrapment syndromes. Definition and classification. Clin Orthop 115:4–5, 1976.
156. Verbiest, H: Neurogenic intermittent claudication in cases with absolute and relative stenosis of the lumbar vertebral canal (ASLC and RSLC) in cases with narrow lumbar intervertebral foramina and in cases with both entities. Clin Neurosurg 21:204, 1972.
157. Jones, RAC and Thomson, JLG: The narrow lumbar canal. A clinical and radiological review. J Bone Joint Surg 50B:595–605, 1968.
158. Huizinga, J, Heiden, JA, and Vinken, PJ: The human lumbar vertebral canal: a biometric study. Proc Roy Acad Sci (Amsterdam) C55:22–33, 1952.
159. Naylor, A: Factors in the development of the spinal stenosis syndrome. J Bone Joint Surg 61B:306–309, 1979.
160. Grabois, S: The treatment of spinal stenosis: Current concepts review. J Bone Joint Surg 62A:308–313, 1980.
161. Keisuke, T, et al: Epidural Pressure and Posture. (Letter) Spine 1:4, 1994.
162. Dommisse, GF: The blood supply of the spinal cord. J Bone Joint Surg 56B:225–235, 1974.
163. Blau, NJ and Ruswort, G: Observations on the blood vessels of the spinal cord and their responses to motor activity. Brain 81:3544–3563, 1958.
164. Mooney, V: Surgical Decision Making: A System Based on Classification and Symptom Chronology. Mayer, TG, Mooney, V, and Gatchel, RJ (eds.): Contemporary Conservative Care for Painful Spinal Disorders. Lea & Febiger, Philadelphia, 1991.

CHAPTER 6
Neck and Upper Back Pain

Pain and subsequent dysfunction issuing from around the neck is seen by clinicians second only to pain and impairment from the low back. Cervical spine pain and impairment involves pain occurring *in* or *from* the neck. The origin of pain associated with tissues of the cervical functional units, along with the functional anatomy of that vertebral segment has been documented.[1,2]

The cervical spine is composed of two major vertebral segments: the upper and lower cervical, each with different functional anatomic structures and different symptoms indicating impairment.

UPPER CERVICAL COMPLEX

Relevant anatomy of the upper cervical spinal complex requires total ligamentous integrity because no bony articular buttressing of the occipito-atlas (O-C1) and atlas-axis (C1-C2) joints exists.[3,4] The atlantoaxial (C1-C2) joint is the most mobile part of the vertebral column and is located between the most immobile joints superiorly (atlantooccipital) (AO) and inferiorly (axis C2-C3).[5]

Of all cervical rotation 50% occurs at the atlantoaxial joint with a concomitant lateral shift of the atlas, whereas 10° to 20° flexion and 25° extension of the occiput occurs at the atlas (Fig. 6–1). Only 10° flexion and 5° extension occurs at the atlantoaxial joint.

Rotation occurs at this joint through activity of the ligamentous encasement of the odontoid process (Figs. 6–2 and 6–3.[6] The transverse ligament (Fig. 6–4) is the largest and strongest of all atlantoaxial ligaments, with a thickness of 7 to 8 mm.[7] The transverse ligament arises from the medial aspects of the lateral masses of the atlas (C1) and passes horizontally behind the odontoid process. A small cruciate ligament ascends from the midportion of

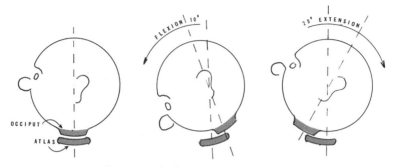

Figure 6–1. Motion at the occipital-atlas joint. Motion at the occipital-atlas joint is essentially flexion-extension with little or no rotation or lateral flexion. The 10 to 20° of flexion and 25° of extension from the midline usually totals 35 to 40° of motion.

the transverse ligament to attach to the occiput and an ascending band that attaches to the body of the axis (see Fig. 6–4) as a *cross* ligament.

Ascending from the superior tip of the odontoid process (dens) are the alar ligaments (see Fig. 6–2), which, strong and rounded, attach to the occipital condyles. They permit axial rotation and limit lateral motion.[8] The alar ligaments cannot prevent dislocation if the transverse ligament is severed. The remaining ligaments (Fig. 6–5) contribute little to the stability of the upper cervical complex.[7]

The upper cervical complex can be delineated radiologically to measure its ligamentous stability using radiographs taken during performance of stress tests.[9,10]

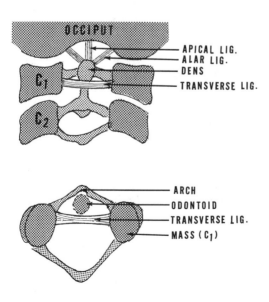

Figure 6–2. Occipital-atlas-axis ligaments. The transverse ligament encloses the odontoid (pons) against a small indenture in the posterior aspect of the arch-permitting rotation. The apical and alar ligaments also stabilize the dens and restrict translatory and rotatory motion.

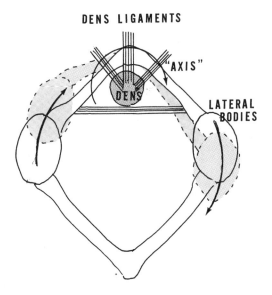

DENS LIGAMENTS

Figure 6–3. Rotational motion of the atlas on the axis. A rotation of approximately 45° to both sides is allowed by translation of the lateral bodies, supported by the transverse ligament (not labeled), and limited by the ligaments attached to the dens, which is the axis of rotation.

Symptoms originating from the upper cervical complex have not been so readily accepted as symptoms from the lower cervical complex have because neuroanatomic structures have only recently been clarified.

Occipital Neuralgia

The first reference to neuralgia of the occiput was in 1821.[11] Initially, it was thought to result from irritation of the nerve at the point of emergence through the upper insertional area of the trapezius muscle, and thus was considered a sequela of fibromyalgia. Deep-lying lesions of the occipitocervical re-

Figure 6–4. Transverse (cross) ligament. Attached from the medial aspects of the bodies of the atlas (C1), the transverse ligament crosses the spinal canal and forms the support of the odontoid (dens) process of the axis (C2). Arising from the superior aspect of this ligament, the vertical ligament ascends and attaches to the foramen magnum and a ligamentous prolongation that descends to attach to the axis (C2). These are **cross ligaments.**

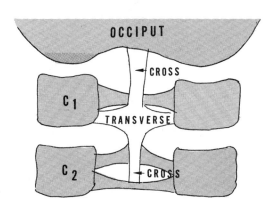

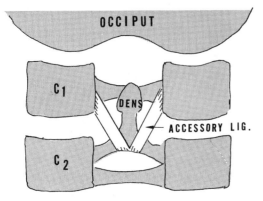

Figure 6–5. Accessory atlanto-axial ligaments. Two ligaments attach from the medial aspects of the bodies of their atlas (C1) and descend to converge and attach on the body of the axis (C2) anterior to the odontoid (dens) process.

gion such as Arnold-Chiari syndrome,[12] primary and metastatic tumors, and certain metabolic disorders such as diabetes have been associated. A cause too often ignored has been occipital neuralgia caused by unilateral C1-C2 arthrosis.[13]

Pain syndromes from vertebral structures have been attributed to irritation of nerve roots; and, in the upper cervical complex, to the cervical dorsal rami of the C2 root (Figs. 6–6 and 6–7).[14] The dermatomal and motomal branches from the upper cervical complex are the C2 and C3 branches.

The C2 and C-3 medial branches run deep to and supply the semispinalis muscle (Fig. 6–8). The greater superior occipital nerve runs transversely and turns abruptly at a right angle bend to ascend rostrally (Fig. 6–9). The greater occipital nerve was previously described as entering the scalp by piercing the trapezius muscle. It is now known, however, that the nerve emerges through an aperture above an aponeurotic sling between the trapezius and the sternocleidomastoid muscle.[15]

Occipital neuralgia is not a disease in the same sense as trigeminal neuralgia[15,16] but it has numerous possible causes. Besides direct nerve compression along its course, a theory evolved that vascular involvement in the upper cervical area causes a sympathetic disorder with leakage of serotonin that initiates the neuralgia,[17,18] due to its proximity to the vertebral artery (Figs. 6–10 and 6–11).

Greater occipital neuralgia is now not considered to be compression between the posterior arch of the atlas and the lamina of the axis nor from compression by the trapezius muscle spasm. Headache from lower cervical spinal lesions has also been proposed,[19–21] but that the pain of occipital neuralgia emanating from articulation of the atlas-axis (C1-C2) is becoming more accepted.

The neuralgia is probably associated with the direct relation the C2 nerve root has with the lateral atlantoaxial joints from which it emerges through soft tissues lying dorsal to the C2 lamina.

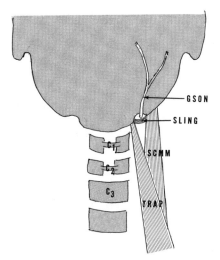

Figure 6–6. Emergence of the greater superior occipital nerve. The greater superior occipital nerve (GSON), primarily the C2 nerve root, emerges in a groove medial to the mastoid process of the occiput. It leaves in an opening between the insertions of the trapezius muscle (TRAP) and the sternocleidomastoid muscle (SCMM). A small fascial sling completes the opening. In some cases the nerve emerges through the trapezius muscle.

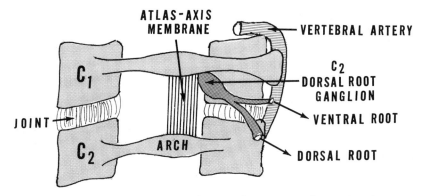

Figure 6–7. Greater superior occipital nerve: the C2 root. The C2 dorsal root ganglion lies under the obliquus inferior muscle (not shown) over the lateral atlantoaxial joint being adherent to the capsule. It emerges lateral to the posterior atlas-axial membrane but does not penetrate it. It proceeds laterally to divide into a dorsal and ventral root.

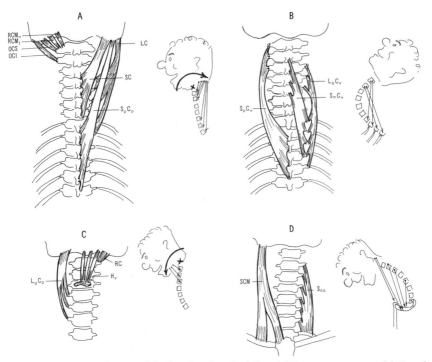

Figure 6–8. Musculature of the head and neck. (*A*) and (*B*) are extensors and (*C*) and (*D*) are flexors. The capital muscles flex and extend the head on the cervical spine and the cervical muscles flex the neck and alter its physiologic curvature. RCM_n = rectus capitis minor; RCM_j = rectus capitis major; OCS = obliquus capitis superior; OCI = obliquus capitis inferior; L_gC_p = longus capitis; RC = rectus capitis anterior; and lateral; H_y = hyoideus and suprahyoid; LC = longissmus capitis; SC = semispinalis capitis; S_pC_v = splenius capitis; L_gC_v = longissmus cervicis; S_mC_v = semispinalis cervicis; SCM = sternocleidomastoid; S_{ca} = scalene medius and anticus.

Cervical neuralgia is therefore not an unexpected result of cervical hyper-extension-hyperflexion injuries especially with a *rotatory component*. The transverse and alar ligaments consist of collagen fibers with few elastic fibers. In the central portion of the transverse ligament, the collagen fibers cross over at a 30° angle, making them susceptible to irreversible damage from external injury. In review of 427 injured spines,[22] most had evidence of ligamentous injury. One result of this ligamentous injury is instability of the upper cervical segment.

Headache as a sequela of upper cervical neuralgia has been propounded. Blockade of the C2 nerve has been of benefit in many post-traumatic headache patients.[23] The C2 cord segment has input from the C1-C2 articulation, and from the periosteum of these two vertebrae as well as their ligaments. The C1 root is not devoid of dorsal root fibers,[24] thus it may

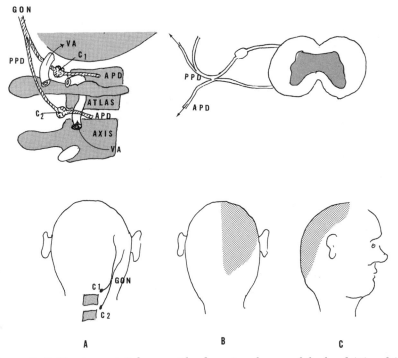

Figure 6–9. Greater occipital nerve. The dermatomal areas of the head (*B*) and (*C*) are subserved by the greater occipital nerve (GON) (*A*). The course of the posterior primary divisions (PPD) of nerve roots C1 and C2 merge to form the greater occipital nerve. Note the relationship to the vertebral artery (VA). The anterior primary divisions (APD) of these roots is shown.

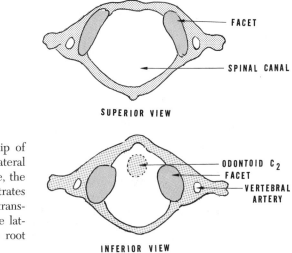

Figure 6–10. Relationship of vertebral artery to the lateral bodies. Viewed from above, the vertebral artery penetrates through a foramen in the transverse process lateral to the lateral body. The C2 nerve root passes close by.

A   B

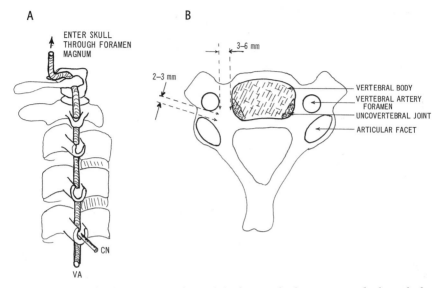

Figure 6–11. Vertebral artery pathway. (*A*) The vertebral artery ascends through the vertebral foramena to angulate at the atlas occipital segment. (*B*) In the lower cervical segments it passes close to the zygapophyseal joints and uncovertebral joints. The distances are marked.

transmit pain from these and from the unmyelinated fibers in the anterior root.

The facet joint between C2-C3 is a transitional zone between the superior zone of rotation and the inferior zone of flexion-extension (Fig. 6–12). It is innervated by the C3 as well as the C2 nerve. Headaches may also arise from lesions of lower cervical segments,[25,26] allegedly from the relationship between the trigeminal nucleus and the ascending fibers of the C1 and C2 levels.

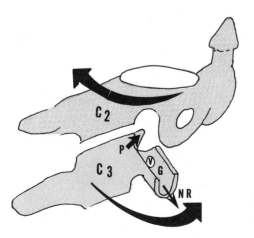

Figure 6–12. Mechanical locking of rotation of C2 on C3. Rotation of C2 on C3 vertebra is mechanically locked by impingement of the facet (F) of C3 on the lateral margin of the foramen of the vertebral artery (V). The C3 nerve root emerges through the gutter (G).

Blockade of the greater superior occipital nerve (GON) is usually effective in relieving headaches of cervical origin because the GON has mostly C2 fibers, whereas blockades of C3, C4, and C5 nerve roots have been ineffectual.[23]

Evaluation of a patient who remains symptomatic with cervical insult after extensive conservative treatment remains difficult. Torn ligaments of the cervical spine usually do not heal spontaneously,[26] but abnormal movement, established by cineradiograms,[27] usually implies ligamentous instability.

Muscular Component of Cervical Pathology

Over a century ago, disruption of the neck muscle was discovered to cause gait disorder.[28] It was rediscovered by Magendie and described by Claude Bernard,[29] when research to determine the cause of ataxia resulting from an incision into the dura to release cerebrospinal fluid was found to cause ataxia after incision of only the cervical muscles.

Neck Muscle Proprioception and Motor Control

Neck muscles have been known to play an important role in control of posture and locomotion. The syndrome came to be known as *cervical nystagmus* or *cervical vertigo*.[30] It often appeared after traumatic injury and even when untreated frequently resolves.[31] Symptoms resemble damage to the vestibular system yet show no clinical evidence of vestibular pathology because many, if not most, patients do not exhibit nystagmus. Unsteady gait may be relieved by local injection of an anesthetic agent into the neck musculature leaving the nystagmus (when present) unchanged.[32]

Vertigo and ataxia are frequently present after an acute cervical sprain from a hyperflexion-hyperextension (*whiplash*) injury,[33] yet remains unrecognized. The mechanism of cervical ataxia remains obscure, yet the research discussed in voluminous articles by Abraham[34] are beginning to shed light. The neck muscle receptors are significantly involved in posture.

In 1897, Sherrington[35] reported that stimulation of the small branches of C2 nerve root caused a profound inhibition of the neck muscles in their role of head support. Postural reflexes were found by Magnus in 1926 to be influenced by C1, C2, and C3 roots to the head muscles.[36] Further studies have provoked experimental ataxia from anesthesia of the upper cervical roots.[37]

The ataxia present appears to result from damage to the more superficial tissues of the neck rather than deeper structures,[38] such as the facet's articulations.

The muscle spindles of the cervical spine appear to be the basis of ataxia when injured[39] but further work remains for confirmation. The presence of ataxia following cervical spine injury demands that a complete neurologic examination be performed, to determine the presence of nystagmus and ataxia and increased symptoms from cervical manipulation. Injection of an anesthetic agent into the tender muscles may also provide confirmation when it produces a diminution or disappearance of the ataxia. The efficacy of wearing a cervical collar following an injury may be explained by this concept as lessening the aggravation of symptoms from excessive cervical movement.

The decerebrate cat was found to have postural reflexes from sensory structures in the neck. These reflexes were postulated to originate in the spindle system (Figs. 6–13 to 6–15) and in the neck muscles in close proximity to the intravertebral joints.[40] Spindle systems perform various functions not yet completely understood, but they undoubtedly contribute to position and joint relationship. Their density varies throughout the body—the high density in small hand muscles is present in order to execute precise fine movements. They are also found in high density in the splenius muscles of the neck exten-

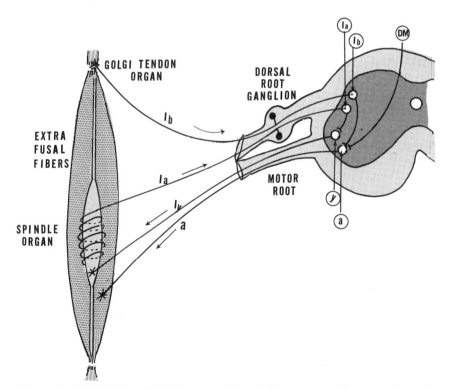

Figure 6–13. Spindle and Golgi systems. The spindle system supplies sensation to the cord through Ia fibers: the Golgi organs through Ib fibers. They end in the gray matter at cells Ia and Ib. The motor fibers to the spindle system are through I gamma fibers. These impulses *reset* the spindle system. The extrafusal fibers are innervated from the anterior horn cells (a) through alpha fibers. Within the cord gray matter are numerous intercommunicating fibers. The upper cortical control is shown as DM.

B   A   C

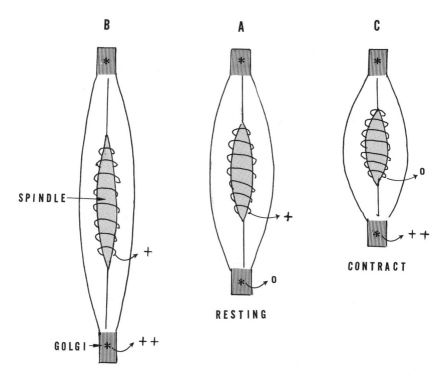

Figure 6–14. Spindle system coordination of muscle length. The length, rate of contraction, and tension created in the muscle is coordinated by the spindle system. (*A*) depicts a resting muscle, which, by its intrinsic elongation, activates the spindle system. (*B*) shows activity engendered in the Golgi organ by passive stretch with no spindle activity. In the actively contracting muscle (*C*), the spindle system is relaxed and the Golgi tendon strongly activated. The spindle and Golgi systems coordinate muscular action. (From Cailliet, R: Neck and Arm Pain, ed 3. FA Davis, Philadelphia, 1991, p 65, with permission.)

sors, which are small intrinsic muscles probably related to the functions of rotation and lateral flexion.

It stands to reason that trauma to the neck can cause a resultant dysfunction of the neck, impairment of posture, and even some ataxia.

Examination of the Upper Cervical Complex

When a patient presents with a history of external trauma invoking abnormal cervical motion, the precise details of the force must be ascertained. The direction of the head at the time of impact is important and so is the aware-

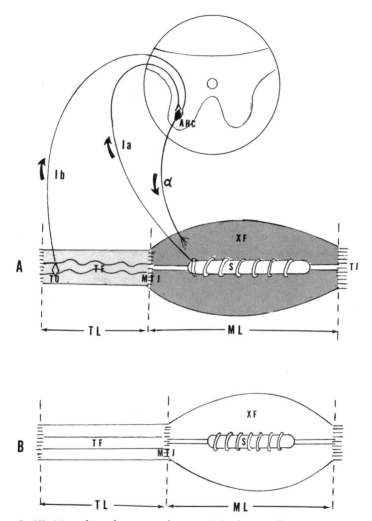

Figure 6–15. Musculotendinous mechanism. (A) The spindle system (S) measures the length of the muscle (ML) and the tendon organs (Golgi) (TO) monitor the tension. Stretching of the spindle system activates the Ia fiber, whereas stretching the tendon organs activates the IB fibers. These influence the anterior horn cell (AHC), which sends motor fiber activity through the alpha fibers to the extrafusal fibers (XF). With the muscle at resting level (A) the tendon fibers (TF) are slightly coiled. When the extrafusal fibers contract (B) the muscle shortens (ML), the tendon elongates (TL) to the degree that the tendon fibers can elongate. The tendon fibrills (TF) uncoil. Excessive muscle contraction can tear the muscle-tendon juncture (MTJ). (From Cailliet, R: Hand Pain and Impairment, ed 4. FA Davis, Philadelphia, 1994, p 163, with permission.)

ness of the impending impact. The former indicates the pathway in which the head has traveled; that is, forward flexion with lateral and rotatory component if the head is slightly turned to one side (Fig. 6–16).

The rotatory component causes a degree of subluxation of the atlas-axis joint (Fig. 6–17) with rotation about the axis of the dens (odontoid process) with the subluxation at the lateral bodies. The presence of the dorsal root ganglion of C2 root being adjacent to the C1-C2 *disk* causes mechanical and chemical irritation of the ganglion with resultant headache in that dermatomal area (Fig. 6–18).

The examination must include determination of limited or painful forward flexion of the head on the cervical spine, impaired lateral flexion and rotation, and finding the sources of unilateral limitation and end point pain. In

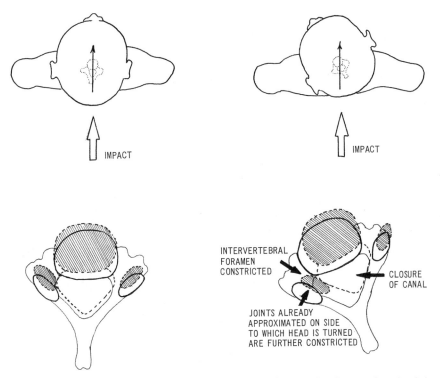

Figure 6–16. Effect of deceleration injury to neck with head turned. (*The left drawing*) Indicates impact on the neck in an anterior-posterior direction. The lower drawing shows the movement of the vertebral bodies and facets from this impact. (*The right drawing*) Indicates impact with the head turned to the left. The lower drawing shows the rotatory component of resultant movement with closure of the left foramen from subluxation of the facets and narrowing of the spinal canal from movement of the lamina. (From Cailliet, R: Neck and Arm Pain, ed 3. FA Davis, Philadelphia, 1991, p 110, with permission.)

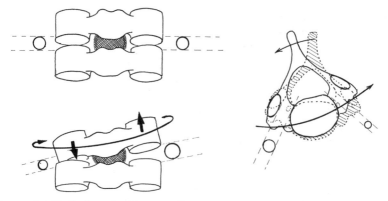

Figure 6–17. Unilateral subluxation from excessive rotation. Excessive rotation with simultaneous lateral flexion causes excessive closure of the foramen (*small circle*) and opening of the contralateral foramen (*larger circle*).

performing the neurologic examination the upper motor neuron must be tested (Hoffmann signs, deep tendon reflexes) as well as dermatomal testing using light touch, pin prick sensation, and testing response to vibration and individual motor strength.

Various structures in the upper cervical area produce neck pain and cervicogenic headache. These include the suboccipital muscles, the C1-C2 nerve roots, C2-C3 disks, upper cervical ligaments, and the three involved synovial joints.

The AO and the atlantoaxial (AA) joints possess nociceptor and sensory afferent nerve fibers from the ventral rami of C1-C2. Distending these joints using a contract medium produces an ipsilateral suboccipital pain pattern.[41]

Motor testing of the upper cervical segment measures the strength of the upper head-neck flexor (capitus flexors) and the upper cervical extensors (capitus extensors).

After discovering a history of ataxia, the patient's gait must be observed

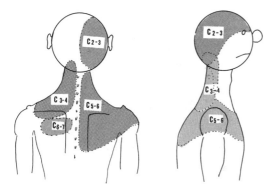

Figure 6–18. Referred zones of cervical root levels (dermatomes). The graphic zones depict the dermatomal referral levels of cervical roots C2 to C7.

during tandem walking, and the finger-nose-finger and one-leg-standing balance tests given.

Vertigo (*dizziness*) is a subjective complaint that may require auditory and vestibular testing as well as testing for nystagmus. Of patients complaining of dizziness after a whiplash cervical injury, 54% to 67% have abnormal electronystagmography (ENG) tests.[42-45]

LOWER CERVICAL
SEGMENT EXAMINATION

After eliciting the history of symptoms, causation, and resultant impairment, the lower cervical segment must be examined. The facets of the lower cervical segment are so vital in determining motion and causation of pain that they deserve specific mention.

The cervical zygapophyseal joints are planar synovial paired joints between the inferior articular process of the superior vertebra and the superior process of the inferior vertebra (Fig. 6–19). The processes (facets) are lined with articular cartilage and are enclosed in a fibrous capsule which is lined with a synovial membrane. Within the capsule are located fibroadipose menisci whose bases are attached to the capsule. They enter the joint space in a tapered form. They contain blood vessels, nerve endings, and are covered with synovium.[46]

The cervical zygapophyseal joints are innervated by articular branches derived from the medial branches of the cervical dorsal rami. The C4-C8 dorsal rami arise from their respective spinal nerves just outside the intervertebral foramina and pass dorsally over the roots of the transverse processes. Beyond the zygopophyseal joints they supply the semispinalis and multifidus muscles.

Encapsulated mechanoreceptors are consistently found in normal cervical

Figure 6–19. Cervical functional unit. A typical cervical functional unit depicts two adjacent vertebrae separated by the intervertebral disk (IVD). The posterior articular processes (facets) are lined with cartilage and enclosed with a capsule that contains fibroadipose menisci (FAM) that are connected to the capsule and insert into the joint. The intervertebral foramen (IVF) is shown through which the nerve roots emerge.

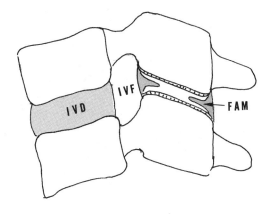

facets[47] which some think indicates position, tension, and pressure, likely factors in initiating protective muscular reflexes in response to pain with resultant limited motion.[48,49]

These receptor endings have a large receptive field allowing one or two nerve endings to monitor the area of each individual facet capsule. These nerve endings have been identified in loose areolar tissue, dense connective tissue, and in the capsule. They may well initiate nociception because substance P immunoreactivity has been identified in the encapsulated receptors of the posterior longitudinal ligaments, periosteum, and encapsulated mechanoreceptors.[50]

The orientation of the zygapophyseal joints resists two types of motion. By facing backward and upward, the superior articular process resists forward and downward motion by preventing displacement and resisting compressive loads. The upper cervical segments are placed more nearly horizontally and so they bear more weight than lower cervical segments.

A typical cervical unit permits flexion-extension, rotation, and lateral flexion. During these motions, the facet surfaces glide on each other to the point of subluxation, in which the leading facet surface loses contact with its opposing facet's surface. At this point the fibroadipose meniscus is drawn out of the joint cavity to cover the exposed articular surface.

During flexion-extension the above mentioned inferior facets move upward and forward over the superior facet below around an arc (Fig. 6–20). Because the plane of the upper cervical segments (C3-C4) are more horizontal they glide (translate) more than the lower segments do and also glide more than they rotate.

During rotation of the cervical spine, the contralateral inferior facet glides upward and medially over its opposed superior facet causing a lateral tilt and lateral flexion of the unit (Fig. 6–21).

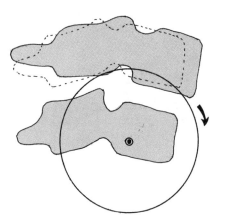

Figure 6–20. Flexion arc of a cervical unit. In forward flexion of the cervical spine, each lower unit flexes about an axis of rotation (*small circle and dot*). The disk deforms as shown and the facets glide forward and separate.

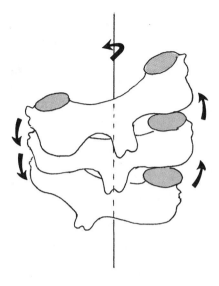

Figure 6-21. Rotation of the cervical spine. Rotation of the cervical spine involves a coupling action with simultaneous lateral flexion (*arrows*), separation of the convex side, and narrowing of the concave side. This occurs because of the angulation of the facet surfaces (*shaded areas*), which undergo a gliding in a forward and upward direction.

Muscle control of the cervical spine dictates the degree of rotation and, in the case of the capsule, limits the range. Posterior and anterior neck muscles fatigue more rapidly in patients with degenerative arthritic changes in the cervical spine, allegedly from nerve ending involvement,[51] so that apparent neck muscle weakness on testing must consider this in older patients.

Increased muscular tension following trauma has been documented to result from release of nociceptor peptides at nerve terminals which are also vasoconstrictive.[52,53] These findings possibly explain the persistent pain and tenderness of the neck and upper shoulder muscles after a whiplash injury. The insertion of these muscles into the occiput may explain, in part, the finding of *tension headaches* in that area.

EXAMINATION OF THE CERVICAL SPINE

A meaningful history should highlight the following:

1. Cervical symptoms as acute, recurrent, or chronic
2. Exact mechanisms of causative factors of the injury
   a. exact external trauma; that is, position of patient's head and neck at time
   b. insidious symptoms from prolonged or repetitive forces considered microtrauma, for example, position, physical stresses, duration of activities, extraneous factors such as emotional stresses, among others.

3. Precise sensation noted by patient at moment of impact or from prolonged postural stresses and the subsequent sensation
   a. description of sensation (character, intensity, and extent)
   b. influence of position or motion upon sensation
4. Exact site of sensation (anatomic as noted by patient and confirmed by examiner)
   a. exclusively in the neck region
   b. exclusively in the upper extremity region but assumed to originate from the neck
   c. both in the neck and the upper extremity
   d. felt in the neck and in the lower extremities with/without bladder and/or bowel symptoms
5. Disability claimed by patient. Inability to function as ascertained to result from impairment
6. Psychologic (emotional) interpretation of the alleged impairment and disability

Objectives of Examination

The examination is the attempt by the examiner to determine the structural, physiologic (i.e., neurologic, orthopedic, vascular), and psychologic aspects of the *impairment*.

Observation of the patient determines the limitations of motions in daily activities such as posture, movement, and restrictions. Attendant grimaces or expressions of pain must be noted. Observations also must denote the malalignment of the body structures in stance, sitting, and lying down. These are the major components elicited in evaluating the *postural* components of motion.

Bony and Soft Tissue Palpation

The patient's neck can be palpated in the supine, seated, or standing position. In the supine position, the neck muscles and the effects of gravity are eliminated.[35] The following major bony structures are palpable:

1. Spinous processes: transverse and posterior superior
2. Facet's joints
3. Mastoid processes

The following soft tissues are palpable:

1. Muscles. Accomplished by the active participation of the patient initiating specific movements and palpating the involved muscles.
2. Ligaments.
3. Nerves.

Subjectivity of impaired nerve function is elicited from the history with findings of symptoms such as tingling, pain, and numbness by alluding to their dermatomal areas. Sensitivity is noted from direct pressure and indicates the precise nerve.

Nerve Function Testing

Motor. This tests with participation by the patient in performing specific motions and determining appropriate muscular activity and thereby also ascertaining the appropriate nerve supply.

Sensory. This determines the dermatomal areas subjectively; but allows objective confirmation using various modalities such as touch, cotton swab, pin prick or scratch, tuning fork, and position sense testing.

Range of Motion Testing

Range-of-motion testing measures integrity of anatomic joint structure and function tested both actively and passively. The term **actively** implies testing motions performed by the patient upon observation and from instructions. In testing range of motion of the cervical spine, the motions flexion, extension, lateral flexion, and rotation are requested and observed (Fig. 6–22).

Passively testing range of motion is measuring motions performed *by* the examiner *on* the patient by movements of the head and neck involving each individual vertebral segment (Fig. 6–23) of both upper and lower cervical segments.

Upper Cervical Measurement. Upper cervical motion: Head flexion, extension, and rotation on the cervical spine. (Occiput atlas–C1 axis–C2) (Fig. 6–24).

Lower Cervical Measurement. Lower cervical motion: Neck flexion, extension, lateral flexion, and rotation of the entire lower cervical spine (C3-C7).

In estimating range of motion, the difference in the "end-point" of one direction versus the opposite end-point is determined (Figs. 6–25 and 6–26). Symptoms (i.e., unpleasant sensations) produced during these motions is noted and recorded. The operative site (segmental level) of the sensation produced (local or referred) is also determined. Knowing that the foramen through which the nerve roots emerge opens and closes during a specific motion (Fig. 6–27) such activity helps to determine the precise level of involvement.

Because it has been generally accepted that the zygapophyseal joints are a source of neck pain, their manual identification is done during clinical testing. Its accuracy has been confirmed both as to location as well as source of pain.[54]

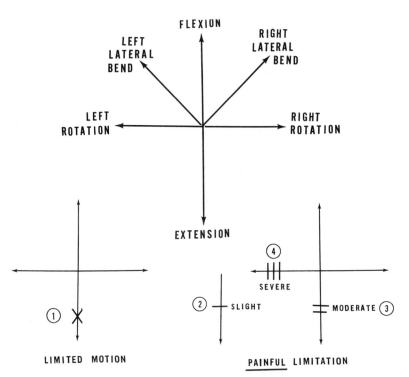

Figure 6–22. Recording range of motion. X indicates mere limitation without pain (1). (2) indicates slight pain whereas (3) and (4) indicate the degree of pain from restricted motion and from which direction of motion the pain occurs.

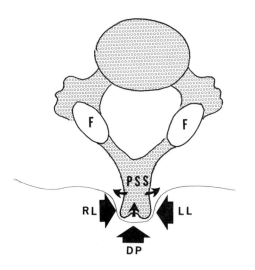

Figure 6–23. Methods of movement of the vertebral segment with direct pressure (DP), right lateral (RL), or left lateral (LL) pressure on the posterior superior spine.

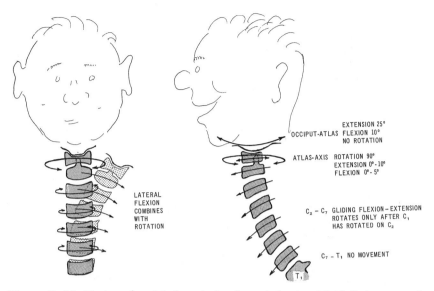

Figure 6–24. Motion of occipital-cervical and cervical spine. The left drawing indicates that lateral flexion is always accompanied with rotation. The right drawing indicates the degrees of motion at each vertebral segment.

The techniques are numerous,[55–59] and are elaborated here. Whether the manual diagnosis of site and operative source of pain is accurate remains controversial, but when compared with testing using medial nerve blocks, such diagnosis proved accurate.[54]

The muscles responsible for active motion are tested for control, strength, and endurance. Doing so requires testing all muscles in both isometric and isokinetic contractions. Repeated contractions indicate endurance. Sensation noted by the patient during contraction may also imply local pain and tenderness.

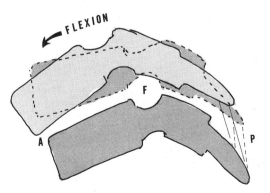

Figure 6–25. Flexion of a functional cervical unit. In forward flexion the superior vertebra glides forward and down approximating the anterior disk space (A) and elongating the posterior ligamentous structures (P) causing the foramen (F) to open.

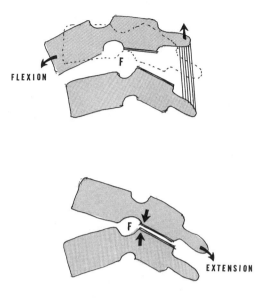

Figure 6–26. Cervical flexion and extension. The upper drawing depicts cervical flexion of a functional unit in which the superior vertebra glides forward and down at the anterior portion. The posterior elements elevate and are limited by the posterior ligaments. The foramen (F) opens. Extension is limited by the superior vertebra gliding backward and down until the facets impinge (*arrows*). The foramen narrows.

Neurologic examination of the head and neck requires testing the sensory, motor, and autonomic nervous systems. The upper cervical nerves (C1-C2-C3) mostly supply sensory neurologic activity to the head. Motor testing of the upper cervical (occipital) area involves the muscles moving the head on the neck. The neurologic examination, both sensory and motor, of the lower

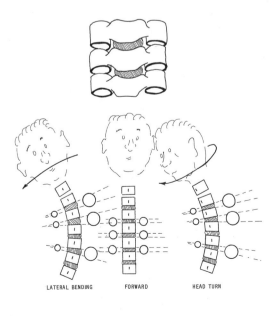

Figure 6–27. Foramenal closure in lateral flexion and rotation of the head and neck. With the head in erect posture (*center drawing*) the foramena are equally opened. In right lateral flexion (*left drawing*) the foramena narrow on the concave side and open on the convex side. In rotation (*right drawing*) the foramena narrow on the side toward which the head turns and open on the contralateral side.

cervical spine (C3-C8) involves observation of the upper extremities, including the musculoskeletal, axillary, radial, median, and ulnar nerves (Figs. 6–28 through 6–32).

The sensory (dermatomal) examination is limited mostly to the hand itself (Fig. 6–33). The details of clinical examination are adequately summarized in another of my works to which the reader is referred.[60]

Confirmation is clinically possible by means of electromyography or nerve conduction velocity studies.

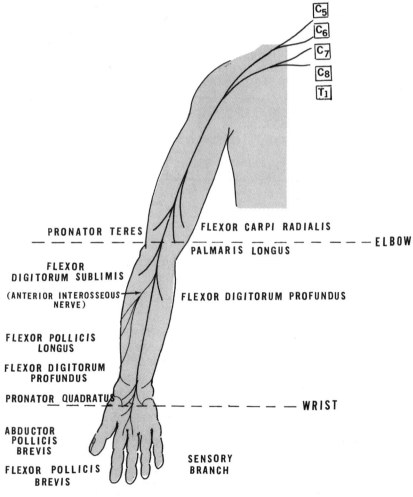

Figure 6–28. Median nerve.

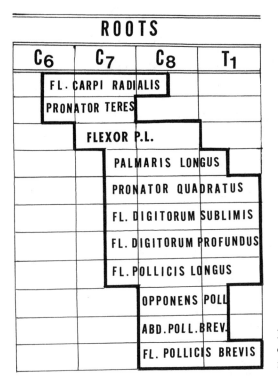

Figure 6–29. Cervical root component of the median nerve.

CLINICAL ENTITIES

Upper Cervical Segment (Occiput–Atlas–Axis)

Most upper cervical segmental symptoms occur after a hyperextension-hyperflexion injury such as a vehicular accident. A translatory force causes the head to hyperflex or hyperextend on the immediate upper cervical vertebrae above cervical segment C3. The resultant "subluxation" has already been discussed. The mechanism has been documented in animal and simulated human models (Figs. 6–34 and 6–35).

The symptoms of subluxation include headache and hypersensitivity of the scalp in the C1, C2, and C3 dermatomes. Palpable tenderness and reproduction of the symptoms of headache can be determined by digital pressure on the emergence site of the greater occipital nerve (see Fig. 6–6). Diagnosis is confirmed by relief from a local injection of an analgesic agent. End-point pain is elicited by active and passive rotation of the head upon the cervical spine which is restricted in one direction.[61]

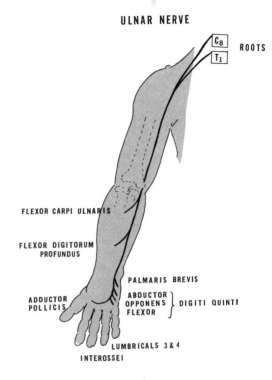

ULNAR NERVE

C₈
T₁
ROOTS

FLEXOR CARPI ULNARIS

FLEXOR DIGITORUM
PROFUNDUS

PALMARIS BREVIS

ADDUCTOR
POLLICIS

ABDUCTOR
OPPONENS } DIGITI QUINTI
FLEXOR

LUMBRICALS 3 & 4

INTEROSSEI

Figure 6–30. The ulnar nerve.

Lower Cervical Segment Pain and Impairment

Neck pain is a poorly understood symptom variously described as *disk disease* or *soft tissue injury pain*.[62,63] Pain is subjectively located in the neck; motion is considered causative or aggravating. Rest and reclining the head are palliative.

Pain is considered to result from disk lesions that are commonly overlooked by the clinician's failure to notice them on radiologic studies. After extension injuries, autopsy studies have revealed anterior rim lesions, posterior disk contusions, herniations, and avulsions.[62]

Rim lesions are a transverse tear in the annulus near its attachment to the vertebral endplate with bleeding into the anterior superior annulus. The anterior longitudinal ligament remains intact (Fig. 6–36).

The evident posterior protrusion results from acute extension injuries with nuclear protrusion posteriorly through annular fissures with protrusion into the anterior epidural space. In severe translatory impacts the disk may be completely avulsed from the vertebral endplate.

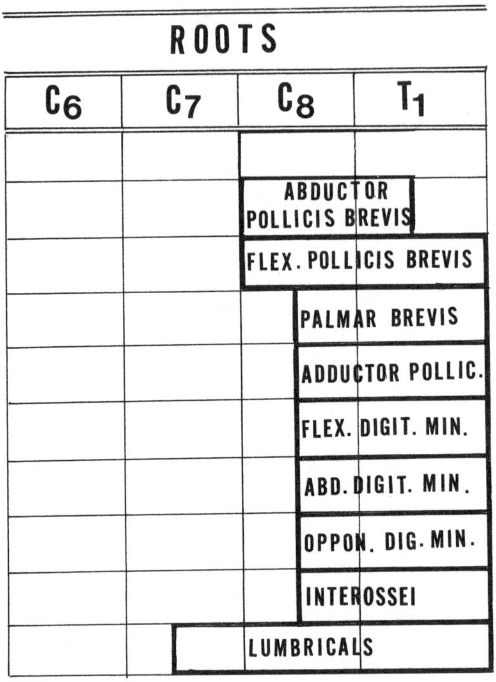

ROOTS

C₆	C₇	C₈	T₁
		ABDUCTOR POLLICIS BREVIS	
		FLEX. POLLICIS BREVIS	
		PALMAR BREVIS	
		ADDUCTOR POLLIC.	
		FLEX. DIGIT. MIN.	
		ABD. DIGIT. MIN.	
		OPPON. DIG. MIN.	
		INTEROSSEI	
	LUMBRICALS		

Figure 6–31. Cervical root component of the ulnar nerve.

Cervical Zygapophyseal Joint Pain

Distension of cervical zygapophyseal joints seen through a contrast medium produces pain characteristic of the pattern complained by the patient.[61] Pain from the C2-C3 joint is perceived in the upper neck and the occipital area (Fig. 6–37). Pain from the C3-C4 joints extends from the upper neck to the levator scapulae muscle. The pain radiating from the C4-C5 forms an angle between the lower neck and the upper shoulder girdle. From the C5-C6 the pain extends from the lower neck over the supraspinatus area and that from the C6-C7 over the blade of the scapula. The areas are large and indistinct but reasonably consistent.

Zygapophyseal joint injuries cause localized pain from bruising of the vascular synovial folds (termed **menisci**). The meniscus of the AO joint may be so bruised it causes a hemorrhage that enfolds the dorsal root ganglion (see Fig. 6–38). Fractures of a facet may occur in an occult manner and thus not be radiologically visualized.

Diagnosis of a facet injury is clinically possible by gentle anterior and posterior palpation and passive motion of each vertebral segment.[62,63] Clinical differential diagnosis of neck pain resulting from a zygapophyseal source rather than from disk pathology remains difficult.[64–67]

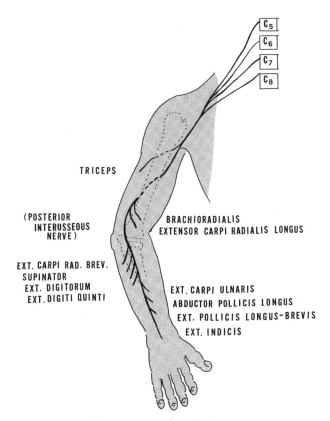

Figure 6-32. The radial nerve.

Provocative discography and cervical zygapophyseal joint blocks[67] revealed that disks alone were symptomatic in 20% of patients tested, zygapophyseal joints were symptomatic in 23%, and in 41%, both were symptomatic. Of these patients, 17% had neither as a cause of pain. These studies did not clarify the *precise* cause of neck pain and a recent study alleges that zygapophyseal joint pain after injury has not been positively ascertained.[68]

Injury to the anterior longitudinal ligament also causes pain.[69] Neck muscles as a source of neck pain after trauma have also been suggested but failed to be confirmed because most limb muscle lesions tend to heal within days or weeks so neck muscles cannot be considered differently.[69]

Vascular changes that result from cervical trauma as a source of pain have not been elucidated yet undoubtedly occur. Hemorrhage from injury to the meniscus of the atlas-axis joint has been mentioned (see Fig. 6-29), but headaches have been attributed to vascular compression of the C2 nerve. These headaches were relieved by injections of anesthetics or by coagulation within the distended veins.[70]

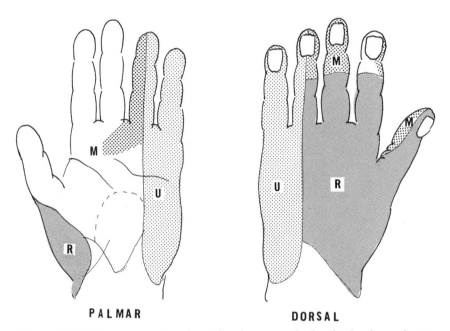

PALMAR   **DORSAL**

Figure 6–33. Sensory mapping of peripheral nerve to the hand. This figure depicts the schematic areas of sensory innervation of the median nerve (M), radial nerve (R), and ulnar nerve (U). The dermatomes of the dorsum of the hand vary as the radial nerve may have either no sensory area or merely a small area over the first dorsal interosseous.

NEUROLOGIC EXAMINATION (NERVES EMANATING FROM CERVICAL SPINE)

The standard upper extremity neurologic examination considers all the nerves subserving the upper extremity. Tests should be done on the deep tendon reflexes, sensory mapping, and individual motor check of myotomes. Compression of the accessible nerves may elicit tenderness and paresthesias.

To ascertain that the deficit discerned originated from the cervical spine requires a history of neck trauma, a history of subjective radiation of pain from neck motions, and physical confirmation of motion creating the radicular symptoms. This examination must bear in mind that extension narrows the foramena, flexion elongates the nerve roots, and lateral flexion causes ipsilateral foramenal closure, as well as rotation to that side. Compression of the head with the head turned and laterally flexed causes radiation of pain down the involved extremity (Fig. 6–39). Traction of the head relieves radicular symptoms (Fig. 6–40).

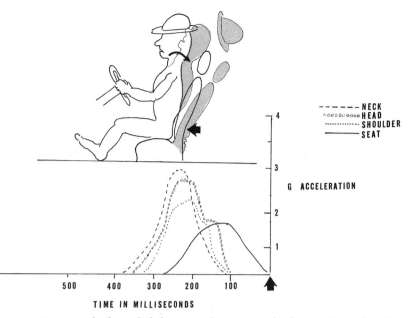

Figure 6–34. Upper body-neck deformation from rear-end collisions. From the effect of a force from the rear, the head, neck, and shoulder deform at different times measured in milliseconds. The major forces (G) are expended within a time frame under 0.5 seconds.

Cervicogenic Headache

The pathophysiologic etiology of recurrent benign headache[71] remains obscure,[72] varying from *tension type* to migraine with or without aura. The cervicogenic headache remains foremost in incidence although it, too, is unclear as to pathomechanics. Edmeads[73] posed the question "can cervical spine disorders cause headache?" He followed with three possible other causes: (1) pain sensitive structures in the neck; (2) identifiable pathologic processes; and (3) identifiable neurologic pathways.

The pain sensitive tissues of the neck have been identified as the zygapophyseal joints, cervical muscles and their attachments, cervical nerve roots, and vertebral arteries. Most headaches radiate from these tissues through the C1 sensory root, C2 sensory roots, tentorial nerves, the C2-C4 cervical roots through the nucleus caudalis of the trigeminal nerve, and tension of the neck muscles, which activates the scalp musculature.

The AO articulation has been proposed as a nociceptor site. Stimulation of the C1 root is difficult due to its proximity to the vertebral artery. C1 is considered to radiate through the mandibular division of the trigeminal.[74] C2 involvement through the greater superior occipital nerve has been discussed. C3

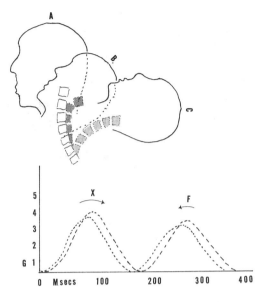

Figure 6–35. Hyperextension injuries from rear-end impact. The effects on the tissue of the cervical spine occur within 300 milliseconds. The head initially extends on the cervical spine (A) to (B) then the remainder of the cervical spine extends (C). X indicates initial extension often followed by reactive flexion (F).

root involvement does not yet enjoy widespread acceptance.[75] Suboccipital musculature also remains unresolved.[76] Vascular pathology has been known to cause pain,[77] such as in pain sensitive intracranial vessels which project to the nucleus caudalis, and then to the thalamus.[77]

The relationship of muscle pain/spasm with vasoconstriction-vasodilatation is an interesting model,[78,79] with the consideration that peripheral noci-

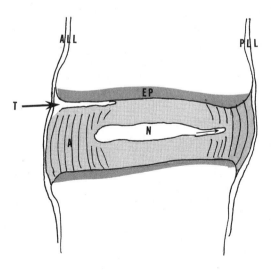

Figure 6–36. Annulus tears and intervertebral disk degeneration. A degenerated disk is depicted showing the nucleus (N) being deformed. A forceful translatory force can tear (T) the outer annular fibers (A) from the vertebral endplate (EP). The anterior longitudinal ligament (ALL) can also be torn from its vertebral attachment. The more distal posterior longitudinal ligament (PLL) does not become involved. This type of disk injury usually occurs from a severe external translatory force.

Figure 6–37. Hemorrhage from meniscus injury. Hemorrhage resulting from a deformed meniscus between the lateral bodies of the atlas and axis encircles and irritates the dorsal root ganglion (DRG) causing pain. The hemorrhage comes from an external injury (see text).

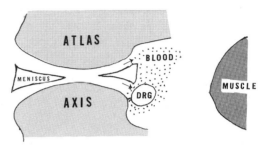

ceptive impulses *trigger* central mechanisms. This concept indicates the value of analgesic injections into the sensitive peripheral tissues in an attempt to abort benign headaches considered to be cervicogenic, although without scientific basis.[80,81]

Hyperextension-Hyperflexion Cervical Injuries: Whiplash Syndrome

This syndrome has been mentioned (see Figs. 6–32 and 6–33), but because it is so common and so controversial it merits additional discussion.[82] The very definition of whiplash remains controversial. The essential elements included in this definition is an injury that results from a motor vehicle accident (MVA), wherein acceleration forces are imposed upon the head and

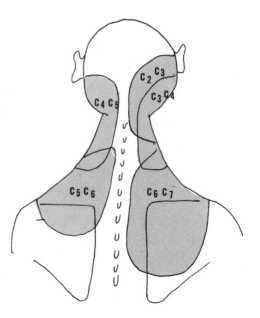

Figure 6–38. Referred pain zones of zygapophyseal joints.

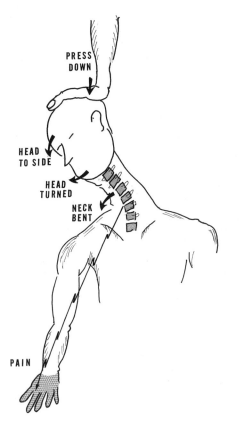

PRESS
DOWN

HEAD
TO SIDE

HEAD
TURNED

NECK
BENT

PAIN

Figure 6–39. Head compression causing radicular signs and symptoms. Downward compression on the head **(Spurling neck compression test)** indicates probable nerve root entrapment. With the head turned and laterally flexed to the side showing symptoms, the head is forced down. Reproduction of radicular symptoms is considered positive in a Spurling test.

neck. Initially it was considered to be the result of a rear end impact collision causing hyperextension of the head and neck followed by *rebound* hyperflexion.

At the time of impact, the vehicle is accelerated forward followed immediately (100 milliseconds) with forward acceleration of the trunk and shoulders of the occupant (see Figs. 6–32 and 6–33). The shoulders travel forward anteriorly under the head causing extension of the neck. The head having been kept immobile, because no force has acted upon it, accelerates forward around the axis of the upper cervical spine in an action of occipital-cervical motion.

The forces involved have been extensively studied and are considerable. A speed of impact at 20 mph (32 km h) initiates an acceleration of 12 Gs.

Assuming that the head is facing directly forward, all forces are linear (sagittal) but this rarely occurs, because some degree of rotation is usually present. This force causes rotation *before* extension occurs,[83] causing stress on the capsules of the zygapophyseal joints, the intervertebral disks, and the alar ligament complex of the upper cervical segment.

Frontal impacts have a different mechanism. These forces rapidly decel-

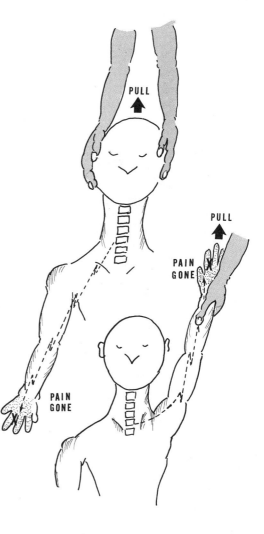

Figure 6–40. Relief of radicular symptoms with manual traction. In a patient with radicular symptoms, manual traction relieves the symptoms if the source of pain is cervical. Elevation and traction of the upper extremity with relief of symptoms may indicate brachial plexus etiology.

erate the vehicle with the body continuing in a forward direction until it is decelerated by the seat belts (if worn) or, if not worn, by the impact on the dashboard of the car.

This force is applied first at the occipitocervical joint because the head is heavy (10 to 12 pounds average). The force is then expended at the C6 joint.[83] The head rotates forward followed by flexion of the neck, extending the posterior neck tissues which are elongated excessively without muscular recoil because the proprioceptors and spindle system do not react rapidly enough.

It has been confirmed that the head accelerates upon the condyles within the first 23 milliseconds after impact. An impact speed of 40 mph (63.5 km h) results in a 90 G force on the vehicle and a 46 G force on the occupant.

The effects upon the axis-atlas complex have been discussed and their symptomatology proposed. The effect upon the lower cervical segments (C3-C7) needs clarification. As well as flexion, extension, and lateral flexion forces, there are also parallel (translatory) forces with segmental motion not occurring around physiologic axes.

Forced Flexion. This force applies compressive forces to the anterior elements (the intervertebral disks and vertebral bodies) and tensile forces to the posterior elements (the zygapophyseal capsules, articular pillars, ligamentum nuchae, and posterior neck muscles). In the upper cervical segment the alar ligaments undergo translatory motion and rotational stress.

Forced Extension. In forced extension, the cervical segments undergo compression of the posterior structures (spinous process and zygapophyseal joints) and tensile forces to the anterior structures (anterior longitudinal ligament, anterior cervical muscles, odontoid process, and the intervertebral disks) Fig. 6–41).

Lateral Forces. These have not been as completely studied as the flexion and extension forces but because some lateral flexion occurs with a slight degree of rotation, these forces can be extrapolated. The coupling that occurs causes compression of the ipsilateral zygapophyseal joints and distraction of the contralateral joints. Joint capsules receive the brunt of the stress, although the intervertebral disk from rotational forces ARS stressed as well.

Shear Forces. Because the impact causes the neck to undergo translatory motion rather than rotation about physiologic axes, these are shear (hori-

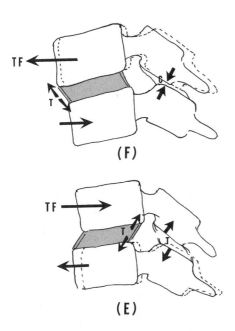

(F)

(E)

Figure 6–41. Effects of horizontal force on cervical disk. (*F*) depicts flexion force with the translatory force (TF) causing the superior vertebra to glide forward. The anterior fibers of the disk undergo tensile force (T), and because of the angulation of the zygapophyseal joints, they undergo compression forces (C). (*E*) is extension with the TFs of the superior vertebra gliding backward on the inferior vertebra. The annular fibers undergo Ts as do the facets and their capsules.

zontal) forces. The resultant motion is articular, through a small excursion, and causes little muscular reaction because muscles are vertically oriented.

The resultant reaction to these shear forces are compression of the surfaces of the zygapophyseal joints and shear stress on the oblique annular fibers of the disk, especially at the fibers' anterior site. The posterior disk is apt to undergo fissuring if the accident victim is old.

Pathology. These tissue changes are now being clarified from animal and cadaveric studies, because most injuries are nonfatal and thus such patients cannot be clinically or pathologically examined. Few patients will require surgery. There are no external clinical signs such as bruising, swelling, or hemorrhage, thus symptoms are subjective. Objective signs are minimal and nonspecific.

The most common lesions noted in the cervical spine after a cervical injury caused by acceleration or deceleration are present in soft tissue—muscle, ligament, joints, capsule, and disk—but may include a pillar fracture of the zygapophyseal joint, tears of the capsule, tears of the longitudinal ligament,[84,85] either anterior or posterior, or both, and tears of the disk annulus.

In the upper cervical segment (O-C1-C2), fracture of the odontoid process and fractures of the laminar and superior processes have been reported.[86,87] Hypermobility of the axis-atlas articulation may result from tear or stretch of the alar ligaments. This can be determined by CT scanning.[88] Fractures of the lower cervical vertebrae may be detected by careful radiologic screening.[89]

Brain Injury. Brain injury to the patient with whiplash has been under reported because the clinical attention has been directed primarily to injury to the cervical spine. A direct relationship exists between brain injury, albeit often subtle, with cervical spine injury.[90–93] The sequelae of brain injury, the so-called postconcussion syndrome, has a voluminous literature that will not be documented here.

Cardinal Symptoms. The most prominent is consistent neck pain—a dull aching sensation initially noted at the base of the head, which is aggravated by movement. In most cases, there is also associated neck stiffness with restriction of movement. Pain may radiate to the head, shoulder, arm, and interscapular areas.

Although referral patterns of various neck tissues have been documented, these patterns do not necessarily document the specific tissue affected, the severity, or the pathology but rather seems to suggest a segmental level.[94] Even given the current proficiency of radiologic studies, computed tomography (CT) and magnetic resonance imaging scanning, the pathology does not ascertain nor confirm the cause of pain in the whiplash patient, although a *fanning* effect (a separation of the spinous processes) has been described on lateral radiologic views.[85]

Elimination of the specific pain by selective analgesic blocks are proving beneficial but are not yet feasible for purposes of clinical diagnosis. These tests include zygapophyseal joint blocks and nerve blocks of the greater occipital nerve and ventral rami of spinal nerves. Cervical discograms have also enjoyed some acceptance, but fail to be diagnostic for the site and cause of pain. They are of clinical value as experimental procedures but are not yet, however, considered routine.

Headache results frequently from a whiplash injury. It is typically occipital, radiating anteriorly into the temporal or occipital region which are subserved by nerve roots C1-C3. Headaches may result from concussion.[95,96] They may also result from injury to the lateral atlantoaxial joint[97,98] which has been discussed earlier in this chapter.

Visual disturbances[99] and dizziness[100-104] have been recorded but explanations for them remain uncertain. Dizziness may result from inner ear dysequilibrium,[105,106] or damage to cervical musculature.

Many patients with whiplash injuries later complain of diminished concentration and of memory disturbances. Neuropsychiatric studies of such victims compared with those of noninjured patients, have shown deficits in attention, concentration and memory,[107] but these findings have been questioned because similar findings have been found in patients with chronic neck and head pain[92,108,109] but without a history of whiplash. Abnormal electroencephalographic (EEG) test results have been found in some patients after significant whiplash injuries.[110,111]

Paresthesia. Numbness and tingling of the hands, especially the two ulnar fingers, along with weakness and reflex changes have frequently been found in patients after suffering whiplash injury. When present without overt neurologic findings these symptoms have been attributed to a thoracic outlet syndrome,[112,113] which is discussed in Chapter 7.

LESIONS OF THE CERVICAL CORD

Injuries of the cervical cord that result in paraplegia or quadriplegia are clinically discernible with upper motor neuron signs: Babinski and Hoffmann signs, hyperactive deep tendon reflexes, spasticity, and clonus, among others. For more subtle injuries of the cervical spine, clinical tests are less specific and thus such injuries often overlooked. Lesions caudal from C4 at the nerve root levels are discernible with dermatomal and myotomal level testing. Above the C4 level, there is a *blind zone* (Fig. 6–42),[114] with lesions in that area being clinically difficult to document. The Shimizu reflex deals with this differential diagnosis. Higher level testing (C1-C4) does not lend itself to the perception of radicular signs. The jaw reflex indicates involvement of the brain stem.[115]

The Shimizu reflex is performed with the patient seated with an elbow bent to 90° angle and the forearm supported. The examiner taps the tip of the spine of the scapula in a caudal direction with a rubber reflex hammer. The reflex involves movement of the scapula from an abrupt stretching of the upper

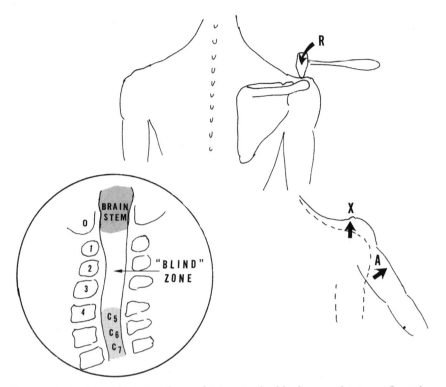

Figure 6–42. Neurologic test for cord injury in the blind zone: Shimizu reflex. The test is performed by striking the outer tip of the scalular spine with a reflex hammer (R). The reflex is elevation of the scapula (X) or abduction of the arm (A). The test determines pathology of the "blind zone" (the nerve roots between C1 and C4 = occiput).

portion of the trapezius muscle. A *positive* test indicating damage to the cord between C1-C4 is indicated by elevation of the scapula and abduction of the humerus, although the latter may not be present.

The presence of *central pain* in spinal cord injuries has been largely overlooked in cervical spine injuries. It may be more prevalent than previously suspected and, in fact, has been totally ignored as an explanation for chronic pain sustained after relatively minor injury.

Treatment of catastrophic spinal cord injuries (SCI) has predominantly been an effort resulting from the early intervention and rehabilitative progress. The resultant pain in SCI has had sparse recognition.[116]

That central spinal cord pain plays a role in chronic whiplash injuries is, although conjectural, still feasible, thus, central pain needs to be clarified. Central spinal cord pain has been differentiated into three categories: (1) mechanical or musculoskeletal pain; (2) radicular pain; or (3) central or *spinal cord dysesthesia pain.*[117] These authors, Brittell and Mariano, do not include psychogenic pain, because it has been rejected in the psychiatric literature. They do emphasize the psychosocial factors that play a role in chronic SCI pain.[118]

Reflex sympathetic dystrophy (RSD) pain[119,120] occurs in a large percentage of patients with SCI. In the patient with an injured cervical cord, the musculoskeletal pain is termed **mechanical** because it is associated with injury to the ligaments, joints, muscles, and even bones caused by a mechanical deformity.

The incidence and prevalence of central pain in SCI patients are influenced by the site, extent (severity) and psychologic, emotional, and environmental factors.

Central pain of spinal cord origin (CCPS) can be caused by a lesion of the cord but the most frequent is trauma[121,122] with pain occurring in from 7.5% to 94% of SCI. Pathologic changes to the cord have been controversial but most have implicated damage to the spinothalamic tracts.[123,124] Pain has usually been steady and spontaneous (burning) rather than intermittent lancinating pain (seen mostly in thoracolumbar lesions).

Summary features of CCPS have been given:[122]*

1. CCPS may be caused by lesions of any degree or pathways at a wide variety of sites in the cord.
2. Trauma is the most common cause.
3. Onset is delayed in 70.1% of patients.
4. Regardless of the causative lesion, pain consists of three common characteristics: steady (96%), intermittent lancinating (31%), and evoked (47%).
5. Steady pain was burning (75%) or dysthetic (26%).
6. CCPS patients may also suffer from deafferentiation, radicular, and musculoskeletal pain.
7. Pain may develop in an area of otherwise complete or clinically inapparent sensory loss.
8. Pain characteristically may change dramatically with time.
9. Pain is relatively resistant to opiates, but does respond fairly well to sodium pentothal.

It was only in 1970 that central pain of spinal cord pathology was recognized,[122] with the following conclusions that lead to include this pain etiology with whiplash injuries to the cervical cord:

---

*Modified from Tasker RR, de Carvalho G, Dostrovsky JO: The History of Central Pain Syndromes, with Observations Concerning Pathophysiology and Treatment. In: Kenneth L. Casey, Ed., Pain and Central Nervous System Disease. The Central Pain Syndromes, Raven Press, New York, 1991, p 41.

1. Pain can be caused by any lesions of the nervous system of any etiology.
2. Pain onset may be delayed.
3. Pain consists of a spontaneous steady (burning or dysesthetic), or evoked character.
4. Pain usually responds poorly to opiates and better to anticonvulsants, antidepressants, or sodium pentothal.
5. Pain may be relieved by proximal or distal sympathetic blockade.

Suspecting the possibility of CCPS in patients who have sustained a whiplash injury insures a correct diagnosis and thus appropriate treatment. This diagnosis has been too frequently neglected.

Treatment Protocols for Cervical Pain

Cervical pain may be related to an acute injury or be an exacerbation of a chronic process. Pain is vaguely localized in a general area and may be associated with specific motions. As with low back pain, cervical pain must be determined to be either strictly local or with radiating symptoms.

Although radicular cervical pain has already been discussed, it behooves the examiner to realize that cervical pain can radiate to the top of the shoulder without necessarily being considered as radiculopathy if there is no attendant radiation of pain into the arm, hand, and fingers. Radiation to the head has been considered as radiculitis emanating from the upper cervical segments.

It should not be surprising that such a poorly understood condition as cervical whiplash has initiated a plethora of therapeutic media. Therapy varies from the acute and the chronic with the former being more accepted. Subjectivity of findings denies careful evaluation so there has been a consequent dearth of controlled trials.

In the acute phase of pain, rest, immobilization, local application of ice followed by heat, and gentle stretching have their benefits. Oral anti-inflammatory medication, if tolerated, is beneficial.

Reassurance by a meaningful explanation and avoidance of frightening terms such as **degenerative disk disease**, **arthritis** or **slipped disk** should be part of therapy. It is well accepted that the patient's comprehension and significance of the symptoms intensify the severity of the pain and can lead to possible chronicity and exaggeration of disability over physical impairment.[125]

Because *spasm* is frequently initiated by localized pain from inflammation which can itself also become a tissue site of pain, this symptom can be managed by application of local ice, heat, massage, gentle stretch, and isometric muscular contractions. Local injection of an analgesic agent into the painful muscle can be considered when local tenderness is pronounced.

Immobilization has been the standard treatment for an acute musculoskeletal injury but whether it is more valid than early mobilization is being questioned.[126] If immobilization is considered, a cervical collar or splint has been the traditional modality. The purpose of such a collar is to hold the head in a comfortable gravity-aligned position and thus to prevent or minimize motion.

A standard cervical collar (Fig. 6–43) is custom made of ¼" to ½" thick felt, cut to mold the neck and jaw of the patient. Because no known orthosis or collar completely eliminates motion, it must be assumed that it merely restricts motion, supports the head in a gravity-aligned posture, and reminds the patient to avoid excessive motion. By being under the chin, it minimizes the need for muscular contraction to overcome the effects of gravity and also limits flexion. The elevation of the collar behind the head limits extension. Plastic collars are now available that are easily applied, easy to keep clean, and cosmetically acceptable (Fig. 6–44). Only when there are neurologic signs and symptoms and a need for significant restriction of motion must a brace be fitted (Fig. 6–45).

As a general rule a collar should be worn constantly for the first week, then wearing time should be gradually decreased, as tolerated. Most soft tissue recovery occurs within 2 weeks. Prolonged immobilization encourages soft tissue contracture, muscular atrophy, and psychologic dependence.

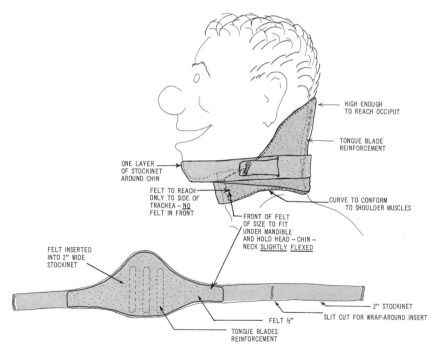

Figure 6–43. Felt cervical collar.

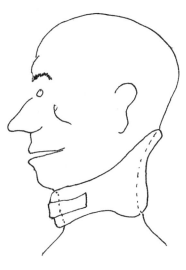

Figure 6–44. Standard plexiglass cervical collar. The fiber glass preformed collar comes in several sizes that need to be fitted to the patient. They are held by a Velcro strap in the front.

Traction has remained popular as a beneficial modality although medical opinions vary. The opinion that traction *distracts* the offending functional units remains questionable. DeSeze and Levernieux[127] determined that 260 lb traction produced a 2 mm separation between the fifth and sixth vertebrae. It took 400 lb traction to produce a 10 mm separation between the fourth cervical and first thoracic vertebra. Such forces are nonphysiologic and intolerable.

Without either subjective or objective radiculitis, the value of traction compared with that using a cervical collar and analgesics has no difference in outcomes.[128]

In treatment of cervical radiculitis, mechanical consideration of nerve root entrapment must be considered in therapy. Decreased cervical lordosis has been postulated as beneficial in consideration of the separation of the posterior elements opening the foramena. Crue[129] reported a 1.5 mm increase in the vertical diameter of the intervertebral foramena between C5 and C6 from 5 lb traction applied with the neck at 20° of flexion and applied for 24 hours. Colachis and Strohm[13] deducted that 30 lb traction at 20° of angulation applied for 7 seconds increased the separation relative to the angle of traction.

The position in which traction is applied is significant. With the head weighing approximately 10 to 12 lb, the supine position eliminates the effect of gravity and thus the muscular contraction of the neck muscles, as well (Fig. 6–46).

In acute cervical injuries, continuous cervical traction for several days is valuable. With subacute or chronic problems, traction for 20 minutes several times daily is beneficial. Manual traction before instituting mechanical traction indicates the tolerance and benefit gained from use of that modality.

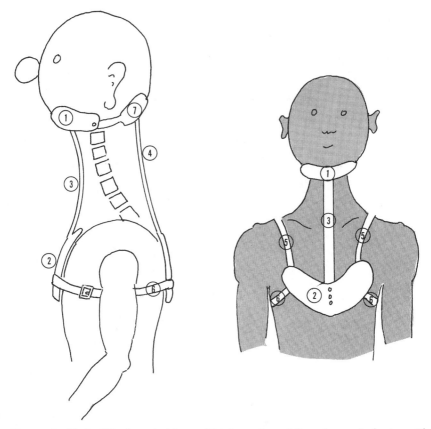

Figure 6–45. Guildford cervical brace. This brace immobilizes the cervical spine with a rest positioned under the chin (1) and an occipital pad (7). A chest pad (2) is connected to an anterior bar (3) that elevates the chin and connects by a strap (6) to the thoracic portion which, by a vertical bar (4), attaches to the occipital pad. The shoulder straps (5) secure the chest pad. All parts can adjust to make the brace customized to the specific patient.

Manipulation or mobilization is prevalent today, but its physiologic benefit has not been proven nor have the indications for this approach been clarified.

Several concepts exist regarding the benefit of manipulation. Efforts are probably directed to the facets, although some advocates indicate that the intervertebral disk is also influenced. Manipulation:

1. *Unlocks* a *jammed* facet joint. This finding is based on the presence of a facet meniscus or an entrapped synovial fold. An entrapped asymmetric facet is also postulated. Restoration of a subluxed facet has also been postulated.

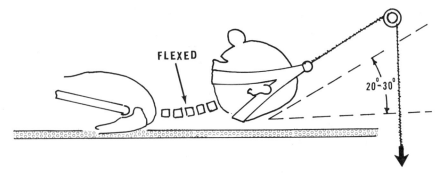

Figure 6–46. Cervical traction is applied to the supine patient causing cervical spine flexion with the angle of pull between 20° and 30°.

2. Allows a neurogenic reaction from manipulation wherein the force alters the spindle system's effect on the muscle, alters the mechanoreceptors in the facets, or has a *central* reaction on reflexes.
3. Elongates the contracted facet capsule or periarticular ligaments.
4. *Centralizes* the nucleus again within the intervertebral disk.

All benefits of manipulation have been subjective with no documented structural changes resulting from the procedure. Serious research has been done to determine the true mechanism of manipulation, because the procedure has significant clinical benefit left to be explored.[131]

Manipulation has been associated with mobilization as a passive procedure to accomplish the benefits stated above. Manipulation requires an abrupt external force, whereas mobilization essentially gradually elongates the constricted tissues. In standard procedures, force is applied in the direction that appears limited but the Maigne's technique differs in that it is applied in the opposite, unrestricted, and painless direction.[132]

Modalities such as ice, heat, ultrasound, massage, and electrical stimulation have their proponents but such therapy should be considered as merely palliative and ancillary to a more active approach. None of these modalities are specific, curative, nor precise and they extend the costs of treatment without benefit. In the presence of myofascial nodularities of muscles with trigger points (TP), a combination of local injection of an analgesic agent followed by passive stretch exercises has some benefit.

Exercise remains the most accepted modality. If range of motion is limited, gentle gradual *active* exercise is indicated. *Active* is stressed because exercise performed *by* the patient is preferable to exercise done *to* the patient. Exercises to strengthen the muscles where a specific weakness is found during a meaningful clinical examination are important. Usually the muscles involved are the short and long flexors.

Isometric exercises should first be initiated, followed soon after by kinetic exercises. Isometric contractions with no joint motion decreases spasm, pain, and atrophy. Isometric exercises should be started early in the management of an acute cervical injury despite pain, because few, if any, contraindications exist. Isometric exercises stretch the joint capsules to a slight but definite degree, compresses the cartilage with benefit, strengthens the ligaments and tendons, and forces out toxic (ischemic) materials from the muscles reflexively contracted by pain and inflammation. They are *active* and initiate the involvement of the patient toward recovery.

Isometric exercise should be followed by active assisted exercises. Because they result in joint movement and change in significant muscle fiber length, they are considered isokinetic. Isokinetic exercises increase strength, endurance, and range of motion. Ultimately resistance should be added to the exercise regimen to increase strength and endurance. Exercises also increase the level of endorphins[133] and minimize chronic pain.[134]

Range-of-motion exercise has been advocated but rarely is it defined or quantitated. A functional pain-free increase in range of motion is desirable but to acquire *complete and extreme* range of motion, albeit physiologic, is not necessary, in fact, it should be avoided because many soft tissues that have been structurally damaged will not tolerate excessive elongation. *Pain free and functionally adequate* should describe the guideline for gradual restoration to greater range of motion from normal daily use accepted at a later stage.

Restoration or institution of physiologic posture is mandatory in all activities of daily living to minimize both tissue stress and any nonphysiologic muscular effort. A *forward head posture*, that is, one ahead of the center of gravity, places excess stress on all cervical spine tissues (Fig. 6–47). The 10 lb head weighs closer to 30 lb when held 3″ in front of the center of gravity. This nonphysiologic posture places excessive demands upon the erector spinae muscles, narrows the foramena, and places force upon the posterior zygapophyseal joints (Fig. 6–48). This posture can result from a depressive state's forming its own *body language*.

Physiologic posture can be taught to the patient by a therapist and then practices by the patient, at first with assistive devices (Fig. 6–49), if necessary until it becomes a *normal* way of life and ensures automatic unconscious implementation. All contributing factors such as occupational demands, emotional and physiologic aspects must be unearthed and addressed.

FACET JOINT INJECTIONS

Cervical zygapophyseal joints, as the major source of pain, have been discussed. Patients frequently receive relief from intra-articular joint injections using either analgesic or steroidal solutions. Many of the *intra-articular injections* given probably do not enter the joints unless administered under fluoroscopic viewing by a person specifically trained in this modality.[135]

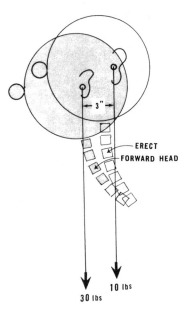

Figure 6–47. With an erect posture, the weight of the head (approximately 10 pounds) is maintained directly above the center of gravity. With the head forward, approximately 3 inches in front of the center of gravity, it adds an estimated 30 pounds of weight on the cervical spine.

Steroids have had no better results than analgesics; neither had benefits lasting longer than a few weeks.[136]

The conclusion of the study summarized with the statement: "Recommend early immobilization and avoiding prolonged use of a cervical collar . . . encouraged to remain functional despite the pain . . . avoid prolonged physical therapy . . . and give up such aggressive therapies such as corticosteroid injections into apophyseal joints now that we have sufficient evidence of their lack of efficacy." At best, recent studies may be summarized to state that an intra-articular analgesic agent injected under fluoroscopic conditions relieving *the* cervical pain may be diagnostic but repeated injections of analgesic and steroids are not justified.[137]

Bogduk claims that imaging and clinical tests to diagnose neck pain are useless,[138] "producing substantial levels of false positive results." Roughly one third of imaging studies reveal *asymptomatic* abnormalities and uncontrolled facet joint injections lead to false positive results in 35% of patients, the same percentage as found using cervical discograms.

The consistency of physical therapy has also been questioned in a recent review[139] varying from place to place and therapist to therapist. Durations of therapy vary from several weeks to months and the number of therapy sessions depend on the geographic region studied and varies also according to the payor. Even an approach as well-documented as the McKenzie approach varies tremendously in its application, despite being *approved and accepted* by the physical therapist.

These recent studies clearly reveal that the mechanism, etiologies, diag-

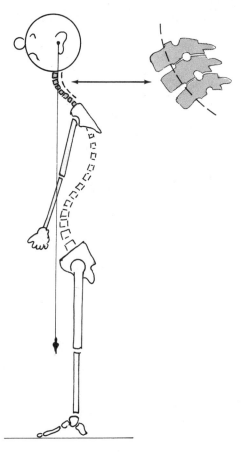

Figure 6–48. Forward head posture of depression. The depressed person has a rounded back and forward posture, which increase cervical lordosis. This increased lordosis approximates the posterior articulations and narrows the intervertebral foramina (*upper right*).

nostic studies, and recommended therapy protocols for neck pain need careful study, honest outcomes assessment, and effective clinical assessment. Treatment of cervical pain after injury remains undeveloped and undocumented; but it may be stated that mobilization is preferred over immobilization and that certain modalities relieve pain better and permit restoration of function earlier.

Chronic neck pain remains an enigma, whereas radicular subjective and objective findings merit conservative treatment. This permits outcomes assessment when evaluated properly.

TEMPOROMANDIBULAR JOINT PAIN

Temporomandibular joint pain, termed **TMJ syndrome**, is a prominent impairing and disabling condition which falls in the category of soft tissue disability.[140,141] The International Association for the Study of Headache has in-

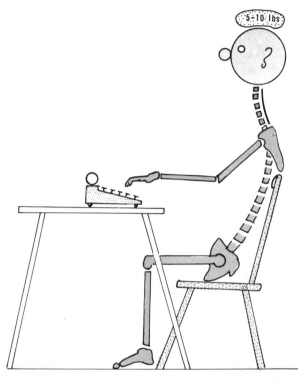

Figure 6–49. Distraction exercise for posture training. With a sandbag weighing 5 to 10 pounds on the head, erect posture is maintained, and cervical lordosis is minimal. The proprioceptive concept of posture is learned with no effort.

cluded temporomandibular disorders in the classification of atypical odontalgia (Table 6–1).[142]

The subdivisions of this classification relate principally to deviations of the disk which include perforation, elongation, and narrowing with or without associated pain (Fig. 6–50).

Pain may result from irritation of any of the tissues contained within the TMJ or the surrounding muscles that activate the joint motion. These muscle disorders are considered prominent in symptomatic TMJ syndrome and include those stated in Table 6–2. The innervation of the TMJ is the auriculotemporal nerve with contributions from the masseter and deep posterior temporal nerve branches of the third (mandibular) division of the trigeminal nerve (Figs. 6–51 and 6–52).

The TMJ is a diarthrodial synovial joint whose motions are delimited by the articular surfaces, the menisci, ligaments, capsules, and muscles. Because the TMJ syndrome may exist *without* organic joint disease or articular dysfunction, the condition is more appropriately termed **myofascial pain**

Table 6–1. TEMPOROMANDIBULAR DISORDERS

Deviation in form
Disk displacement with reduction
Disk displacement without reduction
Inflammation
Hypermobility
Osteoarthritis
Osteoarthropathy
Polyarthritides and connective tissue disorders
 Rheumatoid arthritis
 Psoriatic arthritis
 Ankylosing arthritis
 Systemic lupus erythematosus
 Scleroderma
Fibrous ankylosis
Bony ankylosis
Dislocation

dysfunctional syndrome of the temporomandibular articulation. This controversy refutes the allegation that TMJ syndrome is essentially a meniscal disorder. The meniscal disorder is probably secondary to muscular imbalance.

Within the joint, the cartilages of the glenoid fossa and menisci are fibrocartilagenous and so deform during joint motion (Figs. 6–53 and 6–54).

Pain resulting from TMJ syndrome usually occurs from faulty muscular action, although dental malocclusion can be cause or sequela. Whatever the etiologic mechanism when the articulation becomes deformed by either

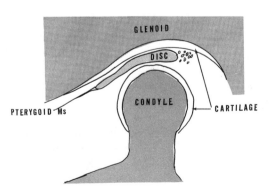

Figure 6–50. The temporomandibular joint. The concavity of the glenoid fossa differs from the convexity of the mandibular condyle by forming an incongruous joint that glides as well as rotates. Both are covered with cartilage that physiologically deforms during motion. The disk is fibrocartilaginous in structure and is held in an elongated manner by the pterygoid muscle. Behind the disk are blood vessels and lymphatic and connective tissues (*small circles*).

Table 6–2. MUSCLE DISORDERS

Myositis
Myofascial pain
Splinting/trismus
Contracture
Hypertrophy

meniscal deformation, tear or entrapment pain and limitation result. Meniscal or cartilage damage results in pain, crepitation, and limited range of motion.

Pain may be noted in the joint or the muscles, which means, intra-articular or extra-articular pain. The functional impairment may be a *locking*, subluxation-limited range from degenerative cartilage changes or capsular thickening.

Diagnosis is a clinical decision because radiologic changes are usually only noted in patients with advanced conditions. The muscle most often affected is the lateral (external) pterygoid; it becomes tender during palpation and the mandible becomes subluxed anteriorly (Fig. 6–55).

History is that of a nocturnal crepitation ("bruxism") with pain and tenderness over the joint and TMJ muscles. Range of motion is limited, both actively and passively (Fig. 6–56).

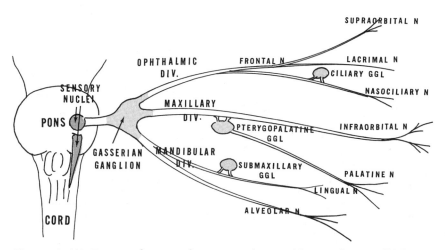

Figure 6–51. Trigeminal nerve. The trigeminal nerve (shown schematically) has its sensory portion within the gasserian ganglion where the peripheral branches synapse with nerves entering the cord via the pons. The trigeminal nerve branches into three major divisions: the ophthalmic, the maxillary, and the mandibular. The sensory areas supplied by the trigeminal nerve included the face and the anterior two thirds of the head (see Fig. 6–52).

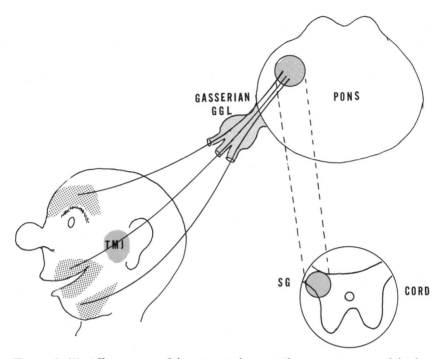

Figure 6–52. Afferent areas of the trigeminal nerve. The sensory regions of the face subserved by branches of the trigeminal nerve through the gasserian ganglion (GLL). These fibers ultimately enter the pons then transmit to the substantia gelatinosa (SG) in the cord gray matter.

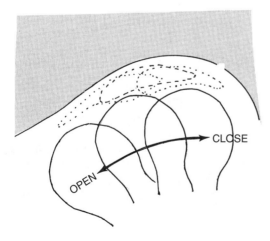

Figure 6–53. Deformation of the disk during jaw opening and closing. The disk deforms (*dotted figure*) rather than moves with the condyle as the jaw opens and closes. The layers of the disk are attached to the glenoid fossa and the condyle. The cartilage is not shown.

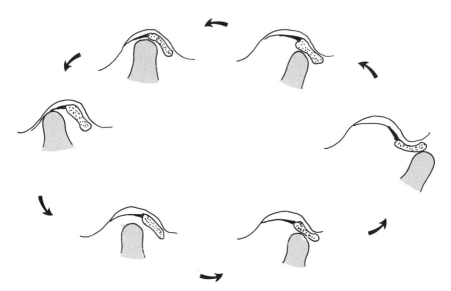

Figure 6–54. Deformation of the TMJ disk during jaw motion. The disk deforms during jaw opening and closing to accommodate the space of the articulation. The disk is held anteriorly by a filament extension of the pterygoid muscle (*dark line emanating from the anterior margin of the disk*). As shown by the *curved arrows*, the condyle glides anteriorly and posteriorly within the fossa during these actions.

Figure 6–55. Lateral (external) pterygoid muscle. The two divisions of the lateral pterygoid muscle lie deep to the zygomatic arch. The muscle originates from the infratemporal crest and the great wing of the sphenoid bone. It attaches to the neck of the condyle and the posterior superior aspect of the ramus of the mandible. Its action is principally protrusion and some lateral motion of the mandible. It has been found to be slightly active during opening of the jaw.

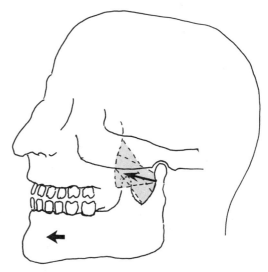

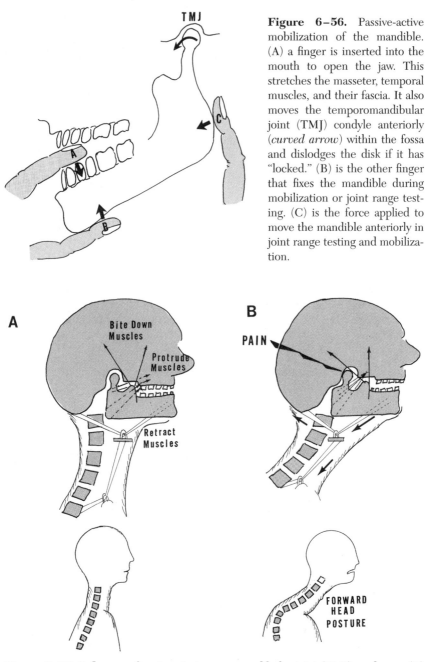

Figure 6–56. Passive-active mobilization of the mandible. (A) a finger is inserted into the mouth to open the jaw. This stretches the masseter, temporal muscles, and their fascia. It also moves the temporomandibular joint (TMJ) condyle anteriorly (*curved arrow*) within the fossa and dislodges the disk if it has "locked." (B) is the other finger that fixes the mandible during mobilization or joint range testing. (C) is the force applied to move the mandible anteriorly in joint range testing and mobilization.

Figure 6–57. Influence of posture in temporomandibular joint (TMJ) syndrome. (A) normal posture and its effect on the bite and TMJ alignment. (B) in the forward head posture the jaw becomes distracted by the hyoid muscles, which cause malignment of the TMJ joint structures.

Injuries to the TMJ have been associated with the cervical whiplash injury,[143-147] although most studies have been retrospective and not prospective. Contrary studies refute this relationship.[148,149] Regardless of the direct relationship of the cervical component and resultant muscular component of whiplash, a postulated concept may cast light on the mechanism (Fig. 6–57).

Management of TMJ syndrome can involve all modalities previously discussed in this text (see Chapter 4); the choice depends on the stage of the disease at which diagnosis is made. In the acute phase, various local measures are employed to relieve pain and muscular spasm; that is, ice, heat, massage, among others. Dental occlusal abnormalities must be addressed (Fig. 6–58) both for immediate relief and to prevent further dental abnormalities. Mobilization and manipulation may be indicated to relieve the *locked* meniscus (see Fig. 6–56), but ultimately the combined neuromusculoskeletal aspect of pain within the cervical spine needs to be addressed.

Many of these treatment modalities are discussed elsewhere in this text but they are emphasized with regard to TMJ in this chapter.

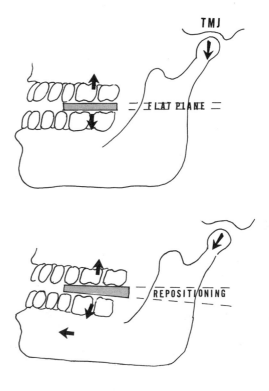

Figure 6–58. Orthosis to open mouth (principle). In the upper drawing the orthosis (splint) is flat planed to open the bite evenly, realign the teeth, and open the temporomandibular joint (TMJ). Besides aligning the teeth, it also overcomes muscular tension and contracture. The lower drawing shows an irregular orthosis to reposition the mandible causing forward movement (*straight arrow*) and opens the bite posteriorly (*curved arrows*).

Flexibility of the cervical spine must be regained by both active and passive exercises. The patient's posture (Fig. 6–59) must be studied and improved (Figs. 6–60 and 6–61). Ergonomics must be evaluated and modified (Figs. 6–62 and 6–63). Neck muscle strengthening exercises must also be initiated after the specific weakness has been determined (Figs. 6–64, 6–65, and 6–66).

Traction, which is a modality used frequently to alleviate cervical pain and

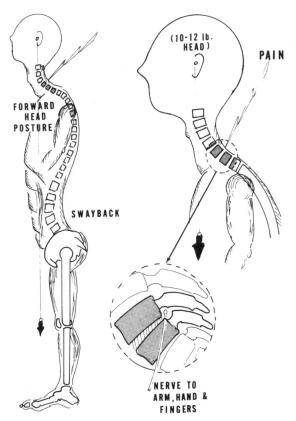

Figure 6–59. Forward head posture. The head normally should be in the direct alignment of the center of gravity from the meatus of the ear. In the forward head posture, the head is ahead of this center, which increases the cervical lordosis as well as the dorsal kyphosis. The foramena of the cervical spine are narrowed causing potential impingement of the nerve roots. The TMJ syndrome is enhanced. (From Cailliet, R: Head and Face Pain Syndromes, ed 1. FA Davis, Philadelphia, 1992, p 161, with permission.)

dysfunction, must be used carefully because most halters (Fig. 6–67) place pressure on the TMJ.

When psychologic tensions are considered to be a major factor in cervical tension or TMJ, appropriate medications, counseling, and stress-management interventions must be initiated.

Text continued on p. 232

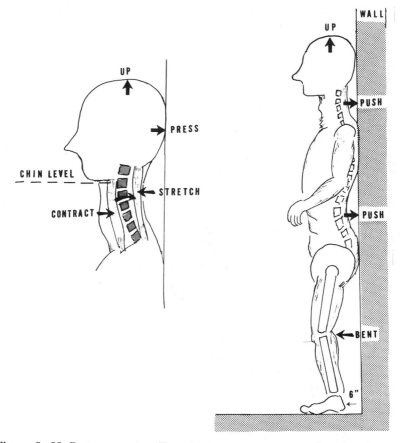

Figure 6–60. Posture exercises. To maintain an erect posture with proper alignments and normal cervical and lumbar curvatures, the person stands with feet several inches from a wall and the neck and low back pressed against the wall decreasing the lordosis. The concept of "standing tall" is also encouraged (*vertical arrow*). The neck flexor muscles must be contracted to decrease the lordosis. (From Cailliet, R: Head and Face Pain Syndromes, ed 1. FA Davis, Philadelphia, 1992, p 166, with permission.)

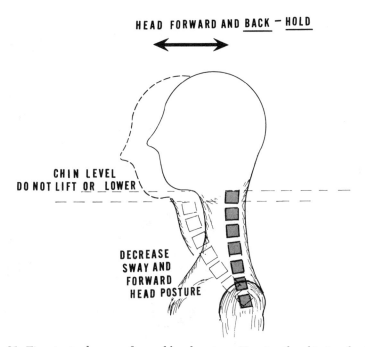

Figure 6–61. Exercise to decrease forward head posture. Keeping the chin in a horizontal line the head is pulled back and up, held there, then released. This decreases the lordosis, contracts the short neck flexors, and stretches the extensors. It also gives the feeling of proper posture. (From Cailliet, R and Gross, L: The Rejuvenation Strategy. Doubleday, New York, 1987, with permission.)

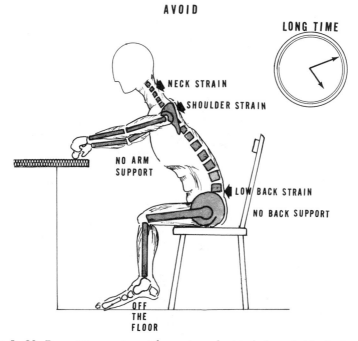

Figure 6–62. Poor sitting posture. The posture depicted above holds the head in a forward posture causing neck muscle strain especially when held for a long time. Brief, frequent breaks from this posture while performing the neck exercises is the remedy. (From Cailliet, R and Gross, L: The Rejuvenation Strategy. Doubleday, New York, 1987, with permission.)

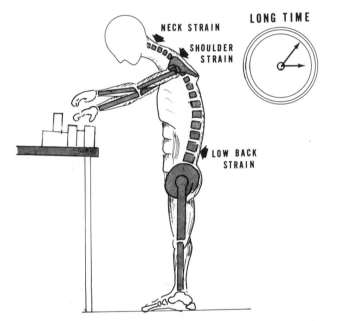

Figure 6–63. Poor standing posture. The posture depicted above holds the head forward, causing neck and upper back muscle strain, especially when held for long periods. Brief frequent breaks from this posture while performing the neck exercises is the remedy. (From Cailliet, R and Gross, L: The Rejuvenation Strategy. Doubleday, New York, 1987, with permission.)

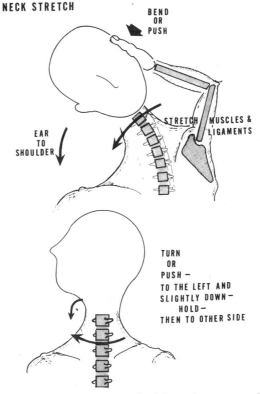

Figure 6–64. Neck exercises to increase flexibility. The exercise depicted is done actively by the person or done to the person by a therapist. This elongates the soft tissues: the muscle, fascia, ligaments, and joint capsules. (From Cailliet, R and Gross, L: The Rejuvenation Strategy. Doubleday, New York, 1987, with permission.)

NECK STRENGTHENING 1

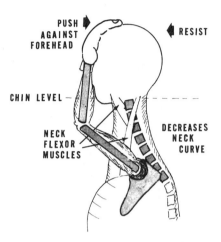

Figure 6–65. Neck exercises to increase strength. The exercise depicted is done actively by the person or done to the person by a therapist. The head is maintained with the chin horizontal and the resistance is increased as tolerated for strength and endurance. (From Cailliet, R and Gross, L: The Rejuvenation Strategy. Doubleday, New York, 1987, with permission.)

NECK STRENGTHENING 2

Figure 6–66. Neck exercises to increase strength. The exercise depicted is done actively by the person or done to the person by a therapist. The head is maintained with the chin horizontal and the resistance is increased as tolerated for strength and endurance. This exercise strengthens the lateral flexors. (From Cailliet, R and Gross, L: The Rejuvenation Strategy. Doubleday, New York, 1987, with permission.)

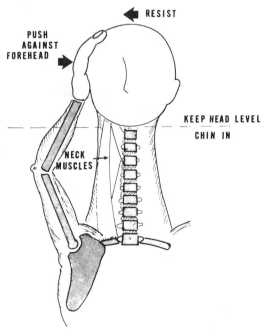

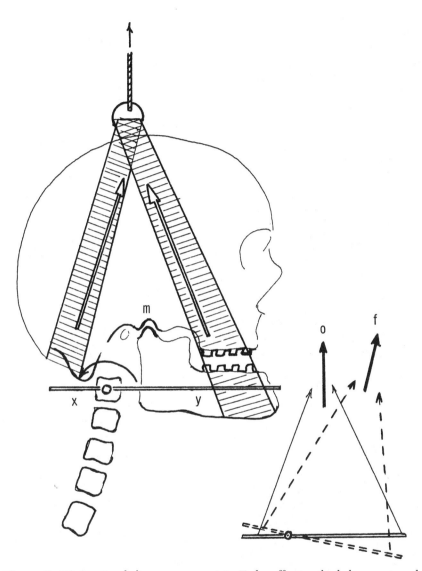

Figure 6–67. Traction halter pressure points. To be effective the halter must apply more pressure at the occiput (x) and less pressure at the chin (y). If the traction is applied incorrectly (o), it places pressure on the TMJ (m). If traction is properly applied (f), the pressure is on the occiput and is less on the mandible. (From Cailliet, R: Neck and Arm Pain, ed 3. FA Davis, Philadelphia, 1991, p 148, with permission.)

UPPER THORACIC PAIN

Although pain in the *upper back* is becoming more frequently seen, its etiology is usually misunderstood. Pain emanating from the thoracic spine is prevalent, but most upper back pains issue from soft tissue in the muscles and ligaments of the upper thorax.

Thoracic spine abnormalities have been minimized but more recently have been found to be wider in variation than expected.[150] Only 29% of asymptomatic patients had normal MRI scanning of the thoracic spine, whereas 60% of these asymptomatic patients were manifesting bulging or herniated thoracic disks, with 54% showing evidence of spinal cord indenture, with 24% showing frank disk herniations, and with 46% having annular tears. These authors concluded that disk herniations are part of the normal aging process of the spine. Of symptomatic patients, 12% had normal results on MRI scan.

Of the tissues in the functional units of the thoracic spine, the facets, so prevalent in the lumbar spine as the site of pain, were also found to be the site of pain in the thoracic spine.[151] In normal volunteers, injection of the thoracic facets is done under fluoroscopic vision. With distention of the articular capsule, there was *no* significant pain beyond a dull local *ache* with vague delineation and a pain perceived superior and inferior to the injected facet. This *vague* pain confirmed sensitivity of the facet capsule, but indicated a mild and vague non radicular distribution.

Recent orthopedic texts[150] even fail to mention thoracic spine pain and impairment, indicating upper thoracic pain is usually derived from paravertebral soft tissue. These are enumerated as thoracic paraspinal muscle syndromes[151] and are included as muscular trigger points.[152] The thoracic paraspinal muscles are long longitudinal muscles in numerous layers.[153]

Trigger points are usually activated and sustained by a overload wherein the muscles sustain an nonphysiologic contraction causing pain and limiting extensibility. Forceful activities such as lifting may be the initiating cause or more sedentary ones, such as prolonged postural activities such as computer use.

In examining patients with these muscular pain syndromes, the trigger points (TP) are located by manual palpation to determine which local pressure causes the pain. These muscular pains are discussed in Chapter 3 on myofascial pain.

REFERENCES

1. Cailliet, R: Neck and Arm Pain, ed 3. FA Davis, Philadelphia, 1991.
2. Cailliet, R: Neck and Upper Arm Pain. In Cailliet, R: Soft Tissue Pain and Disability, ed 2, FA Davis, Philadelphia, 1988, pp 123–169.

3. McKeever, FM: "Atlanto-axoid instability." Surg Clin North Am 48:1375–1390, 1968.
4. Rothman, RH and Simeone, FA: The Spine, vols 1 and 2. WB Saunders, Philadelphia, 1975.
5. Kopis, SE, Perovic, MN, McKusick, V, et al: Congenital atlantoaxial dislocations in various forms of dwarfism. J Bone Joint Surg 54A(6): 1349–1350, 1972.
6. Kapandji IA: The Physiology of Joints, vol 3, ed 2. Churchill Livingstone, Edinburgh, 1974.
7. Panjabi, MM and White, AA: Clinical Biomechanics of the Spine. JB Lippincott, Philadelphia, 1978.
8. Greenberg, AD: Atlanto-axial dislocations. Brain 91:655–684, 1968.
9. Epstein, BS: The Spine: A Radiological Text and Atlas, ed 4. Lea & Febiger, Philadelphia, 1976.
10. Macrae, DL: The significance of abnormalities of the cervical spine. Am J Roentgenology 84:8–25, 1968.
11. Perelson, HN: Occipital nerve tenderness: A sign of headache. South Med J 40:653–656, 1947.
12. Scott, M: Occipital neuralgia. Penn Med 71:85–88, 1968.
13. Ehni, G and Benner, B: Occipital neuralgia and the C1-C2 arthrosis syndrome. J Neurosurg 61:961–965, 1984.
14. Bogduk, N: The clinical anatomy of the cervical dorsal rami. Spine 7:319–330, 1982.
15. Saternus KD: Vertletzungen der Occipito-Atlanto-Axis-Region. Z Orthop Ihre Grenzgebiete 118:442–444, 1981.
16. Cailliet, R: Head and Face Pain. FA Davis, Philadelphia, 1994.
17. Bovim, G, Berg, R, and Dale, LG: Cervicogenic headache: Anesthetic blockades of cervical nerve (C2-C5) and facet joint (C2/C3). Pain 49:315–320, 1992.
18. Jackson, R: Headaches associated with disorders of the cervical spine. Headache 6:175–179, 1967.
19. Sheldon, KW: Headache patterns and cervical nerve root compression—a 15 year study of hospitalization for headache. Headache 6:180–188, 1967.
20. Dugan, MC, Locke, S, and Gallagher, JR: Occipital neuralgia in adolescents and young adults. N Engl J Med 267:1166–1172, 1962.
21. Ehni, G: Extradural spinal cord and nerve root compression from benign lesions of the cervical area. In Youmans, JR (ed): Neurological Surgery, ed 2, vol 4. Philadelphia, WB Saunders, 1982, pp 2574–2612.
22. Schneider, RC: Treatment of cervical spine disease. Cervical herniated nucleus pulposus, spondylitis, and stenosis. In Schneider, RC, Kahn, EA, Cosby, ED, et al (eds): Correlative Neurosurgery. Springfield, Ill, Charles C Thomas, 1982, pp 1094–1174.
23. Kerr, FWL: A mechanism to account for frontal headache in cases of posterior-fossa tumors. J Neurosurg 18:605–609, 1961.
24. Bogduk, N and Marsland, A: On the concept of third occipital headache. J Neurol Neurosurg Psychiatry 49:775–780, 1986.
25. Michler, RP, Bovim, G, and Sjaastad, O: Disorders in the lower cervical spine: A cause of unilateral headache? Headache 31:550–551, 1991.
26. MacNab, I: Acceleration injuries of the cervical spine. J Bone Joint Surg 46A:1797–1799, 1964.
27. Buonocore, E, Hartmen, T, and Nelson, CL: Cineradiograms of cervical spine in diagnosis of soft-tissue injuries. JAMA 198:25–29, 1966.
28. Longet, FA: Sur les troubles qui survient dans l'equilibration, la station et la locomotion des animaux, apres section des parties molles de la nuque. Gaz Med Paris 13:565–567, 1845. Cited in Biemond and De Jong (1969)
29. Bernard, C: An Introduction to the Study of Experimental Medicine. Collier Books, New York, 1961.
30. Weeks, VD and Travell, J: Postural vertigo due to trigger areas in the sternocleidomastoid muscle. J Pediatr 47:315–322, 1955.
31. Cope, S and Ryan, GMS: Cervical and otolith vertigo. J Laryngol Otol 73:113–120, 1959.

32. Gray, LP: Extra labyrinthine vertigo due to cervical muscle lesions. J Laryngol Otol 70:352–361, 1956.

33. Finneson, BE: Diagnosis and Management of Pain Syndromes. WB Saunders, Toronto, 1969.

34. Abraham, VC: Neck muscle proprioception and motor control, proprioception, posture, and emotion. In Garlick, D (ed): Postgraduate Medical Education. Univ So. Wales, 1982, pp 103–120.

35. Sherrington, CS: Decerebrate rigidity and reflex coordination of movements. J Physiol 22:319–332, 1897.

36. Magnus, R: Some results of studies in the physiology of posture (Cameron Prize Lectures). Lancet 211:531–536, 585–588, 1926.

37. Abraham, VC and Falchetto, S: Hind leg ataxia of cervical origin and cervico-lumbar interactions with supratentorial pathway. J Physiol 203:435–447, 1969.

38. Abraham, VC: The physiology of neck muscles: their role in head movement and maintenance of posture. Can J Physiol and Pharmacol 55:332–338, 1977.

39. Abrahams, VC: Sensory and motor specialization in some muscles of the neck. Trends Neurosci 1:24–27, 1981.

40. Richmond, FJR and Abrahams, VC: J Neurophys 42:604–617, 1979.

41. Dreyfuss, P, Michaelson, M, and Fletcher, D: Atlanto-Occipital and Lateral Atlanto-Axial Joint Pain Patterns. Spine 19:1125–1131, 1994.

42. Pang, LQ: The otological aspects of whiplash injuries. Laryngoscope 81:1381–1387, 1971.

43. Compere, WEJ: Electronystagmographic findings in patients with "whiplash" injuries. Laryngoscope 78:1226–1233, 1968.

44. Rubin, W: Whiplash with vestibular involvement. Arch Otolaryngol 97:85–87, 1973.

45. Toglia, JU, Rosenberg, PE and Ronis, ML: Vestibular and audiological aspects of whiplash injury and head trauma. J Forensic Sci 14:219–226, 1969.

46. Lord S, Barnsley L, and Bogduk N: Cervical zygapophyseal joint pain in whiplash. In (ed): Spine: State-of-the-Art Reviews. Cervical flexion-extension/whiplash injuries. Teasell, RW and Shapiro, AP (eds): Vol 7. Hanley & Belfus, Philadelphia, Sept 1993, pp 355–372.

47. Mclain, RF: Mechanoreceptor endings in human cervical facet joints. Spine 19:495–501, 1994.

48. Wyke, B: Articular neurology—a review. Physiotherapy 58:94–99, 1972.

49. Wyke, B and Molina, F: Articular reflexology of the cervical spine. Proceedings 6th International Congress Phys. Medicine, Barcelona, 1972: 61–66.

50. Liesi P, Gronblad M, Korkala O, et al: Substance P: A neuropeptide involved in low back pain. Lancet 1:1328–1329, 1983.

51. Gogia, PP and Sabbahi, MA: Electromyographic analysis of neck muscle fatigue in patients with osteoarthritis of the cervical spine. Spine 19:502–506, 1994.

52. Larsson, S-E, Alund, M, Cai, H, and Oberg, PA: Chronic pain after soft tissue injury of the cervical spine: Trapezius muscle blood flow and electromyography at static loads and fatigue. Pain 57:173–180, 1994.

53. Larsson, S-E, Cai, H, and Oberg, PA: Microcirculation in the upper trapezius muscle during varying levels of static contraction, fatigue and recovery in healthy women. A study using percutaneous laser-doppler flowmetry and surface electromyography. Eur J Appl Physiol 66:483–488, 1993.

54. Jull, G, Bogduk, N, and Marsland, A: The accuracy of manual diagnosis for cervical zygapophyseal joint pain syndrome. Med J Aust 148:233–236, 1988.

55. Bourdillon, JF: Spinal Manipulation, ed 3. London: Heinemann, London, 1982.

56. Grieve, GP: Common Vertebral Joint Problems. Edinburgh: Churchill Livingstone, Edinburgh, 1981.

57. Maitland, GD: Vertebral Manipulation, ed 4. Butterworth, London, 1977.

58. Stoddard, A: Manual of Osteopathic Technique. Hutchinson, London, 1983.

59. Maigne, R: Douleurs d'Origine Vertébrale et Traitements par Manipulation, ed 2. Expansion Scientifique, Paris, 1972.
60. Cailliet, R: Nerve control of the hand. In Cailliet, R: Hand Pain and Impairment, ed 4. FA Davis, Philadelphia, 1994, pp 69–131.
61. Aprill, C, Dwyer, A, and Bogduk, N: Cervical zygapophyseal joint pain patterns. II. A clinical evaluation. Spine 15:458–461, 1990.
62. Taylor, JR and Finch, PM: Neck sprain. Aust Fam Physician 22:1623–1629, 1993.
63. Bogduk, N and Marsland, A: The cervical zygapophysial joints as a source of neck pain. Spine 13:610–617, 1988.
64. Dwyer, A, Aprill, C, and Bogduk, N: Cervical zygapophyseal joint patterns I: A study in normal volunteers. Spine 15:453–457, 1990.
65. Aprill, C, Dwyer, A, and Bogduk, N: Cervical zygapophyseal pain patterns II: A clinical evaluation. Spine 15:458–461, 1988.
66. Davis, SJ, Teresi, LM, Bradley, WG, et al: Cervical spine hyperextension injuries: MR findings. Radiology 180:245–251, 1991.
67. Bogduk, N and Aprill, C: On the nature of neck pain, discography and cervical zygapophysial joint blocks. Pain 54:213–217, 1993.
68. Aprill, C and Bogduk, N: The prevalence of cervical zygapophyseal joint pain: A first approximation. Spine 17:744–747, 1992.
69. Cloward, RB: Cervical discography: A contribution to the etiology and mechanism of neck, shoulder, arm pain. Ann Surg 150:1052–1064, 1959.
70. McNab, I: Acceleration injuries of the cervical spine. J Bone Joint Surg 46A:1797–1798, 1964.
71. Jansen, J, Bardosi, A, Hildebrandt, J, and Lucke, A: Cervicogenic hemicranial attacks associated with vascular irritation or compensation of the nerve root C2. Pain 39:203–212, 1989.
72. Wilson, PR: Cervicogenic headache. APS Journal 1:259–264, 1992.
73. Edmeads, J: The cervical spine and headache. Neurology 38:1874–1878, 1988.
74. Kerr, FWL: Central relationships of trigeminal and cervical primary afferents in the spinal cord and medulla. Brain Res 43:561–572, 1972.
75. Bogduk, N and Marsland, A: On the concept of third occipital headache. J Neurol Neurosurg Psychiatry 49:775–780, 1986.
76. La Rocca, H: Cervical sprain syndrome: Diagnosis, treatment and long term outcome. In Frymoyer, JW (ed): The Adult Spine: Principles and Practice. Raven Press, New York, 1991, p 1051.
77. Janig, W: The sympathetic nervous system in pain: physiology and pathophysiology. In Stanton-Hicks, M (ed): Pain and Sympathetic Nervous System. Klumer Academic, Boston, 1990, p 17.
78. Goadsby, PJ, Jagami, AS, and Lambert, GA: Neural processing of craniovascular pain: A synthesis of the central structures in migraine. Headache 31:365–371, 1991.
79. Jensen, R, Rasmussen, BK, Pedersen, B, et al: Cephalic muscle tenderness and pressure pain threshold in a general population. Pain 48:197–203, 1992.
80. Schoenen, J, Bottin, D, Hardy, F, and Gerard, P: Cephalic and extracephalic pressure pain thresholds in chronic tension-type headache. Pain 47:145–149, 1991.
81. Gawel, MJ and Rothbart, PJ: Occipital nerve block in the management of headache and cervical pain. Cephalalgia 12:9–13, 1992.
82. Barnsley L, Lord S, and Bogduk N: 1. The Pathophysiology of Whiplash. Spine: State-of-the-Art Reviews, Hanley & Belfus, Philadelphia, September, 1993, pp 329–353.
83. Dvorak, J, Panjabi, MM, Gerber, M, and Wichman, W: CT-functional diagnostics of rotatory instability of upper cervical spine. I. An experimental study on cadavers. Spine 12:197–205, 1987.
84. Clemens, HJ and Burow, K: Experimental investigation of injury mechanisms of cervical spine at frontal and rear-frontal vehicle impacts. In Proceeding of the Sixteenth STAPP Car Crash Conference. Society of Automotive Engineers, Warrendale, 1972, pp 76–104.

85. Pintar FA, et al: Biomechanics of human spinal ligaments. In Sances A, et al: (eds): Mechanisms of Head and Spine Trauma. Aloray, Goshen, N.Y., 1986.
86. Gehweiler G, et al: The Radiology of Vertebral Trauma. JB Lippincott, Philadelphia, 1980.
87. Craig, JB and Hodgson, BF: Superior facet fractures of the axis vertebra. Spine 16:875–877, 1991.
88. Seletz, E: Whiplash injuries: Neurophysiological basis for pain and methods of rehabilitation. JAMA 168:1750–1755, 1958.
89. Dvorak, J, Hayek, J, and Zehnder, R: CT-functional diagnostics of rotatory instability of the upper cervical spine. Part 2. An evaluation on healthy adults and patients with suspected instability. Spine 12:726–731, 1987.
90. Abel, MS: Occult traumatic lesions of the cervical vertebrae. Crit Rev Clin Radiol Nucl Med. 6:469–553, 1975.
91. La Rocca, H: Acceleration injuries of the neck. Clin Neurosurg 25:209–217, 1978.
92. Ommaya, AK, Faas, F, and Yarnell, P: Whiplash injury and brain damage: An experimental study. JAMA 204:285–289, 1968.
93. Sano, K, Nakamura, N, Hirakawa, K, and Hashizume, K: Correlative studies of dynamics and pathology of whip-lash and head injuries. Scand J Rehabil Med 4:47–54, 1972.
94. Wickstrom, J, Martinez, J and Rodriquez, R, Jr: The cervical sprain syndrome: Experimental acceleration injuries to the head and neck. In Selzer, ML, Gikas, PW, and Huelke, DF (eds): The Prevention of Highway Injury. Highway Safety Research Institute, Ann Arbor, Mich., 1967, pp 182–187.
95. Bogduk, N: Innervation and pain patterns in the cervical spine. Clin Phys Ther 17:1–13, 1988.
96. Cammack, KV: Whiplash injuries to the neck. Am J Surg 93:663–666, 1957.
97. Gay, JR and Abbott, KH: Common whiplash injuries to the neck. JAMA 152:1698–1704, 1953.
98. Ehni, G and Benner, B: Occipital neuralgia and the C1-2 arthrosis syndrome. J Neurosurg 61:961–965, 1984.
99. McCormick, C: Arthrography of the atlanto-axial (C1-C2) joints: Techniques and results. J Intervent Radiol 2:9–13, 1987.
100. Hidingsson, C, Wenngren, BI, Bring, G, and Toolanen, G: Oculomotor problems after cervical spine injuries. Acta Orthop Scand 60:513–516, 1989.
101. Bring, G and Westman, G: Chronic posttraumatic syndrome after whiplash injury. A pilot study of 22 patients. Scand J Prim Health Care 9:135–141, 1991.
102. Dvorak, J, Valach, L, and Schmid, S: Cervical spine injuries in Switzerland. J Man Med 4:7–16, 1989.
103. Norris, SH and Watt, I: The prognosis of neck injuries resulting from rear-end vehicle collisions. J Bone Joint Surg Br 65:608–611, 1983.
104. Pearce, JM: Whiplash injury: A reappraisal. J Neurol Neurosurg Psychiatry 52:1329–1331, 1989.
105. Pennie, B and Agambar, L: Patterns of injury and recovery in whiplash. Injury 22:57–59, 1991.
106. Chester, JB, Jr: Whiplash, postural control and inner ear. Spine 16:716–720, 1991.
107. Grimm, RJ, Henenway, WG, Lebray, PR, and Black, FO: The perilymph fistula syndrome defined in mild head trauma. Acta Otolaryngol Stockh 464(suppl):1–40, 1989.
108. Kischka, U, Ettlin, T, Heim, S, and Schmid, G: Cerebral symptoms following whiplash injury. Eur Neurol 31:136–140, 1991.
109. Anderson, JM, Kaplan, MS, and Felsenthal, G: Brain injury obscured by chronic pain: A preliminary report. Arch Phys Med Rehabil 71:703–708, 1990.
110. Olsnes, BT: Neurobehavioral findings in whiplash patients with long-lasting symptoms. Acta Neurol Scand 80:584–588, 1989.
111. Torres, F and Shapiro, SK: Electroencephalograms in whiplash injury. Arch Neurol 5:28–35, 1961.

112. Capistrant, TD: Thoracic outlet syndrome in whiplash injury. Ann Surg 185:175–178, 1977.
113. Capistrant, TD: Thoracic outlet syndrome in cervical strain injury. Minn Med 69:13–17, 1986.
114. Shimizu, T, Shimada, H, and Shirakura, K: Scapulohumeral Reflex (Shimizu). Spine 18:2182–2190, 1993.
115. Wartenberg, R: The examination of reflexes. New Book Publishers, Chicago, 1945.
116. Stover, SL and Fine, PR (eds): Spinal cord injuries: facts and figures. University of Alabama Press, Birmingham, 1986.
117. Bonica, JJ: Introduction: Semantic, Epidemiologic, and Educational Issues. In Casey, KL (ed): Pain and Central Nervous Disease: The Central Pain Syndromes. Raven Press, New York, 1991, pp 13–29.
118. Britell, CW and Mariano, AJ: Chronic pain in spinal cord injury. In Walsh, NE (ed.): Physical Medicine and Rehabilitation: State of the Art Reviews—Rehabilitation of Patients with Chronic Pain, vol 5. Henley & Belfus, Philadelphia, 1990, pp 23–34.
119. Davidoff, G, Roth, E, Guarracini, M, et al: Function-limiting dysesthetic pain syndrome among traumatic spinal cord injury patient: a cross sectional study. Pain 29:39–48, 1987.
120. Cailliet, R: Reflex Sympathetic Dystrophy. In Cailliet, R. Pain: Mechanisms and Management, ed 1. FA Davis, Philadelphia, 1993, pp 29–49.
121. Tasker, RR and Dostrovsky, JO: Deafferentiation and central pain. In: Wall, PD and Melzack, R (eds.): Textbook of Pain, ed 2. Churchill Livingstone, Edinburgh, 1989, pp 154–180.
122. Tasker, RR, de Carvalho, G, and Dostrovsky, JO: The history of central pain syndromes, with observations concerning pathophysiology and treatment. In Casey, KL (ed): Pain and Central Nervous System Disease: The Central Pain Syndromes, Raven Press, New York, 1991, pp 31–58.
123. Cassinari, V and Pagni, CA: Central Pain: A Neurosurgical Survey. Harvard University Press, Cambridge, 1969.
124. Pagnii, CA: Central pain due to spinal cord and brain stem damage. In Wall, PD and Melzack, R (eds.): Textbook of Pain, ed 1. Churchill Livingstone, Edinburgh, 1984, pp 481–495.
125. Cailliet, R: Pain: Mechanisms and Management, ed 1, FA Davis, Philadelphia, 1994.
126. Mealy, K, Brennan, H, and Fenelon, GC: Early mobilization of acute whiplash injuries. Br Med J 292:656–657, 1986.
127. DeSeze, S and Levernieux, J: Les tractions vertebrales: Premieres études experimentales et resultats therapeutique d'apres une experience de quatres années. Semaines des Hôpitaux (de Paris) 27:2085–2104, 1951.
128. McKinney, LA, Dornan, JO, and Ryan, M: The role of physiotherapy in the management of acute neck sprains following road-traffic accidents. Arch Emerg Med 6:27–33, 1989.
129. Crue, BJ: Importance of flexion in cervical traction for radiculitis. USAF Med J 8:375–380, 1957.
130. Colachis, SC and Strohm, BR: Cervical traction: Relationship of traction time to varied tractive force with constant angle of pull. Arch Phys Med Rehabil 46:815–819, 1965.
131. Teasell, RW, Shapiro, AP, and Mailis, A: Medical management of whiplash injuries: An overview. Spine: State-of-the-Art Reviews, 7:481–499, 1993.
132. Maigne, R: Orthopedic Medicine. Charles C Thomas, Springfield, Ill, 1973.
133. Francis, KT: The role of endorphins in exercise: A review of current knowledge. Journal of Orthopedic and Sports Therapy 4:169–173, 1983.
134. Fordyce, WE: Exercise and the increase in activity level. In (ed.): Behavioral Methods for Chronic Pain and Illness. CV Mosby, St. Louis, 1976, pp 168–183.
135. Barnsley, L: Common whiplash treatment discredited. Backletter 9:49–50, 1994.
136. Bogduk, N and Aprill, C: On the nature of neck pain, discography and cervical zygapophyseal joint blocks. Pain 54:213–217, 1993.
137. Bogduk, N: Are diagnostic tests for neck pain useless? Backletter 9:51, 1994.

138. Jette, AM: Inconsistency in physical therapy. Backletter 9:49–52, 1994.
139. Costen, JB: A syndrome of ear and sinus problems dependent on disturbed function of the temporomandibular joint. Ann Otol 43:1–15, 1934.
140. Cailliet, R: Temporomandibular joint pain. In Cailliet, R: Head and Face Pain Syndromes. FA Davis, Philadelphia, 1992.
141. Classification and diagnostic criteria for headache disorders: Cranial neuralgias and facial pain. Cephalalgia 8(Suppl 7):1–96, 1988.
142. Frankel, VH: Temporomandibular joint pain syndrome following deceleration injury to the cervical spine. Bull Hosp Joint Dis 26:47–51, 1965.
143. Frankel, VH: Pathomechanics of whiplash injuries to the neck. In Morley, TP (ed.) Current Controversies in Neurosurgery. WB Saunders, Philadelphia, 1976, pp 39–50.
144. Roydhouse, RH: Whiplash and temporomandibular dysfunction. Lancet 1:1394–1395, 1973.
145. Epstein, JB: Temporomandibular disorders, facial pain and headache following motor vehicle accidents. J Can Dent Assoc 58:488–495, 1992.
146. Brooke, RI and Lapoint, HJ: Temporomandibular joint disorders following whiplash. Spine: State-of-the-Art Reviews, 7:443–454, 1993.
147. Garvey, T: Thoracic spine abnormalities. Backletter 9:1–7, 1994.
148. Dreyfuss, P, Tibiletti, C, and Dreyer, SJ: Thoracic zygapophyseal joint pain patterns: A study in normal volunteers. Spine 19:807–811, 1994.
149. Mayer, TG, Mooney, V, and Gatchel, RJ: Contemporary Conservative Care for Painful Spinal Disorders. Lea & Febiger, Philadelphia, 1991.
150. Bonica, JJ and Sola, AF: Chest pain caused by other disorders. In Bonica, JJ (ed.): The Management of Pain, ed 2. Lea & Febiger, Philadelphia, 1990, pp 1133–1135.
151. Travell, JG and Simons, DG: Myofascial Pain and Dysfunction. The Trigger Point Manual. Williams & Wilkins, Baltimore, 1983.

CHAPTER 7

Neurovascular Compression Syndromes

THORACIC OUTLET SYNDROME

Diagnosis of *thoracic outlet syndrome* (TOS) pervades the literature yet remains a poorly understood, based mainly of subjectivity, but very few objective confirmatory signs. The term was first used by Peet and colleagues, in 1956,[1] although the syndrome was described by Adson and Coffee in 1927.[2] The costoclavicular syndrome was described by Falconer and Wedell in 1943,[3] and the hyperabduction syndrome by Wright in 1945.[4] The individual compression syndromes will be discussed, but the generalized term **thoracic outlet syndrome** includes those syndromes which could be caused by neurovascular compression within the thoracic outlet.

The anatomic outlet is located between the first rib, the clavicle, and the scalene muscles. The brachial plexus and the subclavian artery pass between the anterior and medial scalene muscles, the first rib, and the overlying clavicle (Fig. 7–1). This neurovascular bundle progresses downward and passes under the pectoralis minor.

The three scalene muscles originate from the transverse processes of the cervical vertebrae and insert on the first and second ribs (Fig. 7–2).

Because many anatomic structures can impair free passage, TOS has previously been termed **scalene anticus syndrome, cervicodorsal outlet syndrome, hyperabduction syndrome, cervical rib syndrome, clavicocostal syndrome,** and **pectoralis minor syndrome.**

The neural segment of the neurovascular component of TOS implies compression of the brachial plexus (Figs. 7–3 and 7–4) and the subclavian artery (Fig. 7–5).

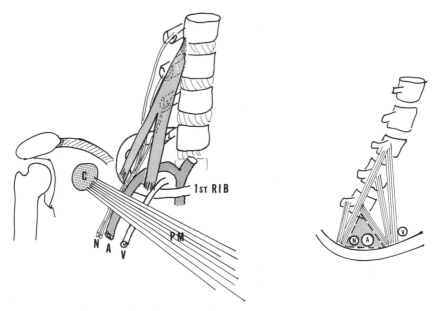

Figure 7–1. The supraclavicular space. The scalene muscles originate from the cervical spine and divide to contain the brachial plexus (N) and the subclavian artery (A). The middle scalene muscle is posterior and the anterior scalene is anterior to the artery. The subclavian vein (V) is anterior to the anterior scalene muscle. After passing over the first rib (not shown) the neurovascular bundle passes under the smaller pectoral muscle (PM). The clavicle covers the neurovascular bundle and lays parallel to the first rib. The coracoid process (C) is the site of attachment of the pectoral muscle.

Symptoms and Signs

Classic TOS originally manifested symptoms from subclavian blood vessels and the lower trunk of the brachial plexus C8-T1 roots. Pain and paresthesias usually appear in the latter dermatomal areas. Pain is generally aggravated, if not initiated, by activities that close the thoracic outlet or place traction on the brachial plexus, for example, carrying heavy objects, working with overhead arm activities or repeating certain physical activities of the arms, which allegedly close the outlet. Cold weather exacerbates the symptoms, as does prolonged severe emotional tension, which affects the structural compressive factors.

Causes of brachial plexus lesions have included:

1. Traumatic, including penetrating lesions
2. Compressive, including mechanical, developmental, or congenital factors

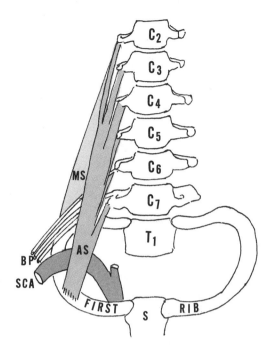

Figure 7–2. Scalene muscles. The anterior (AS) and medial (MS) scalene muscles originate from the transverse processes of the cervical vertebrae (C2, C3, C4, C5, C6, C7, and T1). Both scalenes insert on the first rib. A "tunnel" is formed where the scalenes divide to permit the passage of the brachial plexus (BP) and the subclavian artery (SCA). S is the sternum.

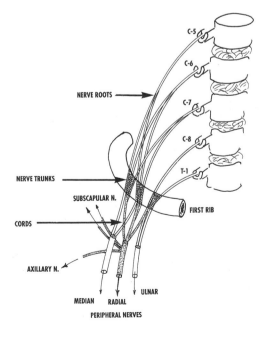

Figure 7–3. Schematic presentation of the brachial plexus. The brachial plexus is composed of the anterior primary rami of roots C5, C6, C7, C8, and T1. The roots emerge from the intervertebral foramen through the scalene muscles. The roots merge into three trunks in the region of the first rib. The trunks become cords via these divisions then divide into peripheral nerves of the upper extremity.

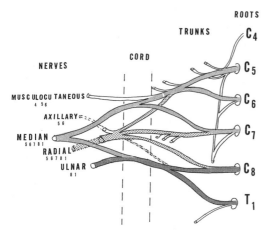

Figure 7–4. Divisions of the roots into the brachial plexus then peripheral nerves.

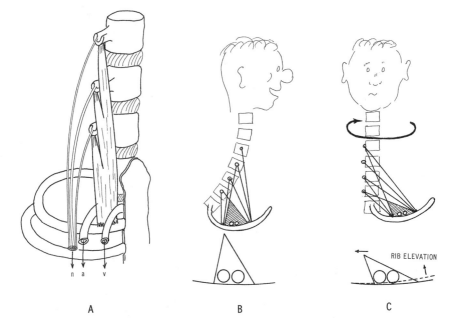

A   B   C

Figure 7–5. Scalene anticus syndrome. (*A*) Relationship of the neurovascular bundle. The subclavian artery (a) passes behind the anterior scalene muscle, loops over the first rib, and is joined by the brachial plexus (n). The artery is separated from the subclavian vein (v) by the anterior scalene muscle. The median scalene muscle (not shown) lies behind the nerve (n). (*B*) The triangle formed by the scalenes and the first rib is depicted. (*C*) As the head turns toward the symptomatic side the triangle deforms and compresses its contents. Deep inspiration elevates the first rib (*dotted line*), which further compresses the bundle.

3. Vascular, including local vascular disease, arteritis, postirradiation fibrosis
4. Infectious, including local abscess
5. Neoplastic lesions, including primary tumors and Pancoast's tumor
6. Miscellaneous, including electrical shock
7. Idiopathic[5]

Many of the above can be understood as compressive forces, but in idiopathic TOS, which is an element of many other clinical syndromes, often no direct causative factor is elicited. Many lesions have been implicated such as that of the cervical rib (extension of the transverse process of lower cervical vertebra), abnormal insertion of the scalene muscles, hypertrophy of both the scalene muscle and bands of Sibson's fascia, yet all of these may be present independently of symptoms. Compression of the brachial plexus may also occur without the characteristic signs and symptoms occurring.

Pain is usually aggravated or initiated by physical activities that compress the outlet. Such pain is usually within a dermatomal pattern (Fig. 7–6), although some patients complain of a vague deep ache in the upper extremity without precise neurologic pattern.

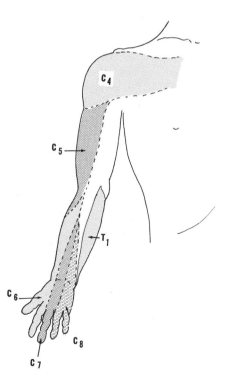

Figure 7–6. Dermatomal areas of the upper extremity. This presents a sensory map of the arm supplied by the cervical nerves C4-T1.

Motor impairment, either subjective or objective, is most common in the intrinsic muscles of the hand. Vasomotor changes are often visualized, but not always characterized by vascular insufficiency. This phenomenon implies that vasomotor symptoms result from involvement of the sympathetic nerve fibers that accompany the blood vessels and not necessarily from mechanical compression of the vessels.

Diagnosis relies primarily on reproducing the symptoms with or without evidence of vascular compression. Inspection and palpation of the supraclavicular space may reveal a fullness or tenderness of the neural structures.

A *positive* Adson test (Fig. 7–7) has been regarded as diagnostic for TOS. The Adson test checks for disappearance of the radial pulse when the patient rotates the head toward the affected side and simultaneously holds a deep inspired breath. The arm may be hanging, elevated, posteriorly flexed, or abducted. The pulse at the wrist is taken during the entire procedure; resultant symptoms are requested of the patient. Because this test measures thoracic outlet closure primarily from the scalene muscles, it tests the *scalene syndrome*. Mere rotation of the head alone does not cause strong tension of the scalene muscles.[6]

Validity of the initial Adson test was questioned because it appeared that the pulse was obliterated when the patient turned the head *away* from the side evincing symptoms.[7,8]

A recent article questioned the pathomechanics of this test, because the test does not take into account hemodynamic changes resulting from deep inspired breath alone.[9] Laser Doppler flowmeter tests were given while performing the test in patients with clinical TOS.[10,11] Using Doppler methods to test circulation in the upper extremity, the blood flow decreases temporarily during deep breathing with return to baseline resulting from neural reflexes.

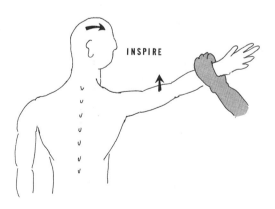

INSPIRE

Figure 7–7. Adson's test. The arm may be held in the dependent position at the side or abducted to 90°. The radial pulse is palpated (*shaded hand of the examiner*). The arm is posteriorly flexed. The patient turns the head toward the tested side and a deep breath is initiated and held to tolerance. The head may also be rotated away from the tested side. A positive test reproduces the symptoms of pain or paresthesia and the pulse is obliterated.

Deep breathing elevates intrathoracic pressure and stimulates the parasympathetic nerves that in turn reduces venous return and cardiac output. These nerve reflexes also decrease the blood flow through the upper extremities.

Obliteration of the radial pulse alone from this maneuver is not diagnostic without reproduction of symptoms, because obliteration occurs in many asymptomatic people.[12] Despite significant anatomic factors considered pertinent to thoracic outlet constriction during the vascular flow tested by the Doppler method,[5] the changes were not significant, nor was body position pertinent. Such test findings indicate a high risk of false positive tests in diagnosing TOS using only the Adson test.

The cause of upper extremity pain varies depending on whether the pain is referred from the cervical spine, or emanates from local lesions.[13] Clinical tests do not distinguish many possible etiologies, for instance cervical distraction,[14] cervical compression,[14] Adson test, upper limb hyperabduction, shoulder abduction,[15] or Lasegue test for the neck.[16] Shoulder abduction and elbow extension produce tension in the short head of the biceps brachii.[17]

To identify arm pain emanating specifically from tension of the brachial plexus, a brachial plexus tension test (BPTT) has been postulated.[18,19] This BPTT strains the brachial (Fig. 7–8) plexus by combining passive shoulder depression, shoulder abduction posterior to the coronal plane, external rotation of the shoulder, elbow extension, forearm supination, and wrist and finger extension. The test is performed with the cervical spine in ipsilateral flexion and with the cervical spine in contralateral flexion. This latter cervical position (CFL) places more tension on the brachial plexus. Pain is elicited from extracervical brachial plexus tension more quickly than with CFL. The BPTT

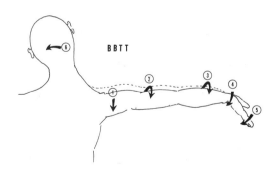

Figure 7–8. Brachial plexus traction test (BPTT). If there is extraspinal inflammation of the brachial plexus the BPTT test confirms its presence. The test is performed in steps: (1) From the neutral position, arm dependent, the shoulder is depressed. The shoulder is then abducted; (2) the upper arm is then externally rotated; (3) the elbow is extended and the forearm supinated; (4) the wrist is extended; (5) the fingers are extended; (6) the head is laterally flexed, first toward the arm then away. A positive BPTT causes the sensation of discomfort in the forearm and in the radial aspect of the hand, thumb, and middle three fingers.

closely resembles the Adson maneuver, indeed without deep inspiration, it is identical.

The BPTT produces tension on the roots of the plexus at the C5, C6, and T1 nerve roots.[20,21] BPTT in asymptomatic patients produced stretch discomfort in the anterior and radial aspects of the forearm, and the radial aspect of the hand, thumb, and middle fingers.[22,23] This further confuses a clear interpretation of pathologic tension signs, as well as patients with TOS, but BPTT does delineate arm pain originating from more proximal nerve tissues.

Radiologic diagnosis also remains vague because revelation of the presence of a cervical rib or abnormality of the first thoracic rib implies but does not confirm an etiology.

Confirmatory diagnostic procedures have emerged. Electromyographic (EMG) conduction studies of the ulnar, median, radial, and musculocutaneous nerves from *above the clavicle* compare those measurements with others distal to the clavicle to reveal a delayed conduction time when the arm is abducted and elevated.[24]

ANTERIOR SCALENE SYNDROME

The brachial plexus and subclavian artery can be compressed as they pass between the anterior and medial scalene muscles, both of which insert on respective tubercles of the first rib (see Fig. 7–2). The posterior scalene inserts upon the second rib. The scalene muscles raise the first rib during deep inspiration. Unilateral rotation of the head turns the face in the opposite direction, that is, turning the head to the right employs the left scalene muscles. Bilateral contraction of the scalene muscles flexes the cervical spine.

The *scalene foramen* is formed by the anterior and medial scalene muscles, the first rib, and the sternocleidomastoid muscle. This space admits the neurovascular bundle; it is approximately 0.4 to 3.5 cm wide.[25] The subclavian artery bends and extends through a sulcus in the first rib.

The anterior scalene syndrome is also termed **cervical rib syndrome.**[26–31] Normally the space (tunnel) is adequate to allow the passage without neurovascular encroachment. Postural abnormalities have been implicated in increasing the tension of the bundle as it passes over the first rib.

The human thorax has its greatest diameter during lateral dimension. Thoracic abnormality increases the tension upon the neurovascular bundle.[32] Poor posture manifested in dorsal kyphotic abnormalities causes downward anterior rotation of the shoulder and increases the distance that the neurovascular bundle must travel.

It is conceivable, although not yet confirmed that prolonged abnormal posture causes hypertrophy of the scalene muscles,[33,34] which causes a narrowing of the thoracic outlet.

Symptoms and Signs

Pain in the fingers, hand, and forearm and possibly the shoulder are frequent findings. Paresthesia and hyperesthesia (numbness and tingling) occur in the dermatomal distribution of the eighth cervical and first thoracic nerve roots. Depending on the degree of vascular compression, there may be sensations of coldness and weakness and objective confirmation of skin color changes.

The examination may reveal paresis and slight atrophy of the hypothenar and interosseous muscles.[35]

The *specific* diagnosis makes incumbent a *positive* Adson sign. The usual sign requires obliteration of the radial pulse and reproduction of the symptoms with the arm abducted (either elevated above heart level when termed the **signe de plateau** by the French), or below that level, with the neck extended and the head turned toward the side being tested, when deep inspiration is simultaneously requested of the patient (see Fig. 7–6). The pulse returns rapidly when performing this test in a normal person, but more slowly in one whose test results are positive. Hypertrophied or taut scalene muscles may be palpated in the supraclavicular fossa and compared with the opposite side.

Treatment

Conservative therapy of TOS should be administered for an extended period before more drastic measures such as arteriography, venography, or surgical exploration are considered. Such conservative measures include improvement in posture,[36] modification of those work-related postural habits that cause prolonged dorsal kyphosis, or those that require prolonged carrying of heavy objects with the arms extended at the side. The scapular muscles must be strengthened (Figs. 7–9 and 7–10). This reinforcement is done both standing and sitting—it increases strength and endurance. With weight being borne gradually the shoulders are slowly elevated and lowered with increasing frequency of lifts. Standing and sitting lifts are preferably done using a proper posture to avoid a head forward position.[36]

If it is determined that the scalene muscles and their fascia are thickened, they can be lengthened with cervical traction done manually by a therapist initially and ultimately by a machine. This treatment is essentially what is advocated in treating cervical discogenic disease.

In the presence of a cervical rib, a damaged or deformed clavicle, or a congenital defective scalene muscle that proves to be a mechanical factor in disease resulting from TOS, surgical correction is indicated. Abnormal elongation of the lower cervical transverse process termed **cervical rib** was originally considered to be a likely cause but because it was present from birth without symptoms, it is now being questioned as being solely responsible for

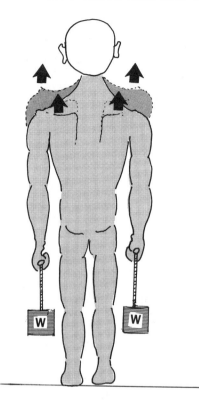

Figure 7–9. Scapular elevation exercise. With proper posture both arms are elevated at the shoulder blade, held, and slowly lowered. Increasing weights (W) are used and the elbows must be held extended.

this syndrome. At present, neither the ideal surgical procedure nor the best time for intervention has been uniformly accepted.[37,38]

COSTOCLAVICULAR SYNDROME

A variant of TOS is the **costoclavicular syndrome** in which the neurovascular bundle is compressed between the clavicle and the first rib.[39] The triangular costoclavicular space has the following boundaries: anteriorly, the medial portion of the clavicle and the subclavius muscle; posteriorly and medially, the anterior third of the first rib into which insert the scalene muscles.

When the costoclavicular space narrows, neurovascular tissues are compromised. The narrowing can result from congenital abnormalities of any of these tissues. Raising one's arm overhead rotates the clavicle posteriorly, thus causing a possible mechanical narrowing resulting from curvature of the clavicle. Deep inspiration elevates the first rib and completes the narrowing.

The test diagnostic for costoclavicular neurovascular compression is to place the patient in an exaggeratedly military stance with shoulders held back

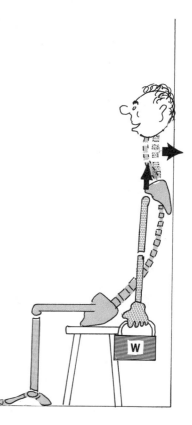

Figure 7–10. Scapular elevation exercise and seated posture training. Patient is seated on a stool with back and head to the wall. The cervical lordosis is diminished by pressing neck to the wall. In this position the extended arms holding weights (W) are slowly elevated and circumducted.

and then, having the patient take and hold a deep breath, the patient's shoulders are forced downward manually.

Symptoms and Signs

Largely similar to those seen with scalene syndrome; the paresthesia and hyperesthesia are present in the lower dermatomal areas of C8-T1. Venous compression may lead to transient or permanent edema. When symptoms are prominent, venography may identify the situation.[39]

Treatment

Treatment is as given with the scalene syndrome but when pain persists, surgical relief may be had from removal of a pseudoarthrosis of the clavicle, an exhuberant callous from a previous fracture, or even removal of the first rib.

HYPERABDUCTION SYNDROME

Prolonged repetitive hyperabduction of the arm may cause compression of the neurovascular bundle under the pectoralis minor muscle (Fig. 7–11). Symptoms are similar to those seen with the scalene syndrome, but in this syndrome, they are reproduced by hyperabduction of the arms to an overhead position of 180°.

Leaving the supraclavicular space, the neurovascular bundle (brachial plexus, subclavian artery, and subclavian vein) pass under the pectoralis minor muscle, which attaches to the coracoid process. As the arm is elevated overhead, the bundle is stretched around the fulcrum of the pectoralis minor tendon, the coracoid process, and against the humeral head.[32] Overhead arm elevation concurrently elevates the clavicle and narrows the costoclavicular fossa.

Treatment

Treatment of this syndrome is essentially having the patient avoid hyperabduction, thus requiring a change in the workplace or occupational habits. Persistence of symptoms may require resection of the pectoralis minor tendon.

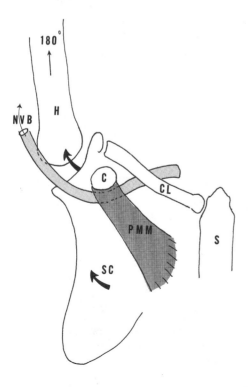

Figure 7–11. Hyperabduction syndrome. As the humerus (H) in the arm elevates overhead to 180° the scapula (SC) externally rotates (*curved arrow*) about the acromioclavicular joint (clavicle) (CL) thus also rotating the coracoid process (C). Tension is placed on the pectoralis minor muscle (PMM), which mechanically compresses the neurovascular bundle (NVB). S is the sternum. The ribs have not been drawn.

BRACHIAL PLEXUS INJURIES

Besides the compression syndrome already discussed, injuries to the brachial plexus are common and difficult to diagnose because the complex anatomy involved. These injuries require proper diagnosis (neuropraxia, axonotmesis, neuromesis are possible signs) must be made to determine treatment and prognosis. (See the discussion of nerve regeneration in Chapter 1.)

The fascial attachments of the plexus between the cervical roots and the axilla render it vulnerable to injury at fixed points along its course (Fig. 7–12). Brachial plexus lesions can be classified as supraclavicular or infraclavicular.[40]

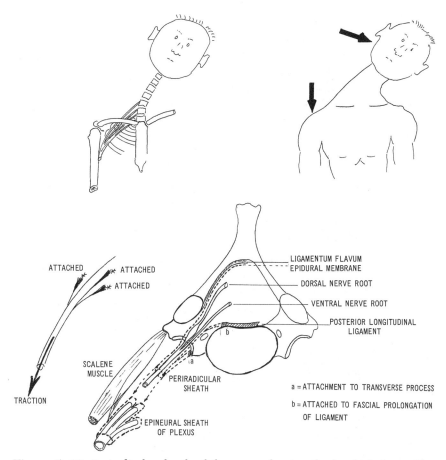

Figure 7–12. Periradicular sheath of the nerves forming the brachial plexus. The epidural membrane of the spinal canal continues along the nerve roots through the foramena to form the periradicular sheath. This continues downward to form the epidural sheath of the plexus. The scalene muscles attach to the brachial plexus.

The former have a guarded prognosis, whereas with the latter, up to 90% recover function.

The brachial plexus receives contribution from five nerve roots: C5, C6, C7, C8, and T1. Some anatomists have also claimed roots from C3 and C4.[41] The plexus passes under the clavicle at the level of the cords (Fig. 7–13), thus injury to the supraclavicular portion of the plexus involves the nerve portion before the cords. Injury at or below the level of the clavicle involves the plexus at the level of or below the cords.

Although three trunks are formed from the five roots, only the C7 root forms the middle trunk. Each trunk separates into anterior and posterior divisions (see dotted lines in Fig. 7–12). Two major nerves do not enter trunks; the dorsal scapular and long thoracic, which originate from C5 and C6 and are purely motor; the former to the levator scapula and rhomboids and the latter to the serratus anterior. Injury to these nerves cause a "winging" of the scapula. The suprascapular nerve which originates at Erb's point in the upper trunk (C5, C6) supplies the supraspinatus and infraspinatus muscles.

Traction injuries are most ominous to the brachial plexus because they damage the neurolemmal sheaths which repair themselves by scarring and thus injure intraneural blood vessels. Supraclavicular injuries are further divided into those involving preganglionic and postganglionic sites. The former are proximal to the dorsal root ganglion located within the intervertebral formena and the latter distal to the ganglion (Fig. 7–14). The dorsal and ventral roots coalesce within the intervertebral foramen to form the spinal nerve.

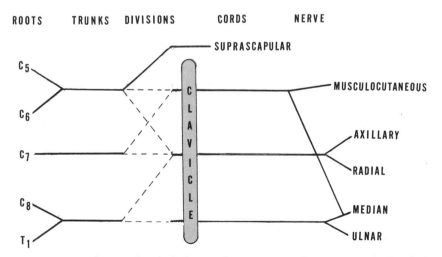

Figure 7–13. Schematic brachial plexus. The nerve roots that comprise the brachial plexus are essentially C5 to T1, which form three trunks, then divisions, cords into nerves. The clavicle is shown as the demarcating anatomic site.

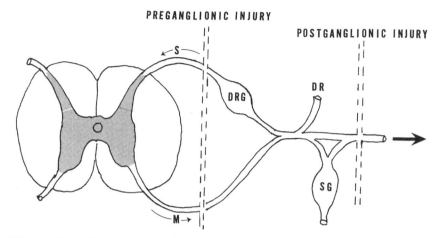

Figure 7–14. Microanatomy of sites for preganglionic and postganglionic injuries. The gray matter of the cord is shown with its afferent sensory (S) and efferent motor (M) fibers. The preganglionic injury is proximal to the dorsal root ganglion (DRG). The dorsal ramus (DR) innervates the paravertebral muscles. SG indicates the sympathetic ganglion. Postganglionic injuries invoke any nerve tissue distal to the DRG.

Preganglionic injuries are those proximal to the dorsal root ganglion, thus indicating physical disruption and avulsion of the root from the spinal cord with no prospect of reattachment or recovery. Postganglionic injuries usually occur distal to the takeoff of the peripheral nerve, to the dorsal ramus to the paracervical muscles, and to the sympathetic ganglion.

Plexus lesions are most often incomplete and characterized by weakness, muscle atrophy, reflex changes, sensory changes, and sympathetic dysfunction. Pain is usually constant and severe, located above the elbow, and aggravated by arm movement.[42] If from a nontraumatic cause, that is, tumor or injection injury, weakness can be experienced without pain or sensory changes. Sensory changes are patchy and incomplete and sympathetic involvement is rare except with attendant involvement of T1.

The following findings are indicative of preganglionic disruption:

Denervation of the paracervical muscles (as determined by electromyographic [EMG] studies)

Winging of the scapula (resulting from paresis of the rhomboids and serratus muscles)

Horner's syndrome (tetrad of anhidrosis, miosis, enophthalmus, and ptosis)

Poor response to histamine test (subcutaneous injection of histamine which normally forms a wheal, flare, and erythema). Cervical myelography often reveals an outpouching of the meninges to form a menigocele.

Recovery from a preganglionic disruption is almost totally hopeless, whereas recovery from postganglionic injury is possible,[43] and may even benefit from surgical intervention.[44,45]

LESIONS OF THE TRUNK

Upper Plexus (Trunk) Lesions

Damage involving the fifth and sixth cervical roots is the most commonly seen and is usually incomplete. The muscles normally involved are the deltoid, biceps, brachioradialis and brachialis and less frequently, the supraspinatus and subscapularis. Weakness is manifested by shoulder abduction, external rotation, elbow flexion, and forearm supination. Sensation is often unaffected.

Middle Plexus (Trunk) Lesions

This lesion is rare except from penetrating injuries. This lesion is characterized by triceps paralysis. The brachioradialis is not affected. A sensory deficit of the back of the forearm or radial aspect of the dorsum of the hand may be present.

Lower Plexus (Trunk) Lesion

Certain lesions of the eighth cervical and the first thoracic roots cause paralysis and atrophy of the flexors of the forearm and the intrinsic muscles of the hand. Sensation may be normal. Horner's syndrome occurs if the significant T1 root involvement is diagnostic of Horner's syndrome.

LESIONS OF THE CORDS

Signs and Symptoms

Lateral cord lesions cause weakness of the muscles innervated by the musculocutaneous nerve and the lateral head of the median nerve. Flexion and pronation of the forearm are weak. Sensory deficit is mild and limited to a small area on the radial aspect of the forearm.

Medial cord lesions produce weakness of the muscles innervated by the ulnar nerve and the medial head of the median nerve. Sensory loss is present in the medial cutaneous nerve of the forearm and arm. The lesion is essentially a combination of median and ulnar nerve lesions.

Posterior cord lesion produce weakness of the deltoid (axillary n.) and wrist and finger extensor (radial). The anatomy depicted in Figure 7–12 helps the diagnosis.

Therapy

Treatment is largely symptomatic and tailored to the individual patient's needs. Appropriate splinting is valuable; physical therapy may probably speed the recovery of motor weakness. Surgical intervention with neurolysis following penetrating injuries has mixed acceptance. Bonney's exhaustive study of severe supraclavicular traction injuries found mediocre results from therapy or surgical intervention.[46]

BRACHIAL PLEXUS COMPRESSION

Compression of the brachial plexus often elicits pain at the point of compression even though no brachial plexus pathology is present. A recent article[47] reveals that this test can indicate a cervical root lesion when there is also radiation of pain into the shoulder, that is, an upper extremity when *other* cervical radicular tests are equivocal (Fig. 7–15).

Associated tests are discussed in Chapter 6, and include:

1. Referral of radicular pain on neck extension (Jackson's sign)
2. Spurling's sign (axial compression)[47]
3. Lhermitte's sign (electric shock-like pain on neck flexion)[48,49]
4. Brachial plexus compression (BP test)

The BP test consists of pressure applied from the examiner's thumb over the brachial plexus which refers pain into the shoulder and upper extremity. Radiation must occur for the test to be considered *positive*.

In a differential diagnosis of radicular pain, a lesion of the cervical spine must be differentiated from one resulting from a brachial plexus lesion. Electromyographic studies assist in confirmation as do magnetic resonance imaging studies of the cervical spine.

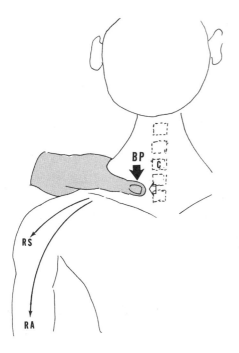

Figure 7–15. Brachial plexus pressure sign in radiculopathy. Digital pressure over the brachial plexus (BP) in the event of a cervical (C) root entrapment (*open arrow*) causes radiation of pain or paresthesia into the shoulder (RS) or down the arm (RA) for a positive sign.

REFERENCES

1. Tsairis, P: Brachial Plexus Neuropathies. In Dyke, PJ, Thomas, PK, and Lambert, EH (eds): Peripheral Neuropathy, Vol 1. WB Saunders, Philadelphia, 1975, pp 659–681.
2. Adson, AW: The gross pathology of brachial plexus injuries. Surg Gynecol Obstet 34:351, 1922.
3. Bonney, G: Prognosis in traction lesions of the brachial plexus. J Bone Joint Surg Br 41:4, 1959.
4. Coran, AG, Simon, A, Heimberg, F, and Beberman, N: Avulsion injury of the brachial plexus. Am J Surg 115:840, 1968.
5. Loeser, JD: Cervicobrachial neuralgia. In JJ Bonica, JS (ed.): The Management of Pain, vol 1. Lea & Febiger, Philadelphia, 1990, pp 868–881.
6. Imagama, T: Mechanism of vascular test in thoracic outlet syndrome. In Orthopedics and Traumatology. Vol 27, No 4, pp 559–563, 1978.
7. Wood, WW: Personal experiences with surgical treatment of 250 cases of cervicobrachial neurovascular compression syndrome. J Int Coll Surg 44:273–283, 1965.
8. Wright,IS: The neurovascular syndrome produced by hyperabduction of the arms. Am Heart J 29:1–19.
9. Kitamura T, Takagi K, Yamaga M, et al: Problems with Adson's test: The influence of deep breathing, Neuro-orthopedics 15:15–24, 1993.
10. Bolton, B, Carmichael, EA, and Sturup, G: Vaso-constriction following deep inspiration. J Physiol 86:83–94, 1936.
11. Hachulla, E, et al: Etude clinique, vélocimetrique et radiologique de la traverse thoracique-brachiale. Revue de Médecine Interne:19–24, 1990.

12. Gage, M and Parnell, H: Scalene anticus syndrome. Am J Surg 73:253–268, 1947.
13. Selvaratnum, PJ, Matyas, TA, and Glasgow, EF: Noninvasive discrimination of brachial plexus involvement in upper limb pain. Spine 19:26–33, 1994.
14. Viikari-Juntura, E, Porras, M, and Laasonen, EM: Validity of clinical tests in the diagnosis of root compression in cervical disc disease. Spine 14:253–257, 1989.
15. Davidson, RI, Dunn, EJ, and Metzmaker, JN: The shoulder abduction test in the diagnosis of radicular pain in cervical extradural compressive monoradiculopathies. Spine 6:441–445, 1981.
16. Frykholm, R: Cervical nerve root compression resulting from disc degeneration and root sleeve fibrosis: a clinical investigation. Acta Chir Scand (suppl):160, 1951.
17. Ginn, K: An investigation of tension development in upper limb soft tissues during upper limb tension test. Proceedings of the International Federation of Orthopaedic Manipulative Therapists, New York, 1988, pp 25–26.
18. Kenneally, M, Rubenach, H, and Elvey, RL: The upper limb tension test: the SLR test of the arm: physical therapy of the cervical and thoracic spine. In Grant, R (ed.): Clin Phys Ther 17:167–194, 1988.
19. Elvey, RL: Brachial plexus tension test and pathoanatomical origin of arm pain. In Idczak, RM, Dewhurst, D, Glasgow, EF, et al (eds.): Aspects of manipulative therapy. Proceedings of a Multidisciplinary International Conference of Manipulative Therapy. Melbourne, Victoria: August 1979. Lincoln Institute of Health Sciences, New York, 1980, pp 105–110.
20. Elvey, RL: Brachial plexus tension test and the pathoanatomical origin or arm pain. In Glasgow, EF, Twomey, LT, Scull, ER, and Kleynhans, AM, (eds.): Aspects of Manipulative Therapy, ed 2. Melbourne: Churchill Livingstone Melbourne, 1985, pp 116–122.
21. Selvaratnam, PJ, Glasgow, EF, and Matyas, TA: The strain at the nerve roots of the brachial plexus (abstr). J Anat 161:260, 1988.
22. Pullos, J: The upper limb tension test (abstr). Aust J Physiotherapy 32:258–259, 1986.
23. Pullos, J: The upper limb tension test. Department of Physiotherapy, University of Queensland, St Lucia, Queensland, 1986 (unpublished).
24. Urschel, HC, Wood, RE, and Paulson, DL: Objective diagnosis (ulnar nerve conduction velocity) and current therapy of the thoracic outlet. Ann Thorac Surg 12:608–620, 1971.
25. Turner, JWA: Acute brachial radiculitis. BMJ 2:592, 1944.
26. Tsaris, P, Dyk, PJ, and Mulder, DW: Natural history of brachial plexus neuropathy: report of 99 patients. Arch neurol 27:109, 1972.
27. Murphey, F, Hartung, W, and Kirklin, JW: Myelographic demonstration of avulsing injury of the brachial plexus. Am J Roentgenol Radium Ther 58:102, 1947.
28. Harris, W: The Morphology of the Brachial Plexus. Oxford University Press, London, 1939.
29. Magee, KR, and DeJong, RN: Paralytic brachial neuritis. JAMA 174:1258, 1960.
30. Roos, DB: Experience with first rib resection for thoracic outlet syndrome. Ann Surg 173:429, 1971.
31. Seddon, HJ: Lesions of individual nerves: upper limb. In Surgical Disorders of the Peripheral Nerves. Williams & Wilkins, Baltimore, 1972.
32. Walshe, F: Disease of the Nervous System, ed. 10. Livingstone, Edinburgh, 1963.
33. Hall, CD: Neurovascular syndromes at the thoracic outlet. In Hadler, NM (ed): Clinical Concepts in Regional Musculoskeletal Illness. New York, Grune & Stratton, 1987, pp 227–244.
34. Sallstrom, J and Schmidt, H: Cervicobrachial disorders in certain occupations, with special reference to compression in the thoracic outlet. Am J Ind Med 6:45–52, 1984.
35. Cailliet, R: Nerve control of the hand. In Cailliet, R: Hand Pain and Impairment, ed 4. FA Davis, Philadelphia, 1994, pp 69–131.
36. Cailliet, R: Posture. In Cailliet, R: Neck and Arm Pain, ed 3. FA Davis, Philadelphia, 1991, pp 43–50.
37. Woodsmith, FG: Post-operative brachial plexus paralysis. BMJ 1:1115, 1952.
38. White, JC and Sweet, WH: Pain and the Neurosurgeon. Springfield Il, Charles C. Thomas, 1969, pp 560–565.

39. Naffziger, HC: The scalene syndrome. Surg Gynecol Obstet 64:119, 1937.
40. McCann, PD and Bindelglass, DF: The brachial plexus: Clinical anatomy. Orthop Rev 20:413–419, 1991.
41. Kerr, AT: The brachial plexus of nerves in man: The variations in its formation and branches. Am J Anat 23:285–395, 1918.
42. Rogers, L: Upper-limb pain due to lesions of the thoracic outlet. The scalene syndrome, cervical rib and costoclavicular compression. BMJ 2:956, 1949.
43. Leffort, RD: Brachial Plexus Injuries. New York, Churchill Livingstone, 1985.
44. Jamieson, A and Huges, S: The role of surgery in the management of closed injuries to the brachial plexus. Clin Orthop 147:210–215, 1980.
45. Kline, DG, Hacket, ER, and Happel, LH: Surgery for lesions of the brachial plexus. Arch Neurol 43:170–181, 1986.
46. Uchihara, T, Furukawa, T, and Tsukagoshi, H: Compression of brachial plexus as a diagnostic test of cervical cord lesion. Spine 19:2170–2173, 1994.
47. Spurling, RG and Scoville, VB: Lateral rupture of the cervical intervertebral discs. Surg Gynecol Obstet 78:350–358, 1944.
48. Lhermitte, J, Bollack, J, and Nicolas, M: Les douleurs à type de décharge électrique consecutives à la flexion céphalique dans la sclérose en plaque: Un cas de forme sensitive de la sclérose multiple. Rev Neurol (Paris) 39:56–62, 1924.
49. Gutrecht, JA: Lhermitte's sign—from observation to eponym. Arch Neurol 46:557–558, 1989.

CHAPTER 8

Shoulder Pain and Impairment

Shoulder pain and disability is an outstanding example of **soft tissue pain** because the tissues capable of causing pain and impairment in this entity are predominantly tendinous, capsular, and synovial.

The shoulder complex is made up of seven joints each essential to normal function, but also thus capable of being the site of pain and impairment. As in most extremities, understanding of normal *functional anatomy* is essential to perform a meaningful examination, elicit a discerning history, and request confirmatory diagnostic procedures.

The shoulder girdle includes the following joints:

1. glenohumeral
2. suprahumeral
3. acromioclavicular
4. claviculosternal
5. scapulocostal
6. sternocostal
7. costovertebral
8. bicipital-humeral

All have a role in upper extremity activity in which the shoulder places the hand into its functional position.

GLENOHUMERAL JOINT

This is probably the most important shoulder complex joint, as well as the site of most pain and impairment. It is a complex incongruous articulation which demands gliding and spinning motion (Fig. 8–1), rather than merely ro-

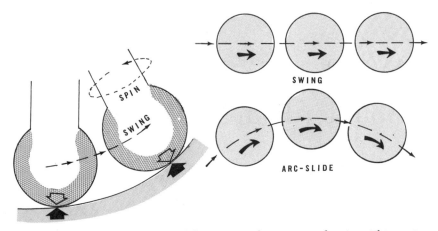

Figure 8–1. Joint motion. A joint sliding in one plane is termed **swing.** This motion has no rotation or spin. If there is simultaneous spin the motion is termed **arc slide,** which is the motion at the glenohumeral joint.

tation about a fixed axis (Fig. 8–2). This structure makes the stability of the joint depend on the supporting soft tissues.

The base of the joint is the concave glenoid fossa which is located at the lateral tip of the scapula (Fig. 8–3). The fossa is pear shaped and shallow, allowing little *seating* of the head of the humerus. It is deepened by a lip (glenoid labrum) to which is attached the glenohumeral capsule.

The head of the humerus is held within the glenoid fossa against the forces of gravity predominantly by muscles, the supraspinatus, to a lesser degree by the angulation of the fossa, and by the superior aspect of the capsule (Fig. 8–4). The supraspinatus muscle, originating within the supraspinatus fossa of the scapula attaches to the greater tuberosity of the humerus. It performs its function by preventing the downward subluxation of the humerus by virtue of its tone (Fig. 8–5).

Movement of the glenohumeral joint is done by the rotator cuff muscles (Fig. 8–6), so called because they rotate the head within the glenoid fossa. Rotation is that of abduction, that is, forward and backward flexion and external-internal rotation. The motions of the upper extremity demand appropriate glenohumeral motion (Fig. 8–7).

The motion of the arm requires action at all joints of the complex. The humerus can abduct only about 90°, when the greater tuberosity abuts against the overhanging acromium. To minimize this obstruction and to permit the arm to abduct further and thus ultimately reach the overhead position, the humerus externally rotates, causing the greater tuberosity to pass *behind* the acromium. To achieve the overhead arm motion, the scapula initially supports the arm, then gradually rotates about the chest

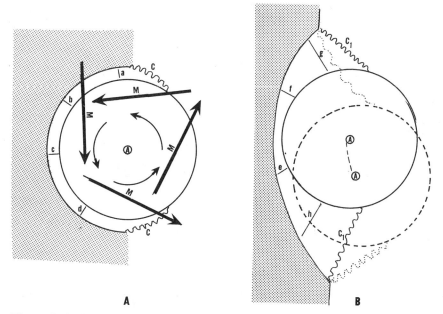

A   **B**

Figure 8–2. Congruity versus incongruity in joints. (A) In a congruent joint, the concave and convex surfaces are symmetric. The articular surfaces are equidistant at all points along their circumferences ($a = b = c = d$, and so on). In rotation movement occurs about a fixed axis (A). Muscular action (M) is that of symmetric movement about this fixed axis and is needed for motion not stability. The capsule (C) has symmetric elongation. (B) Incongruous joints have asymmetrical articular surfaces. The concave surface is elongated, whereas the convex surface is more circular, causing the surfaces to differ in their relationships ($g > f$, $e > h$). As the joint moves, the axis (A) of rotation shifts (A) and the articular surfaces glide rather than roll as the congruous joint does. The muscles of this type of joint stabilize the joint as well as move it. The capsule varies in its length.

wall and causes the acromium to be elevated, thus allowing the humerus greater movement. Movement of the scapula demands rotation about the acromioclavicular joint and rotation of the clavicle about the sternoclavicular joint.

Muscular Action

Muscular activity to initiate shoulder movement is well coordinated. The supraspinatus muscle maintains isometric contraction to hold the humerus within the glenoid fossa. The deltoid merely exhibits tonus and the scapula is

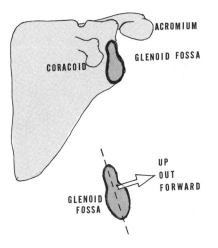

Figure 8–3. The glenoid fossa. The glenoid fossa is at the superior lateral end of the scapula. It is ovoid, shallow, and faces upward, outward, and forward when the scapula is dependent.

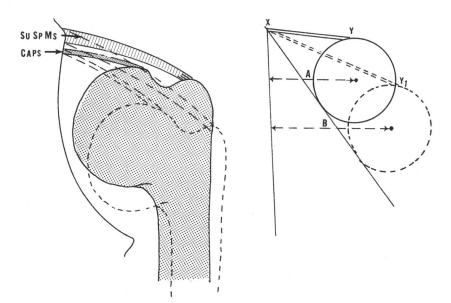

Figure 8–4. Structures supporting the dependent humerus. As the glenoid fossa faces upward, outward, and forward, it is in an inclined position. Gravity tends to cause the rounded head of the humerus to glide down. The supraspinatus (Su), infraspinatus (Sp), teres minor muscle (MS), and the superior aspect of the capsule (Caps) prevents this glide. The structures mentioned (X-Y) prevent elongation (X-Y₁) and prevent the axis (A) from sliding outward (B).

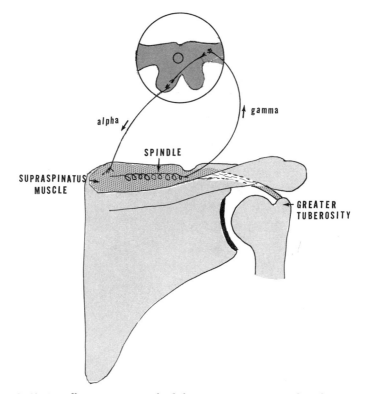

Figure 8–5. Spindle system control of the supraspinatus muscle. The tone of the supraspinatus muscle is controlled by the tension on the spindle system, which ensures appropriate contraction of the muscle.

passively supported by the scapuloclavicular ligaments (Fig. 8–8) and isometrically held by the trapezius and serratus anterior.

As motion begins, the supraspinatus, infraspinatus, and teres minor muscles contract and cause gradual abduction and forward flexion. After a few degrees of motion, the deltoid muscle contracts to increase the desired motion. The scapula initially remains isotonic, but with further abduction or forward flexion, the scapula begins isometric contraction and moves about its acromioclavicular articulation in a graduated degree of motion.

In abduction, the humerus externally rotates to place the greater tuberosity behind the acromium. This results from the synchronous activities of the supraspinatus, infraspinatus, and teres minor. The internal rotators, the sub-

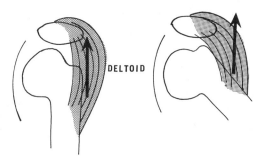

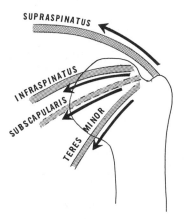

Figure 8–6. Rotator cuff muscles. The humerus is activated by the rotator cuff muscles and the deltoid in a synchronous manner. The lower drawing shows the rotator muscles, which abduct or flex the humerus (*large arrow*) and is ultimately joined by the deltoid (*upper drawing*).

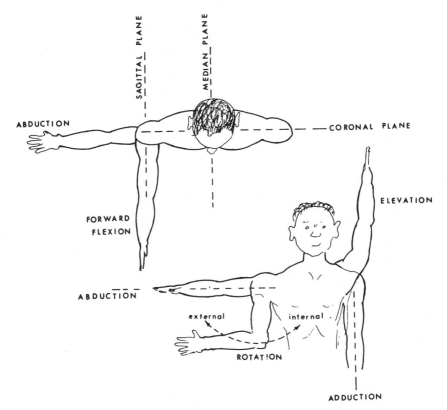

Figure 8–7. The planes of motion of the shoulder and upper arm. The upper drawing is a view from above, and the lower drawing is a view from the front. (From Cailliet, R: Shoulder Pain, ed 3. FA Davis, Philadelphia, 1991, p 29, with permission.)

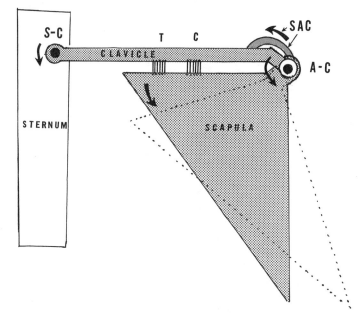

Figure 8–8. Static support of the scapula by the claviculoscapular ligaments. The clavicle acts as a strut from the sternum at the sternoclavicular joint (S-C). The scapula articulates at the acromioclavicular joint (A-C). Because of its eccentrically distributed weight, the scapula could rotate about the A-C joint (*small arrow*) but is restrained by the claviculoscapular ligaments: the trapezium (T) and the conoid (C) ligaments. The superior acromioclavicular ligament (SAC) also adds support.

scapularis, pectoralis, and latissmus dorsi muscles are quiet (Figs. 8–9 and 8–10).

The biceps tendon plays a passive role in that it does not actively move within the bicipital groove but passively depresses the head of the humerus as the head of the humerus descends within the glenoid fossa during active abduction and forward flexion of the arm. When there has been faulty motion of the glenohumeral joint, the biceps tendon can also be inflamed and become a site of nociception.

The glenohumeral capsule originates from the glenoid labrum and attaches to the upper aspect of the humerus. In the static dependent arm, it prevents downward motion. As abduction and forward flexion occurs, the inferior folds elongate and the superior folds contract (Fig. 8–11).

Normal shoulder action is a pain-free synchronous activity of rotator cuff muscles which must be well conditioned and used in a coordinated neuromuscular manner observing the scapulohumeral rhythm. The capsule

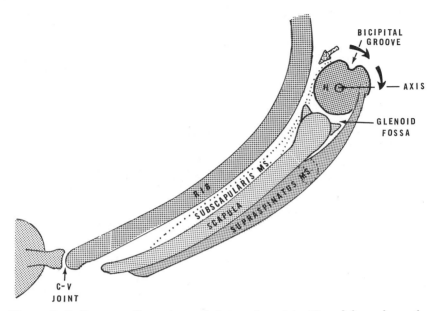

Figure 8–9. Rotator cuff muscles at their scapular origin. Viewed from above, the subscapular muscle is contained between the rib cage and the scapula. It is an internal rotator (*speckled arrow*) of the humerus (H). The supraspinatus muscles are located on the external surface of the scapula and are external rotators (*dark arrows*). The costovertebral joint (C-V) is shown.

must be flexible and intact and the bursal walls well lubricated. The articular cartilaginous surfaces must be adequate to permit articular movement. When any of these functions are deficient, pain and dysfunction result in disability.

Pathogenic Factors

Dysfunction and pain occur with inappropriate neuromusculoskeletal function, or excessive activities lead to repetitive trauma and attrition or also from a traumatic external force. The tissues that maintain normal function but are the sites of nociception are depicted in Figure 8–12.

All related tissues are compacted in a narrow space requiring coordinated action and good lubrication. Daily frequent motion occurs within the fibro-osseous case (Fig. 8–13).

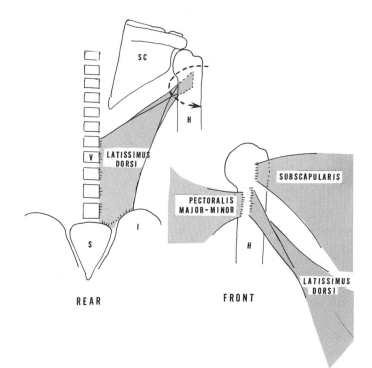

Figure 8–10. The internal rotators of the humerus. The muscles that internally rotate the humerus (H) are shown. The latissimus dorsi originates from the ischium (I) and sacrum (S) and passes anteriorly to the humerus, which articulates about the glenoid fossa of the scapula (SC). Viewed from the front are the pectoralis, subscapularis, and the latissimus dorsi muscles.

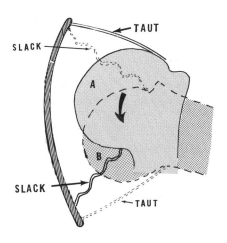

Figure 8–11. The glenohumeral capsule. With the arm dependent (A) the humerus is supported by a taut superior cable. The inferior capsule is slack. As the arm abducts, the head descends on the glenoid fossa (B) and the inferior capsule becomes taut. If the inferior capsule becomes contracted, a *frozen shoulder* results.

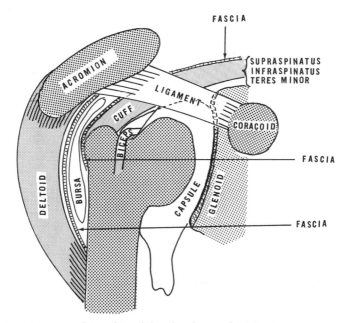

Figure 8–12. Tissue relationship of the glenohumeral joint. Numerous tissues, many of which are nociceptive, are contained within a relatively small space. Because of the amount of motion, lubrication is mandatory and is afforded by the subdeltoid bursa and the capsule with their synovial fluids.

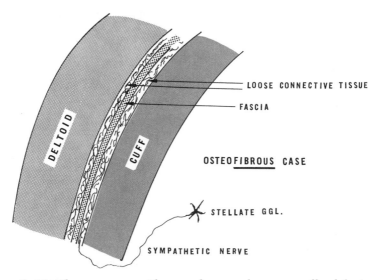

Figure 8–13. Fibroosseous case. The space between the rotator cuff and the inner aspect of the deltoid is termed the **osteofibrous,** in which is contained fascia and loose connective tissue. It is here that the *frozen shoulder* results from inflammation and disuse.

History and Examination

A direct fall on the outstretched arm is a definite case of external force that can cause tissue damage. The history must elicit the exact manner and position of the arm at the moment of trauma. The resultant injury can afflict any or many of the tissues (Fig. 8–14) within the shoulder complex. A meaningful examination, including radiologic studies, is diagnostic. Faulty neuromuscular or repetitive minor trauma requires taking a more precise history, because many are not recognized by the patient.

Faulty neuromuscular activity indicates that the scapulohumeral rhythm has been violated. The arm has abducted and elevated without adequate external rotation. Repetitive activities such as occur in today's athletic leisure activi-

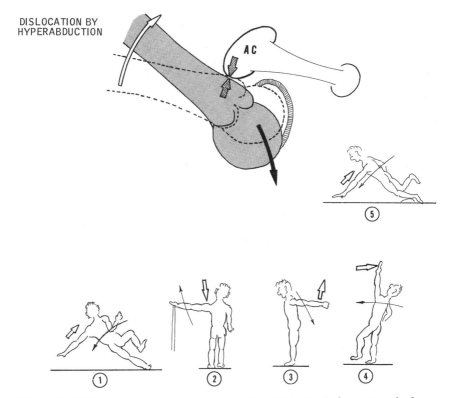

Figure 8–14. Injury on an outstretched arm. Direct injuries to the outstretched arm are shown by arrows in (1), (2), (3), and (4). A direct fall, (5), is a common cause of dislocation as shown in the larger drawing. The humerus impinges on the overhanging acromium (AC) (*two stippled arrows*) and dislocates inferiorly (*large curved dark arrow*).

ties and certain occupations are responsible for many repetitive trauma (Figs. 8–15 to 8–18).

The acromium may be in a faulty position because defective posture (Fig. 8–19) has a propensity for causing degenerative cuff disease (Fig. 8–20). The position of the body during work at a computer is generally detrimental.

Diagnostic Procedures

The patient localizes the site of pain, which can be corroborated by precise manual palpation. Movements and positions of the arm that cause or relieve pain can be elicited.

With injury to the rotator cuff, the glenohumeral activity is impaired. The nature of a painful arc is elicited (Fig. 8–21) and glenohumeral abduction is impaired with the scapular phase occurring in the absence of glenohumeral rotation (Fig. 8–22). This is termed **shrugging abduction.**

If a rotator cuff is torn, abduction and external rotation are not possible. If the arm is passively abducted it can be held momentarily by the deltoid but ultimately, because the supraspinatus muscle is not connected, it will drop (Fig. 8–23). If a capsular tear has been suspected the *apprehension* test often proves diagnostically positive (Fig. 8–24).

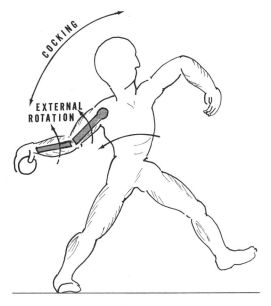

Figure 8–15. Pitching trauma. The repetitive action of abduction, external rotation, overhead elevation, and violent muscular force is a cause of repetitive trauma to the glenohumeral joint.

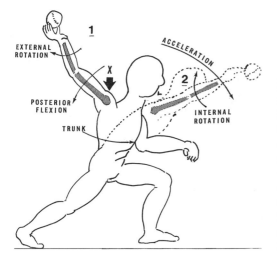

Figure 8–16. Repetitive trauma: mechanisms in pitching. The cocking (see Fig. 8–15), which places the arm in an elevated, posteriorly flexed, and externally rotated position (1) is followed by forceful downward acceleration and internal rotation (2). These motions all occur within the confines of the glenohumeral joint (X).

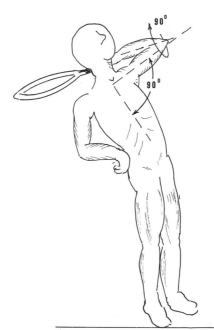

Figure 8–17. Shoulder trauma in tennis. In serving or overhead action, the shoulder is abducted (90°) externally rotated (90°) then descends forcefully into internal rotation and adduction.

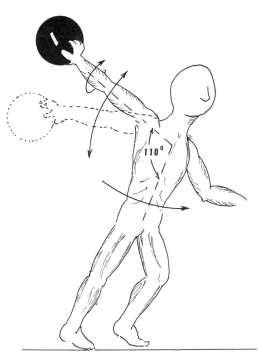

Figure 8–18. Bowling shoulder trauma. When bowling, the arm with a large weight at the end of the fulcrum is posteriorly placed and internally rotated, then descends (110°) with simultaneous external rotation and traction on the glenohumeral joint.

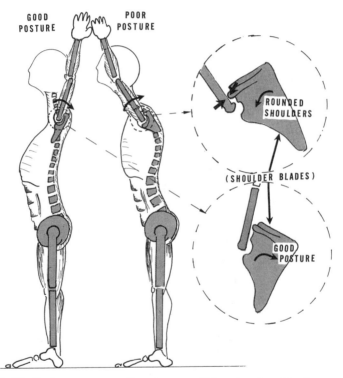

Figure 8–19. Faulty posture predisposing to cuff deterioration. Good posture positions the scapula so that overhead arm elevation does not impinge against the overhanging acromium (*lower dotted circle*). Rounded shoulder posture (poor posture) impinges the humerus against the acromium (*upper dotted circle*).

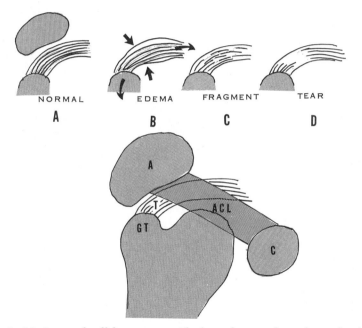

Figure 8–20. Stages of cuff degeneration. The large drawing shows the tendon (T) attaching to the greater tuberosity of the humerus (GT), which resides under the overhanging acromium (A), and shows the acromiocoracoid ligament (ACL), which connects the acromium to the coracoid process (C). The normal tendon (A) shows parallel intact collagen, fibers which, when traumatized, undergo edematous separation (B) of the fibers. Some fibers ultimately fragment (C) and tear (D).

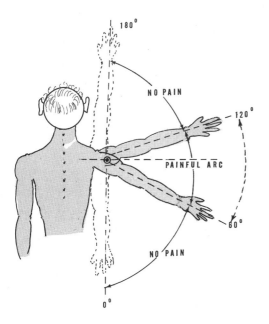

Figure 8–21. Painful arc. In acute tendinitis the arm can abduct to 60° without significant pain. Pain is present in the range from 60° to 120° of abduction (the painful arc). Because the humerus has externally rotated placing the greater tuberosity behind the acromium, the remaining elevation to 180° is painless, if no capsular contraction is present.

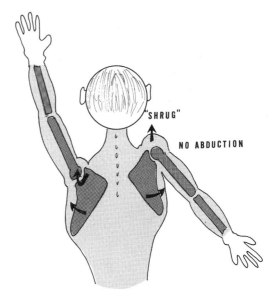

Figure 8–22. Shrugging abduction. With a tendinitis or partial cuff tear, abduction of the arm at the glenohumeral joint is limited, thus initiating only the scapular phase of abduction, which *shrugs* the shoulder.

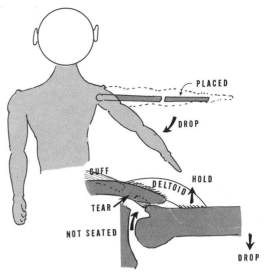

Figure 8–23. Drop sign of rotator cuff tear. In a complete tear of the rotator cuff, the arm, passively abducted, can be held momentarily and weakly by the deltoid muscles. Without stabilization of the humerus within the glenoid fossa by the cuff muscles, the arm gradually drops. This is a clinical sign of complete cuff tear.

Most soft tissue injuries of the shoulder can be diagnosed by a careful history and appropriate examination. For instance, a rotator cuff injury, which is common, can be estimated as being tendinitis, a partial tear, or a total tear. The shrugging mechanism with a painful arc indicates tendon inflammation with the possibility of some torn fibers. Both cause the same symptoms and findings. With a complete tear, active abduction is impossible and passively holding the abducted arm as placed is impossible, as is external rotation.

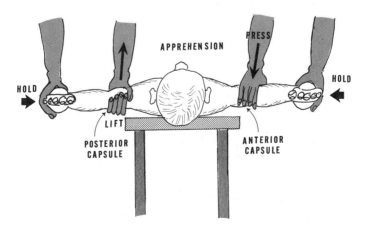

Figure 8–24. Apprehension test for capsular tear. By placing the supine patient with abducted and supported arms, a capsular tear can be suspected when elevation (testing the posterior capsule) or depression (testing the anterior capsule) of the humerus causes pain and apprehension in the patient.

There are *subtle* signs of minor adhesive capsulitis (Fig. 8–25), which can be missed with only a cursory examination.

Missing these subtle signs frequently denies the patient proper diagnosis and appropriate treatment. Slight limitations of capsular elasticity prevents proper glenohumeral action with pain being elicited at the end point of all shoulder joint motion, whether passive or active.

As the patient has an otherwise normal examination, a possible psychologic diagnosis is overemphasized and proper treatment will not be instituted.

As has well been established in neurophysiologic studies, painful afferent impulses from articular tissues, of which the capsule is one, inhibit proper neuromuscular strength and the arm is noted to be *weak* (see Chap. 3). Strengthening exercises are fraught with failure as long as there is end-point pain from stretching a constricted capsule, albeit minor pain.

Diagnostic procedures today are well established. Arthrography reveals

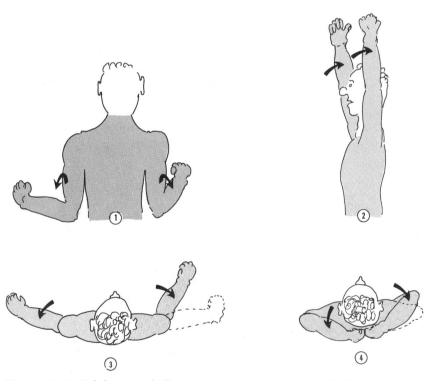

Figure 8–25. Subtle signs of adhesive capsulitis. In early signs of adhesive capsulitis the person (*1*) cannot externally rotate the affected arm as compared with the normal side. This can be viewed from above (*3*). Viewed from the side, the affected arm does not elevate posteriorly as the normal arm does (*2*). Placing the hands behind the head and posteriorly moving the arms backwards is limited on the affected side (*4*).

tears and their extent. Computed tomographic (CT) scans and magnetic resonance imaging also have value as has arthroscopic evaluation.

Treatment

After a precise examination provides an accurate diagnosis, proper treatment ensues.

1. Immediate rest and support of the shoulder is accomplished by the application of ice and support by a sling for a few days. Oral anti-inflammatory medication may be of value.
2. A significant residual impairment is the *frozen shoulder*: adhesive capsulitis or adhesive bursitis (Fig. 8–26). Pendular exercise that passively
   stretches the capsule without initiating muscular activity should be
   started immediately (Fig. 8–27).

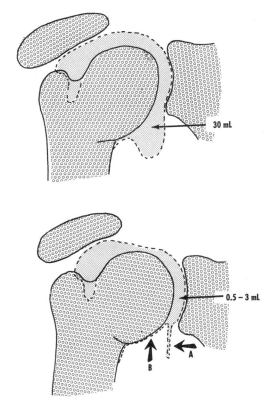

Figure 8–26. Adhesive capsulitis. A normal capsule has a
capacity of at least 30 mL of
fluid. In adhesive capsulitis,
which adheres the inferior aspect of the capsule (A) and adheres to the head of the
humerus (B), the volume decreases to as little as 0.5 to 3
mL.

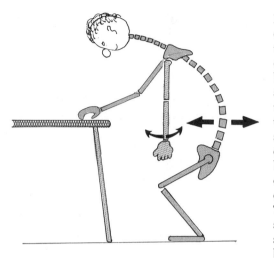

Figure 8–27. Pendular exercises. If acute adhesive capsulitis is suspected from acute tendinitis, pendular exercise should be started early. The objective is an active-passive range-of-motion exercise where the arm is **totally dependent** and is swung in all directions by an oscillating action of the entire body. Because no shoulder muscular action is allowed, the exercise to the shoulder is passive. The knees are bent to minimize stress on the low back and to supply the oscillation of the body.

3. Intra-articular injection of an analgesic agent and use of soluble steroids both have their advocates (Fig. 8–28).
4. Posture must be corrected.
5. As soon as tolerated, active exercises should be started. These address the range of motion and strengthening the rotator cuff muscles. Most exercises can be performed without equipment. Physical therapy is needed only for instruction and supervision, because most such regimens need to be done frequently, daily, gently, and progressively. They may be preceded with application of heat and followed by ice if residual discomfort occurs (Figs. 8–29 to 8–33).

Strengthening exercises emphasize the external rotators (supraspinatus, infraspinatus, and teres minor). They can be done with any elastic graded type of equipment (Figs. 8–34 and 8–35).

If frozen shoulder develops, treatment is more difficult. Manipulative *breaking* of adhesions appears most successful. For meaningful therapy, the patient must be evaluated preoperatively to ascertain the levels of perseverance, tolerance to pain, and cooperation to be expected postoperatively.

Before manipulation, an extensive exercise program to ensure maximum range of motion and strength of involved muscles is instituted. This ensures that the postoperative exercises are well understood, and that they will actually increase the range and strength.

Also before manipulation, intra-articular injection and a local anesthetic,

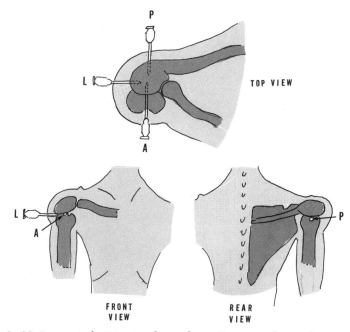

Figure 8–28. Intraarticular injection for tendinitis. Injection of an analgesic agent and possibly a steroid is performed using any of three routes: anterior (A), laterally (L), or posteriorly (P). Palpation of the bony landmarks indicates the site and avoidance of striking bone is mandated as is aspiration before injection.

preferably a long-acting one and a solution of deprohydrocortisone should be given. This minimizes postmanipulation pain and prevents readhesion.

The manipulation, done under anesthesia, is followed by splinting in the abducted externally rotated position. The manipulative procedure must be done with a short lever arm and minimal abrupt force to avoid fracture or dislocation of the humerus. Immediately after manipulation, active exercise must be initiated. The splint is gradually decreased in abduction and ultimately removed.

Brisement also has its advocates where an intra-articular injection of an analgesic agent (Fig. 8–36) and a steroid is followed by a forceful injection of 30 to 40 mL of solution that ruptures the capsular adhesions mechanically. The same postoperative regimen is needed as after manipulation.

Ergonomically, the patient's professional and athletic activities that may have caused or aggravated the shoulder or may have incurred repetitive trauma must be evaluated and either modified or eliminated. An excellent dissertation on workplace evaluation and modification is available (Vern-Putz Anderson).

Text continued on p. 289

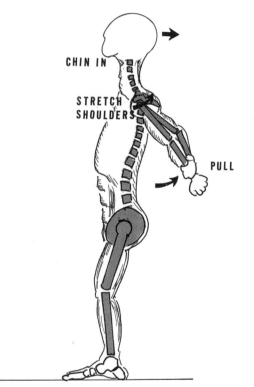

HEAD UP & BACK

CHIN IN

STRETCH SHOULDERS

PULL

THE ONE MINUTE BREAK: SHOULDER STRETCH 1

Figure 8–29. One-minute break: shoulder stretch. Daily exercises done frequently, hence termed *one-minute break*, are to maintain full range of shoulder range. Assuming proper posture, the affected arm is moved posteriorly by the normal arm: gently and periodically.

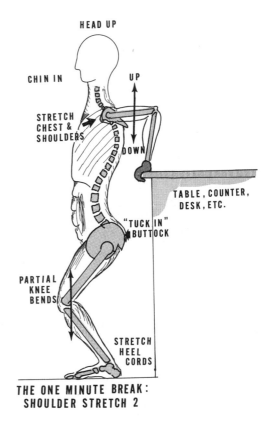

HEAD UP

CHIN IN

STRETCH CHEST & SHOULDERS

UP

DOWN

TABLE, COUNTER, DESK, ETC.

"TUCK IN" BUTTOCK

PARTIAL KNEE BENDS

STRETCH HEEL CORDS

THE ONE MINUTE BREAK: SHOULDER STRETCH 2

Figure 8–30. One-minute break: shoulder stretch 2. Using a convenient piece of furniture of proper height, the patient places both hands posteriorly on the surface and does gentle repeated deep knee bends, assuming proper posture during the exercise.

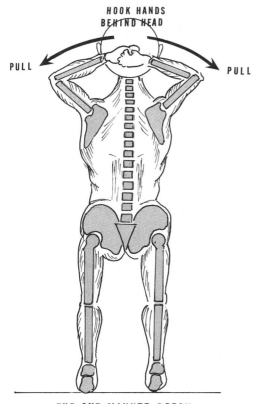

THE ONE MINUTE BREAK:
SHOULDER STRETCH 3

Figure 8–31. One-minute break: shoulder stretch 3. In the standing position, both hands are hooked behind the head and pulls the other hand to both sides slowly, gently, and repeatedly to full range as tolerated.

Figure 8–32. Internal rotator stretch with weight. In the seated position with arm supported on a table and elbow flexed 90°, a weight in the hand causes stretch of the rotators when allowed to descend outward. In an additional exercise (not shown in drawing) with the weight on the table and the arm internally rotated, the external rotators are strengthened by bringing the weight to the vertical position.

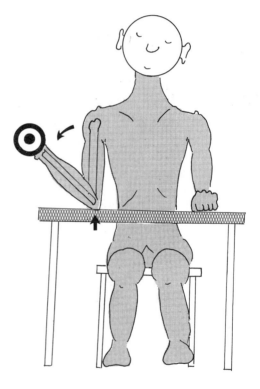

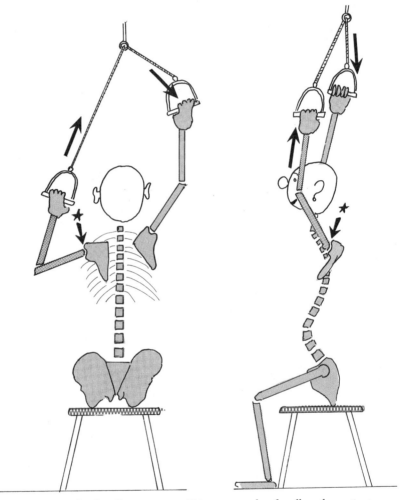

Figure 8–33. Overhead pulley exercises. Using an overhead pulley, the patient uses the normal side to exert the force to increase the shoulder range of motion (*star*). By changing the position under the overhead pulley, the direction of motion is also altered (*right drawing*).

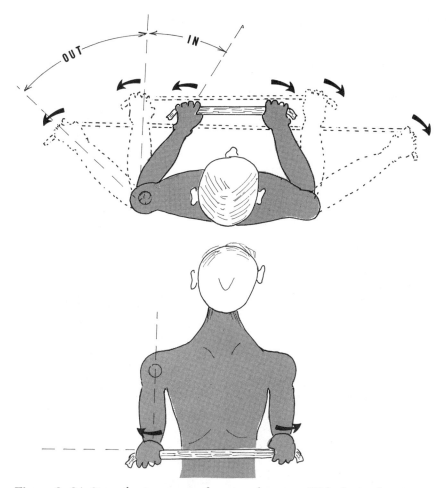

Figure 8–34. Strengthening exercise for external rotators. With elastic of varying resistance, the external rotators of both shoulders can be strengthened as depicted in the drawing. Increasing the length of the elastic adds external rotation range.

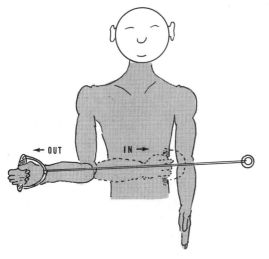

Figure 8–35. Unilateral exercise for external rotator. Tying an elastic to a fixed object allows the person to strengthen the external rotators. The length of the elastic or changing position of the elastic changes the area of strengthening (range of motion).

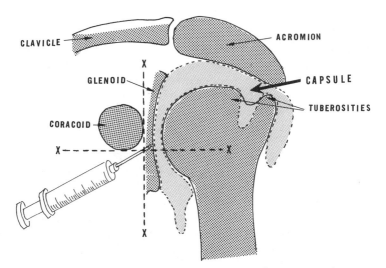

Figure 8–36. Intraarticular injection for brisement. Performing an arthrogram injection to determine that the capsule has been entered (as shown in drawing), the first syringe is replaced with a syringe holding 40 mL of a long-acting analgesic agent and steroid and is slowly but forcefully injected into the joint, causing a tearing of the adhesions (brisement). Postoperative therapy is mandated (see text).

SHOULDER DISLOCATION

The most painful and disabling injury to the shoulder is dislocation of the glenohumeral joint. Most dislocations occur anteriorly (Fig. 8–37) but there are four types of dislocation (Fig. 8–38).

Reduction of the dislocation has universally been the Kocher manipulation (Fig. 8–39).

In this brief discussion of shoulder injuries obviously all lesions cannot be discussed in detail but if recognized the enclosed bibliography can assist the provider with a source of information to assure the injured patient receives appropriate care and avoids ineffectual treatment modalities.

ACROMIOCLAVICULAR JOINT

Among the shoulder complex joints, a frequent site of pain and impairment is the acromioclavicular joint (AC). The commonest cause is direct trauma from above or in front. A direct frontal blow, such as occurs in an auto accident where the arm held flexed forward to avoid impact may injure the AC joint.

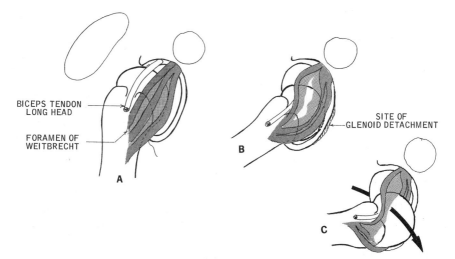

BICEPS TENDON
LONG HEAD

FORAMEN OF
WEITBRECHT

SITE OF
GLENOID DETACHMENT

A

B

C

Figure 8–37. Anterior dislocation mechanism. The anterior capsule and the glenohumeral ligaments medial to the biceps tendon form an avenue (A) for dislocation of the head of the humerus. The labrum of the glenoid may also be torn (B) and (C).

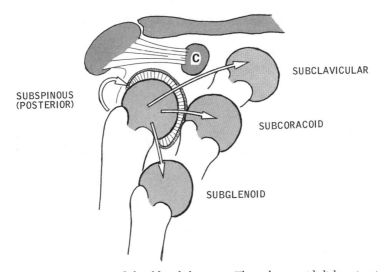

Figure 8–38. Four types of shoulder dislocation. The subcoracoid dislocation is the most frequent and the subspinous (posterior) is the least frequent. The designated type is the position of the humeral head in relation to the glenoid at the time of diagnosis.

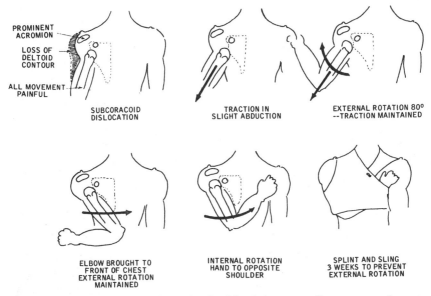

Figure 8–39. Kocher manipulation for shoulder dislocation. All movements shown in sequence should be done smoothly and gently. Traction on the upper arm should be maintained constantly during the maneuver. Once reduced, the arm is splinted for 3 weeks to prevent redislocation. (From Cailliet, R: Shoulder Pain, ed 3. FA Davis, Philadelphia, 1991, p 143, with permission.)

In normal scapulohumeral abduction or overhead elevation, the clavicle rotates about the acromium during the scapular phase. In elevation of the scapula also produces movement in the AC joint. Crepitation and localized pain are elicited by this motion (Fig. 8–40).

The acromioclavicular joint is not a true synovial joint, but rather a synarthrosis with both ends of the bones joined by fibrous tissue that gradually degenerates and forms a meniscus (Fig. 8–41). The outer edge of the clavicle is convex, articulating with the concave aspect of the acromium. This configuration allows rotation.

Direct trauma causes varying degree of tearing of the fibers of the joint, which causes instability of this joint in shoulder motions. Examination provides findings of localized pain and tenderness in any shoulder motion causing AC motion. Crepitation may be palpated.

Radiographs are often diagnostic, especially when a suspected dislocation and weight-bearing arm radiologic view reveals subluxation. Local injection of an analgesic agent into the joint is diagnostic.

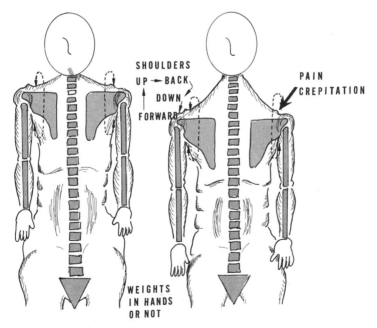

Figure 8–40. Scapular elevation and circumduction testing the acromioclavicular (AC) joint. Asking the patient to elevate and circumduct the shoulder girdle and then palpating the AC joint will elicit tenderness and crepitation in the advent of AC pathology.

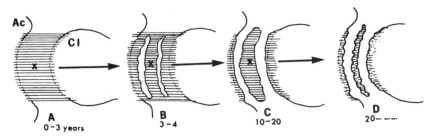

Figure 8–41. Acromioclavicular meniscus. The acromioclavicular meniscus is an evolutionary development. (A) From birth to age 2 years there is a fibrous bridge (X) that joins the acromium (Ac) to the clavicle (Cl). (B) From age 3 to 4 years cavities form within the body of the bridge. (C) During the first two decades, the central fibers form a meniscus that gradually thins (D) from age 20 to ultimately disappear completely by age 60. (From Cailliet, R: Shoulder Pain, ed 3. FA Davis, Philadelphia, 1991, p 39, with permission.)

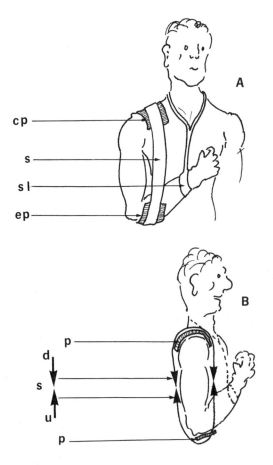

Figure 8–42. Immobilization treatment of the acromioclavicular (AC) joint. (A) The AC joint can be immobilized by strapping (s) as shown. Pressure points are avoided by felt inserts (cp) (p) and (ep). The hand and forearm are supported by a sling (sl). (B) The arrows depict the direction (d = down) and (u = up) of support afforded by this sling method. The elevation (u) approximates the AC joint as the pad (p) lowers the clavicle.

Treatment is usually nonsurgical, because most surgical repairs are ineffective. Local injection of an analgesic agent with or without steroids is useful to diminish pain. Immobilization of the joint by wrapping it with a figure-eight bandage pulls the shoulder backwards and upwards (Fig. 8–42). If the trauma has torn the coracoclavicular ligaments (see Fig. 8–8), however, surgical repair is indicated.

STERNOCLAVICULAR JOINT

Pain and impairment may occur from injury to the sternoclavicular joint (Fig. 8–43), but is relatively rare. The joint is formed by the inner edge of the clavicle's joining a fossa on the superior lateral margin of the sternum and the cartilage of the first rib. A small disk is present between these bones and strong ligamentous support.

Diagnosis is made by findings of localized pain and tenderness at that site and by crepitation on shoulder girdle motion. Treatment is local, as it is in the AC joint.

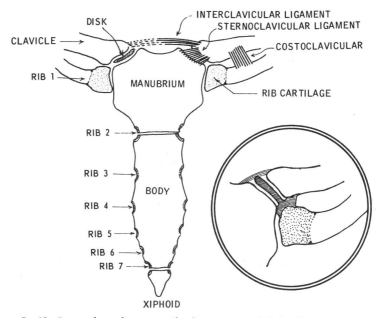

Figure 8–43. Sternoclavicular joint. The ligaments and disk of the sternoclavicular joint are shown. In the circle, the meniscus is depicted between the sternum, the clavicle, and the first rib. (From Cailliet, R: Shoulder Pain, ed 3. FA Davis, Philadelphia, 1991, p 43, with permission.)

BIBLIOGRAPHY

Instead of references, this chapter has a list of recommended readings.

Adams, JC: Review of 180 cases of recurrent dislocations of the shoulder. J Bone Joint Surg 30(B):26, 1948.

Allman, FL: Fractures and ligamentous injuries of the clavicle and its articulations. J Bone Joint Surg 49(A):774, 1967.

Andren, L and Lundberg, BJ: Treatment of rigid shoulders by joint distention during arthrography. Acta Orthop Scand 36:45, 1965.

Bateman, JE: The diagnosis and treatment of rupture of the rotator cuff. Surg Clin North Am 43:1523, 1963.

Bjelle, A, Hagsberg, M, and Michaelsson, G: Clinical and ergonomic factors in prolonged shoulder pain among industrial workers. Scand J Work Environ Health 5:205, 1979.

Cailliet, R: Shoulder Pain, ed 3. FA Davis, Philadelphia, 1991.

Codman, EA: The Shoulder. Thomas Todd, Boston, 1934.

Cook, DA and Heiner, JP: Acromioclavicular Joint Injuries. A Review Paper. Orthop Rev XIX:510–516, 1990.

DePalma, AF: Surgery of the Shoulder, ed 2. JB Lippincott, Philadelphia, 1973.

DePalma, AF: Surgical anatomy of the rotator cuff and natural history of degenerative periarthritis. Surg Clin North Am, 43:1507, 1963.

Grey, RG: The natural history of "ideopathic" frozen shoulder. J Bone Joint Surg 60A:564, 1978.

Hagberg, M: Work load and fatigue in repetitive arm elevations. Ergonomics 24:543, 1981.

Hagberg, M: Shoulder pain-pathogenesis. In Hadler, NM: Clinical Concepts in Regional Musculoskeletal Illness. Grune & Stratton, New York, 1987, p 191.

MacNab, I: Rotator cuff tendinitis. Ann R Coll Surg Engl 53:271, 1973.

McGregor, L: Rotation at the shoulder: Critical inquiry. Br J Surg 24:425, 1937.

Moseley, HF: Shoulder Lesions, ed 3. Churchill Livingstone, Edinburgh, 1969.

Moseley, HF: Athletic injuries to the shoulder region. Am J Surg 98:401, 1959.

Neer, CS: Impingement lesions. Clin Orthop 173:70, 1983.

Neer, CS: Frozen shoulder. In Neer, CS (ed): Shoulder Reconstruction. WB Saunders, Philadelphia, 1990, pp 422–427.

Neviaser, JS: Adhesive capsulitis of the shoulder. J Bone Joint Surg 27:2,211.

Neviaser, RJ: Treating patients with rotator cuff tears. J Musculoskeletal Med 17, 1985.

Noah, J and Ramesh, G: Rotator cuff injuries in the throwing athlete. Orthopedic Review 17:1091, 1988.

Rizk, TE, Christopher, RP, Pinals, RS, and Frix, P: Adhesive capsulitis (frozen shoulder): A new approach to its management. Arch Phys Med Rehabil 64:29, 1983.

Simmonds, FA: Shoulder pain with particular reference to the "frozen" shoulder. J Bone Joint Surg 31B:426, 1949.

Simon, WH: Soft tissue disorders of the shoulder: Frozen shoulder, calcific tendinitis and bicipital tendinitis. Symposium on surgery of the shoulder. Orthop Clin North Am 6:521, 1975.

Turek, SJ: The painful and stiff shoulder. J Int Coll Surg 22(6):695, 1954.

Vern, PA (ed.): Cumulative trauma disorders. A manual for musculoskeletal diseases of the upper limbs. Taylor & Francis, Bristol, PA, 1988.

CHAPTER 9

Elbow Pain

Elbow pain, as a soft tissue injury, is common and frequently disabling. Because of the complexity of the joint, it is a potentially severe disability that is often refractory to what seems appropriate care.

The elbow joint consists of three articulations: the *humeroulnar*, the *capitular radial* (radiohumeral), and the *radioulnar* (Fig. 9–1). The humeroulnar joint permits flexion extension; the other two allow pronation and supination.

Two major collateral ligaments stabilize the elbow—an anterior band and a posterior band. The anterior arises from the medial epicondyle and attaches to the medial side of the coronoid process of the ulna. This is the major stabilizing ligament of the elbow. The posterior band is thinner; it restricts elbow motion when the elbow is flexed at an angle exceeding 90°.

The following muscles act on the elbow: the brachialis, the long and short heads of the biceps, and the triceps. Many forearm muscles originate at the elbow—the flexor group from the medial epicondyle and the extensor group from the lateral epicondyle (Fig. 9–2).

TRAUMA

Trauma to the elbow may result in major impairment and disability, because it hinders functional use of the hand and fingers and causes pain as well. Sprains, which are examples of dislocation (subluxation), injure the ligaments and the joint capsules. They become clinically evident from a meaningful history and physical examination. Results of radiologic examination can eliminate the possibility of bony injury.

Examination and treatment of fractures are beyond the scope of this text but when fractures are diagnosed or even suspected, should such patients im-

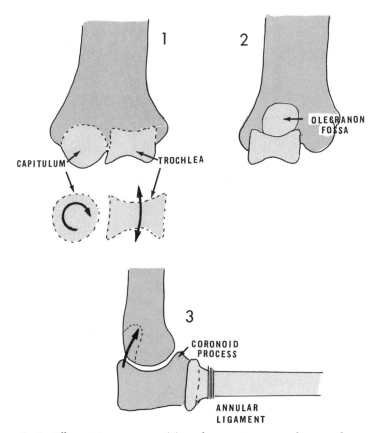

Figure 9–1. Elbow joint anatomy. (*1*) is the anterior view showing the rounded sphere of the capitulum, on which the radius rotates, and the spoon-shaped trochlea, about which the ulna flexes and extends. (*2*) is the posterior view showing the olecranon fossa, into which enters the posterior (olecranon) portion of the ulna, which enters on full elbow extension. (*3*) is the lateral view showing the ulna (*dark shade*) and the radius (*light shade*). The radius rotates about the annular ligament in pronation and supination.

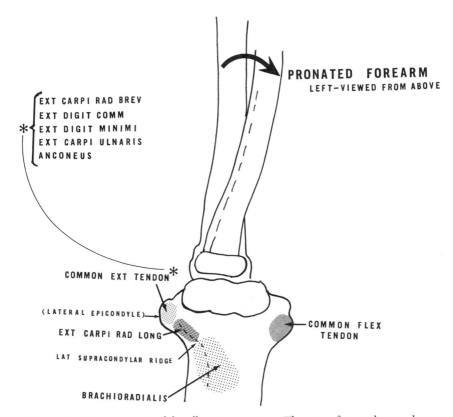

Figure 9–2. Bony aspects of the elbow in pronation. The sites of muscular attachment are shown.

mediately be referred to an orthopedic surgeon because the sequelae of untreated or improperly treated elbow fractures are ominous.

NERVE DAMAGE

Ulnar Nerve

The ulnar nerve's being superficial in the olecranon fossa makes it subject to direct trauma. The groove is behind the medial condyle. The enclosed nerve is covered by a fibrous sheath termed the **arcuate ligament,** which forms the cubital tunnel (Fig. 9–3). Because the sensory fibers of ulnar nerves are more superficial than those of the motor fibers, sensory symptoms are more prevalent.[1]

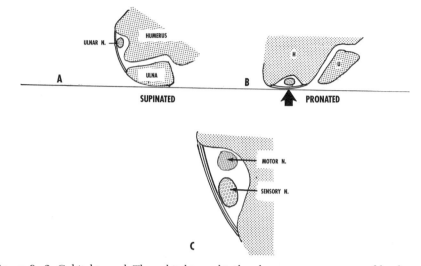

Figure 9–3. Cubital tunnel. The cubital tunnel is the olecranon groove covered by the arcuate ligament, which contains the ulnar nerve. The sensory nerve is more superficial (*C*). (*A*) The supinated forearm position removes the potential of direct pressure on the nerve whereas (*B*) the pronated position directly exposes the nerve to pressure (*arrow*).

Initial symptoms of ulnar nerve pressure or trauma include paresthesia (numbness and tingling) of the ulnar nerve dermatomes of the hand, specifically the ulnar half of the fourth finger and the entire fifth finger (Fig. 9–4). The differential diagnosis with findings of paresthesia and paresis of the ring finger and little finger includes the possibility of cervical discogenic disease, thoracic outlet compression, or pressure of the ulnar nerve at the wrist.

Treatment is conservatively managed by avoiding direct pressure to the cubital canal by wearing a sponge pad over the elbow and also by avoiding excessive elbow flexion. Surgical transplantation is usually avoided because it has been determined that conservative management is just as effective.[2]

Radial Nerve

The radial nerve is subject to entrapment within its passage at the elbow (Fig. 9–5). As it passes the lateral condyle of the humerus, it travels below the origin of the short radial extensor muscle by means of a fibrous band that stretches from the epicondyle to the deep fascia of the volar surface of the forearm.

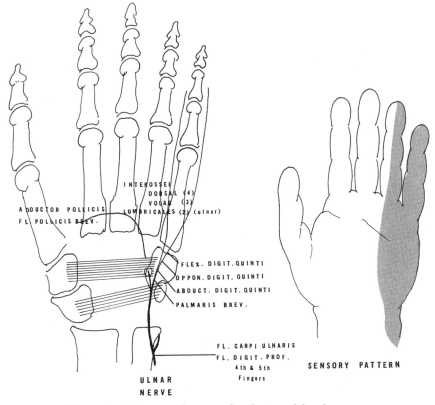

Figure 9–4. Motor and sensory distribution of the ulnar nerve.

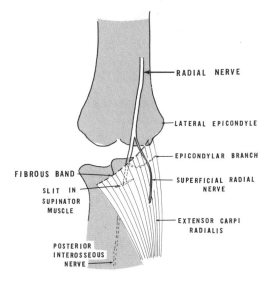

Figure 9–5. Course of the radial nerve. The deep nerve passes under the fibrous band, which is the origin of the short radial extensor muscles. Before it passes under the band, it branches into the superficial radial nerve. A small recurrent branch proceeds to the lateral epicondyle.

The radial nerve divides at this point into a deep branch and a superficial branch. The superficial branch allows sensation to be perceived at the lateral aspect of the forearm. The deep branch ultimately becomes the posterior interosseous nerve that supplies the motor functions of wrist (Fig. 9–6) and finger dorsiflexion (Fig. 9–7).

Forceful repeated contraction of these muscles tightens the fibrous band and compresses the nerve. Pain is perceived over the lateral epicondyle, and so the syndrome somewhat resembles *tennis elbow*.

Treatment begins with avoidance of muscular activities that aggravate the symptoms. This includes action involving forceful repeated wrist and finger extension with wrist supination. Wearing a splint to restrain the wrist in neutral position is valuable. Local injection of an analgesic agent and soluable steroid can also be useful. Persistent symptoms may require surgical intervention to release the fibrous band.

Baseball Elbow

As can be seen in conditions involving pitching trauma (see Figs. 8–15 and 8–16), tennis trauma (see Fig. 8–17), and bowling trauma (Fig. 8–18), the elbow undergoes repeated and excessive extension-flexion with simultaneous rapid pronation-supination. The end point of these athletic activity motions usually causes collateral ligamentous and capsular stress as well as repeated forceful contraction of the biceps, triceps, and brachialis along with forceful contraction of the forearm muscles that attach to the condyles.

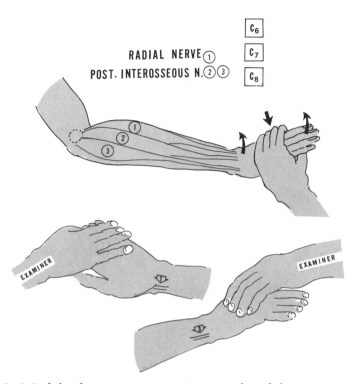

Figure 9–6. Radial and posterior interosseous nerves. The radial nerve contains roots from C6, C7, and C8. The upper drawing shows resistance in testing the nerve by contraction of (*1*) extensor carpi radialis, (*2*) extensor digitorum communis, and (*3*) extensor carpi ulnaris. *Arrow 1* in the middle figure indicates the tendon of the extensor carpi radialis and *arrow 3* indicates the tendon of extensor carpi ulnaris.

Figure 9–7. Finger extensor test of the radial nerve. This nerve contains roots C7 and C8. The extensor digitorum communis (*X*) originates from the lateral epicondyle. The tendons are seen at the dorsum of the wrist (*arrow 2*). In testing the function of the radial nerve, the examiner resists extension of all four finger extensors.

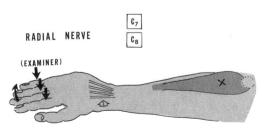

Treatment is initial rest and local analgesic applications of ice followed by heat. Review of the patient's athletic activities may reveal faulty neuromusculoskeletal activity patterns that can be corrected or modified.

Epicondylalgia

The condition more commonly termed **tennis elbow** is a frequent sports-related activity, but currently it is also seen in workplace-related pain and disability. The term "epicondylalgia" was suggested by Ferre in 1897[3] as the pathology was not always inflammatory,[4] nor degenerative.[5] The mechanism by which epicondylitis occurs and its pathology remain enigmas. Trauma has been considered as the major factor in causing the syndrome. The concept advanced by the author as related to joints[6] also applies here:[6]

1. Abnormal tension on a normal joint.
2. Normal tension on an abnormal joint.
3. Normal stress on a normal joint when that joint is neither prepared nor accustomed to the particular activity.

Repetitive trauma fits into classifications (1) and (3).

That epicondylalgia is truly a syndrome is apparent because many etiologies, concepts, and mechanisms must be considered.

An early hypothesis[7] was that epicondylalgia was a traction injury to the periosteum from the muscles that attach to the lateral epicondyle (Fig. 9–8). Treatment[8] consisted of detaching the tendons from their sites of attachment, although evidence of periostitis has never been confirmed.[5,9]

Bursitis under the tendon has been described,[10,11] but it suggested that the granulation tissue reported[9] was responsible for the clinical situation. This *bursa* was also similar to the described meniscus.[12,13] Mills[14] considered the presence of a fibrotic stenosis of the orbicular ligament as causing a syndrome requiring surgical removal.[15,16]

A tear in the proximal body of the extensor muscle group was also considered as a cause for epicondylar symptoms (Fig. 9–9).[17,18] Radicular pain resulting from compression of the radial nerve (Fig. 9–10) has been postulated and many clinicians advocate decompressing this nerve within the radial tunnel as either a primary approach or in conjunction with other procedures.[19–27]

Regardless of the actual pathology, numerous mechanisms cause the syndrome. Repetitive trauma or acute trauma, either occupational or professional, are frequent causes of this syndrome.[28–31]

An epicondylalgia of cervical origin has also been postulated, although this is contrary to local traumatic mechanisms. This concept alleges that a lesion of C5-C6 with irritation of the C6 nerve root involves the anterior face of

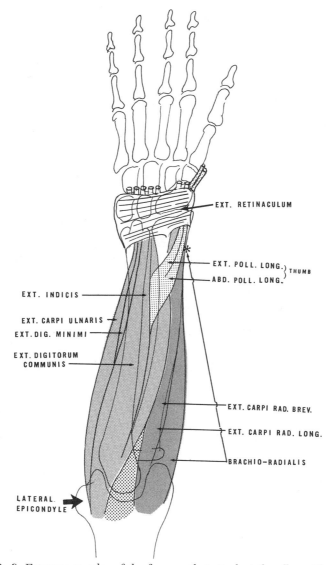

Figure 9–8. Extensor muscles of the forearm that attach at the elbow. The extensor group is emphasized at its origin from the lateral epicondyle, which is the site of epicondylitis ("tennis elbow").

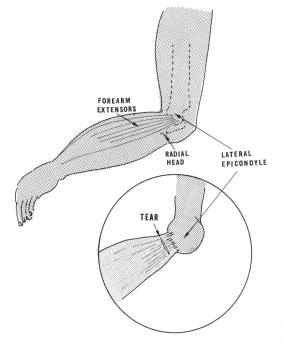

Figure 9–9. Lateral epicondylitis: "tennis elbow." At the origin site of the extensor muscle from the lateral epicondyle (see Fig. 9–3), microscopic tears may occur, causing pain and impairment.

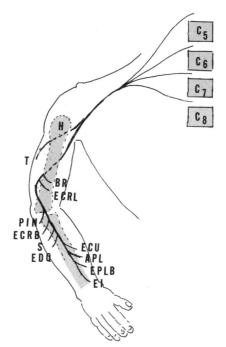

Figure 9–10. The radial nerve, emerging from roots C5–C8, enters the arm to pass behind the humerus (H) and then down the anterior-lateral aspect of the forearm to innervate the following muscles: triceps (T), brachioradialis (BR), extensor carpi radialis longus (ECRL), posterior interosseous nerve (PIN), extensor carpi radialis brevis (ECRB), supinator (S), extensor digiti quinti (EDQ), extensor carpi ulnaris (ECU), abductor pollicis longus (APL), extensor pollicis longus-brevis (EPLB), and extensor indicis (EI).

the epicondyle.[32] Electromyographic studies have revealed a cervical lesion in patients whose conditions remain resistant to local treatment.[33–37]

Diagnosis. The condition rarely appears before age 20 or after age 60, and is most common in patients between 35 and 50 years old. It occurs equally in men and women but is more prevalent in the dominant arm. Local tenderness is present at the anterolateral face of the epicondyle. This is also the site of the radial head, the orbicular ligament, and the radial nerve or its branches.

Aggravation, if not initiation, of pain on wrist and finger extension and forearm supination. Weakness of prehension resulting from pain may be present. The test for radial nerve function measures the strength of the wrist extensors (see Fig. 9–6), supinator (Fig. 9–11), the abductor pollicis longus, and the extensor pollicis longus (Fig. 9–12).

The procedure rarely wakes the patient, which is not the case with rotator cuff injuries.[38] If the causative factor is cervical radiculitis, neck position during the night may aggravate the condition. In the presence of cervical radiculitis, neck positions may initiate pain and local tenderness over the cervical foramen of C5-C6 may be palpated.

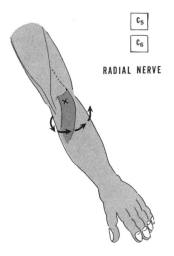

C_5

C_6

RADIAL NERVE

Figure 9–11. Radial nerve: the supinator test. The supinator muscle is innervated by the radial nerve with roots from C5 to C6. The supinator muscle originates from the lateral epicondyle and inserts on the dorsal lateral surface of the upper third of the radius. It supinates the forearm (*curved arrows*).

Treatment involving complete local rest of the elbow is effective during the immediate acute phase, but not when the pain persists or becomes chronic. Local ice is initially effective, as are oral nonsteroidal anti-inflammatory medications. A splint to limit wrist motions is also partially effective.[39–41]

Local injection into the lateral epicondylar region of maximum tenderness suggests local pathology, although referred cervical pain may also be ameliorated by a local injection into the referred site. Manipulation to complete the tear of the extensor musculature from its attachment site has been proposed (Fig. 9–13).[42]

RADIAL NERVE
(POST. INTEROSSEOUS NERVE)

C_7

C_8

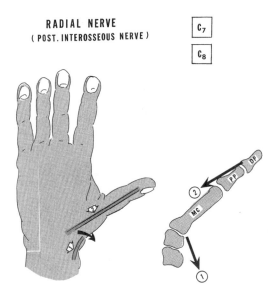

Figure 9–12. Abductor pollicis longus and extensor pollicis longus: test of radial nerve. The abductor pollicis longus tendon (*arrow 1*), the extensor pollicis longus (*arrow 2*), and their muscles are innervated by the posterior interosseous nerve. Abduction of the thumb (*1*) and extension of the distal phalanx (*2*) are tested by the examiner.

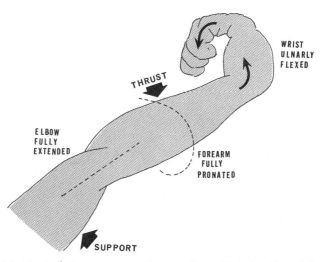

Figure 9–13. Manipulation treatment of tennis elbow. With the elbow fully extended, the forearm fully pronated, and the wrist and fingers fully flexed, the upper arm is supported and a *brisk thrust* is placed on the lower arm to further extend and pronate it. This maneuver is thought to complete the tear that may be present in the extensor musculature.

A recent neuromusculoskeletal theory has posited that the mechanism of carpal tunnel syndrome[43] is similar to that seen with tennis elbow. The musculoskeletal function of the elbow that involves central coordination (agonist-antagonists) of the wrist flexors and extensors originating at the elbow are the result of breakdown within the peripheral inhibitory mechanism.

Instead of relaxation of the antagonists during contraction of the agonists, there is also cocontraction with both agonist-antagonist contracting simultaneously, thus causing a breakdown at the musculoskeletal attachments. The resultant pathology, such as tearing at the muscle tendon periosteum site or increased tautness of the fibrous band entrapping the radial nerve, is the result of this cocontraction. The cause of central breakdown may be assumed to be fatigue as well as faulty neuromuscular activity. The cervical radicular component also implies that the postures and tensions of many activities leading to epicondylitis play a role in this situation.

REFERENCES

1. Payan, J: Anterior transportation of the ulnar nerve: An electrophysiological study. J Neurol Neurosurg Psychiatry 33:157–165, 1970.
2. Wadsworth, TG and Williams, JR: Cubital tunnel external compression syndrome. Br Med J 3:662–666, 1973.

3. Maestracci, D and Acquaviva, E: Épicondylitis, Épicondylalgie. Med du Sport 49: 35–37, 1975.
4. Nicholas, JA and Hershman, EB: The Upper Extremity in Sports Medicine. CV Mosby, St. Louis, 1990.
5. Unthoff, HK, et al: L'épicondylite externe (tennis elbow) Union Med Can 107:684–688, 1978.
6. Cailliet, R: Shoulder Pain, ed 1. FA Davis, Philadelphia, 1976.
7. Hotchkiss, RN: Common disorders of the elbow in athletes and musicians. Hand Clin 6:507, 1990.
8. Whiteside, JA and Andrews, JR: Common elbow problems in the recreational athlete. J Musculoskel Med 6:17, 1989.
9. Kivi, T: The etiology and conservative treatment of humeral epicondylitis. Scand J Rehab Med 15:37, 1982.
10. Osgood, RB: Radiohumeral bursitis, epicondylitis, epicondylalgia (tennis elbow). A personal experience. Arch Surg 4:420–433, 1922.
11. Dittrich, RJ: Radiohumeral bursitis (tennis elbow). Report of two cases. Am J Surg 7:411–414, 1929.
12. Goes, H and De Silva, O: The radio-humeral "meniscus" and its relationship to tennis elbow. Arch Interam Rheum 3:582–599, 1960.
13. Tucker, WE: Tennis elbow treated by De Goes operation. Proc Roy Soc Med 57:95, 1964.
14. Mills, GP: The treatment of tennis elbow. Br Med J 1:12–13, 1928.
15. Preiser, G: Ueber "Epicondylitis Humeri". Dtsh Med Wochenschr 36:712–715, 1910.
16. Newman, JH and Goodfellow, JW: Fibrillation of head of radius: As one cause of tennis elbow. Br Med J 2:328–330, 1975.
17. Clado, S: Tennis-Arm. Le Progrés Medical 16:273, 1902.
18. Cyriax JH: The pathology and treatment of tennis elbow. J Bone Joint Surg 18B:921–940, 1936.
19. Cailliet, R: Radial nerve. In Cailliet, R: Hand Pain and Impairment, ed 4. FA Davis, Philadelphia, 1994, pp 100–101.
20. Winckworth, CE: Tennis elbow. Br Med J 2:7–8, 1883.
21. Capener, N: The vulnerability of the posterior interosseous nerve of the forearm. J Bone Joint Surg 48B:770–773, 1966.
22. Kopell, HP and Thompson, WAL: Peripheral Entrapment Neuropathies. Williams & Wilkins, Baltimore, 1963.
23. Sharrard, WJW: Posterior Interosseous Neuritis. J Bone Joint Surg 48B:777–780, 1966.
24. Somerville, EW: Pain in the upper limb. J Bone Joint Surg 45B:621–623, 1963.
25. Spinner, M: Injuries of the Major Branches of Peripheral Nerves of the Forearm, ed 2. WB Saunders, Philadelphia, 1978.
26. Boles, NC and Maudsley, RH: Radial tunnel syndrome. J Bone Joint Surg 54B:499–508, 1972.
27. Kaplan, EBL: Treatment of tennis elbow (epicondylitis) by denervation. J Bone Joint Surg 41A:147–151, 1959.
28. Saudan, Y: Nonsurgical treatment of the acute and chronic epicondylitis (tennis elbow). Ther Umsch 34:81–87, 1977.
29. Lapidus, PW and Guidotti, FP: Lateral and medial epicondylitis of the humerus. Industr Med Surg 39:171–173, 1970.
30. Wall JL: Tennis elbow. Industr Med Surg 29:173–178, 1960.
31. DeLoore, JJ: Epicondylitis radialis. J Belge Rheum Med Phys 25:254–262, 1970.
32. Maigne, R: Épicondylalgies, rachis cervical et articulation huméro-radialis. Am Med Phys 3:299–311, 1960.
33. Illouz, G and Limon, J: L'épicondylalgie. Étude de 130 cas. Note préliminaire sur l'élctrodiagnostic. Ann Med Phys 17:214–224, 1974.

34. Gunn, GC and Milbrandt, WE: Tennis elbow and cervical spine. Can Med Assoc J 114:803–809, 1976.

35. Bence, Y, et al: Les épicondylalgies rebelles: Intertitre de l'étude électromyographique. Ann Phys Med 21:80–98, 1978.

36. Meerschaert, JR, et al: Tennis elbow associated with decreased shoulder internal rotation and cervical radiculopathy. Arch Phys Med Rehabil 56:553, 1975.

37. Iselin, M: Influence of the vertebral column on epicondylitis. Ther Umsch 34:88–91, 1977.

38. Cailliet, R: Shoulder Pain, ed 2. FA Davis, Philadelphia, 1981.

39. Tanaka, S and McGlothlin, JD: A conceptual model to assess musculoskeletal stress of manual work for establishment of quantitative guidelines to prevent hand and wrist cummulative trauma disorders (CTD). In Mital, A (ed): Advances in Industrial Ergonomics and Safety. Tayler & Francis, London, 1989, pp 419–425.

40. Vadeboncoeur, R: Les cervico-brachialgies et leur traitment. Union Med Can 105:741–745, 1976.

41. Froimson, AI: Treatment of tennis elbow with forearm support hand. J Bone Joint Surg 53A:183–184, 1971.

42. Cyriax, JH: Textbook of Orthopaedic Medicine, Vol 2, ed 8. Williams & Wilkins, Baltimore, 1971.

43. Masear, VR, Hayes, JM, and Hyde, AG: An industrial cause of carpal tunnel syndrome. J Hand Surg 11A:222–227, 1986.

CHAPTER 10

Wrist and Hand Pain

Of all the soft tissue injuries the hand presents the greatest disability when impaired. Loss of dexterity or impairment causes significant problems with activities of daily living and many occupations.

Pain is a frequent symptom, as is loss of function. Numerous tissues in the wrist and hand are subject to painful impairment and disability. Accurate diagnosis demands a knowledge of functional anatomy, a meaningful history, and a precise examination.

The hand is an *organ* of grasp as well as one of fine movement, with exquisite sensation and delicate discrimination. A large portion of the brain controls the function of the hand, indicating its ultimate development and training.

Restoration of function is the ultimate goal of treatment and is based on understanding the neuromusculoskeletal nature of the hand. Early care is paramount as prolonged immobilization is detrimental and reconstructive surgery still limited.

Although all aspects of hand injury will be discussed, depth will be limited by the available space. The major clinical syndromes will, however, be emphasized.

CARPAL TUNNEL SYNDROME

The carpal tunnel is a narrow fibro-osseous opening through which traverse six structures: the flexor pollicis longus tendon, four flexor digitorum profundus tendons, and the median nerve (Fig. 10–1). The distal volar skin crease of the wrist (Fig. 10–2) is the proximal border of the canal. The tunnel itself extends approximately 3 centimeters.

The roof of the carpal tunnel is the transverse carpal ligament, which

310

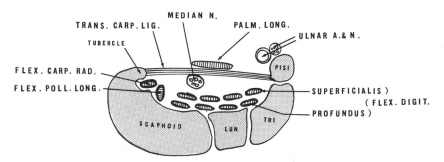

Figure 10–1. Contents of carpal tunnel. The tunnel contains the deep and superficial long finger flexor tendons, the tendons of the long flexor muscles of the thumb, the ulnar flexor muscle of the wrist, and the median nerve.

comprises two bands: one from the hook of the hamate bone extending to the tubercle of the trapezium and another, more proximal, that extends from the tubercle of the navicular (scaphoid) bone to the pisiform bone (Fig. 10–3). The floor of the tunnel is occupied by the carpal bones of the hand.

Carpal tunnel syndrome (CTS) occurs when the median nerve is compressed within these anatomic structures. The syndrome can be divided into three categories[1]: (1) increased volume of the contents of the tunnel; (2) enlargement of the median nerve; and (3) decreased cross-sectional area within the tunnel. The increased contents are considered to cause tendinitis and tenosynovitis in most symptomatic patients.[2] Enlargement of the nerve is rare

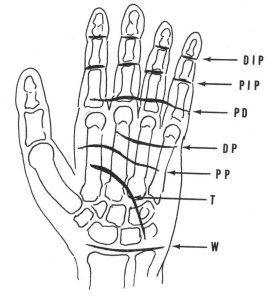

Figure 10–2. Palmar creases and their bony landmarks. DIP = distal interphalangeal crease; PIP = proximal interphalangeal crease; PD = palmar digital crease; DP = distal palmar crease; PP = proximal palmar crease; T = thenar crease; W = wrist crease.

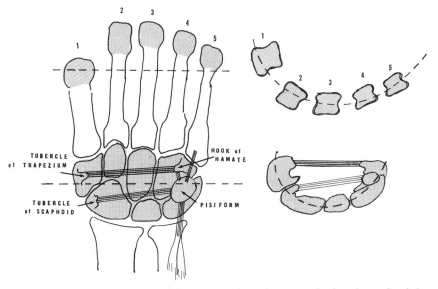

Figure 10–3. Transverse carpal ligaments. These ligaments bridge the arch of the carpal rows to form a tunnel. The proximal band extends from the tubercle of the navicular bone to the pisiform bone. The distal band extends from the tubercle of the trapezium to the hook of the hamate bone.

and decreased cross sectional area in the tunnel, without rheumatoid arthritis, is also infrequently seen. Surgical intervention in patients with CTS has revealed thickened and edematous synovial sheaths of the enclosed tendons.[2] Most people have a minor tenosynovitis of the tendons within the tunnel but to a lesser degree than people with symptomatic CTS.[3]

The biomechanics of the carpal tunnel tendons (flexor digitorum profundus, flexor digitorum superficialis, and the flexor pollicis longus) is that they move in the manner of a belt around a pulley[4,5] with the transverse carpal ligamants acting as the fulcrum. Flexion and extension of the wrist causes these tendons to be displaced against or past the ligaments (Fig. 10–4).

The power grip or repeated finger flexion with wrist stabilization, which is so common in many workplace activities, involves simultaneous wrist extension and active finger flexor contraction. This action increases load on the flexor tendons; this leads to degenerative, and possibly inflammatory, changes in the tendons. Normally the coefficient of friction is minimal, but with increased muscular action and repetitive motions, friction undoubtedly increases.

The transverse carpal ligament is an important component of the digital flexor pulley system. Its action in the tunnel causes those problems that lead to the syndrome. Its removal or modification in the treatment of the

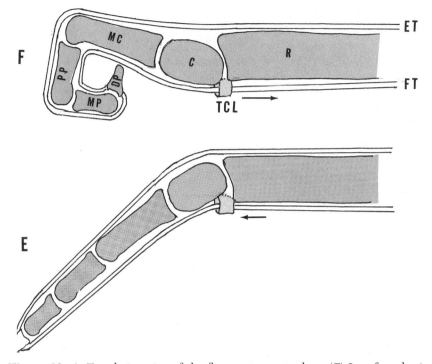

Figure 10–4. Tenodesis action of the flexor-extensor tendons. (*F*) In a forced grip (flexion of the hand), force is generated by tenodesis action with the wrist being slightly extended, which causes the flexor tendons (FT) to elongate and thus have greater tension. (*E*) With the hand extended the flexor tendons have less tension from the carpal bones' (C) being slightly flexed on the radius (R). The transverse carpal ligament (TCL) acts like a pulley preventing the flexor tendons from bowing. Repeated flexion-extension (opening and closing the fist) causes repeated movement within the transverse carpal ligament pulley and increases friction. ET = the extensor tendons; MC = metacarpals; PP = proximal phalanx; MP = middle phalanx; and DP = distal phalanx.

syndrome adds undesirable, as well as remedial, factors. It also plays a large causative role in the syndrome, which must be considered in prevention, and cure.

The flexor tendon pulley assures maximul flexion force of the joints with minimal excursion of the tendons.[6] Both definite flexion weakness and an inability to touch the fingers to the palm with the wrist fully flexed are present. Flexion decreases with wrist flexion at 20° and is fully lost with the wrist flexed to 40°.

Maximum muscle strength occurs at resting length. Passive stretching of 40% loses strength.[7-9] The closer to the center of rotation of a joint the tendon passes the less distance that tendon must traverse but with attendant loss of mechanical efficiency. This is the *rule of the moment arm*. The greater the moment arm, the greater its mechanical efficiency, but also the longer the excursion is. The flexor pulley system at the transverse carpal ligament minimizes the moment arm's decreasing the extent of tendon excursion,[10] which in turn allows the muscle to remain closer to its resting stage.

The flexor pulley system of the metacarpophalangeal, proximal interphalangeal, and distal interphalangeal joints have been extensively described[11] as performing with the efficacy of a pulley system (Fig. 10–5). The effects of surgery on the transverse carpal ligament in the treatment of CTS have been extensively discussed[12–16] (e.g., claiming a residual grip

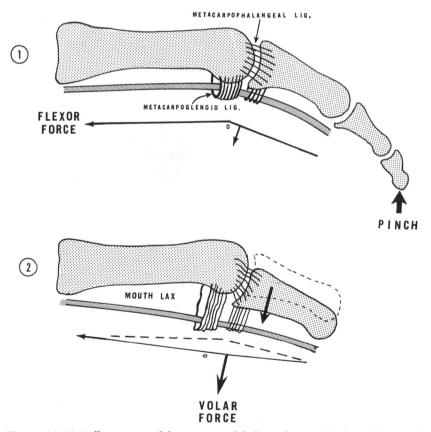

Figure 10–5. Pulley system of the metacarpalphalangeal joint. (*1*) shows the normal pulley assembly fulcrums of the flexor tendons during a forceful pinch. (*2*) In a condition such as rheumatoid arthritis, which weakens the flexor pulley, the alignment of the flexor tendon loses its efficiency and exerts a volar force from the bowing.

weakness, bow stringing of the flexor tendons, and collapse of the transverse arch).

Pathophysiology of Nerve Compression

Those flexor tendon factors in CTS that cause compression of the median nerve, the primary locus of impairment and disability, have been studied. Low-grade peripheral nerve compression reduces epineural blood flow (Fig. 10–6). Axonal transport is impaired (Fig. 10–7). With segmental axonal compression (see Figs. 1–9 and 1–10), the endoneural (Fig. 10–8) fluid pressure is increased with resultant paresthesia.

Clinically, patients with early CTS experience numbness and tingling in the distribution of the median nerve (Fig. 10–9). Early abnormalities are noted in vibration tests and in the Semmes-Weinstein monofilament testing (Fig. 10–10).

Experimentally, pressure changes have been determined within the carpal tunnel depending on wrist positions (Figs. 10–11 and 10–12). Applying pressure of 50 mm Hg for two hours causes endoneural edema.[17] Clinically, median nerve compression of 60 mm Hg can cause complete sensory conduction block.[18] Pressure changes resulting in median nerve ischemia have been postulated as the major cause of carpal tunnel syndrome, which has led to specific therapeutic approaches. Of the three postulated causes of CTS, this increased volume of the contents of the carpal tunnel[19] has the greatest number of proponents, but what increases the contents remains unclear.

Tenosynovitis brought about by repetitive trauma is most often implicated.[2,20–23] Visible synovial thickening has been reported by some, yet denied by others. Fuchs, Nathan, and Myers[24] who found inflammation infrequent in their research series noted that those patients who did show inflammation (10%) had significantly impaired conduction time.

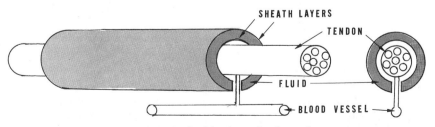

Figure 10–6. The blood supply of a tendon.

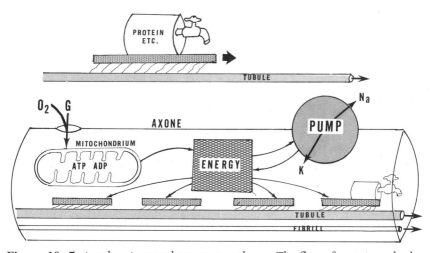

Figure 10–7. Axoplasmic neural transport: a theory. The flow of protein and other derivatives begins with the entry of glucose (G) into the mitochondria through metabolism of adenosine-triphosphate (ATP), which transmits the energy to the sodium pump. This pump regulates the balance of sodium (Na) and potassium (K) and determines nerve activity. The transport filaments move along the axon by oscillation and carry the nutritive protein elements along the nerve pathways. (Data from Ochs, S: Axoplasmic transport: A basis for neural pathology. In Dyck, PJ, Thomas, PK, and Lambert, EH: Peripheral Neuropathy, Vol 1, WB Saunders, Philadelphia, 1975, pp 213–230.)

These researchers did find edema as did others, and to a greater degree than has been established in controls. Faithfull, Moir, and Ireland[25] observed "the usual microscopic finding in the typical carpal tunnel syndrome is one of oedema [sic]". The question arises whether the edema is inflammatory, which can be asked because inflammatory cells are found in fewer than 7% of patients with edema.

Venous congestion resulting from hyptonia during sleep was considered a likely precursor to anoxic capillary endothelial damage and edema in CTS.[26]

Tenosynovitis in itself is not a major factor in CTS, but edema is. Repetitive tendon excursions from sustained and possibly improper muscular tension are important factors. Because the pulley mechanism of the transverse carpal ligament is a physiologic mechanism and so not a major cause in CTS, therefore the attempts to remove or elongate the tendon surgically to increase the volume of the carpal tunnel should be used only as a last resort.

Carpal tunnel release immediately reduces the pressure within the carpal tunnel. Knowing that various positions of the wrist change the intracarpal tunnel pressures (wrist flexion greater than flexion[27] as well as sustained extension

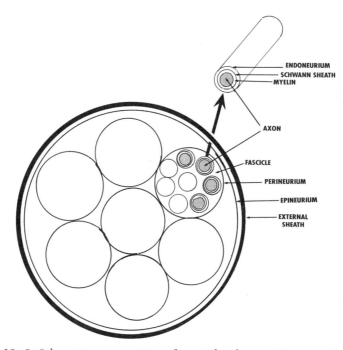

ENDONEURIUM
SCHWANN SHEATH
MYELIN

AXON

FASCICLE

PERINEURIUM

EPINEURIUM

EXTERNAL
SHEATH

Figure 10–8. Schematic representation of a peripheral nerve. A cross section shows the axons (*upper drawing*) grouped into a fascicle. Each axon is surrounded by myelin enclosed within a sheath of Schwann. This sheath is coated by endometrium. A group of fascicles is contained within a sheath of perineureum, which is grouped within a sheath of epineureum. The entire nerve is covered by an external sheath.

leading to nerve ischemia) must be addressed in initiating a treatment protocol. The long-range effects of high pressure on a nerve is well known, but the effects of lower pressure, as measured in CTS, suggest the disturbance of function is rapidly reversible and indicate that vascular insufficiency, rather that morphologic changes, occur in the nerve as a result of this amount of pressure.[28]

Long-term pressure impairs microvascular flow with gradual leakage of proteins through the walls of the venules causing epineural edema: the *primum mobile* in CTS (Fig. 10–13).

Treatment

Early intervention after diagnosis of CTS is preferred with gratifying results and avoidance of surgery. CTS develops over a period of months; it is initiated by edema, which is reversible. This edema likely results from me-

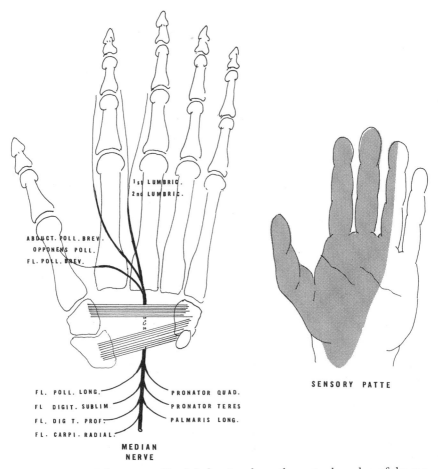

Figure 10–9. Median nerve. The left drawing shows the motor branches of the median nerve and the right drawing shows the sensory (dermatomal) pattern.

chanical tendon friction from repetitive mechanical activities in which wrist motions coupled with certain finger flexor[1] activities are the major type. Tendon action for maximum force indicates significant finger flexor forces with sustained wrist extension position. Friction over the transverse carpal ligament increases and thereby causes *inflammation* with resultant edema of the median nerve.

After symptoms occur (paresthesia, numbness, and weakness), significant edema can be assumed to be present. If early signs are noted or if the patient

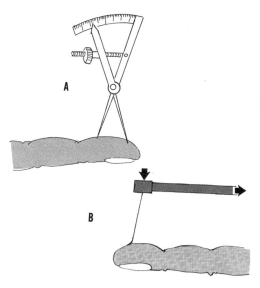

Figure 10–10. Light touch testing. (A) The caliper two-point test and (B) the Semmes-Weinstein monofilament discrimination test both measure sensory perceptions in peripheral nerve function. A measures two point discrimination and B measures light palpation discrimination.

is occupationally susceptible early testing of median nerve conduction time is indicated. The early signs are:

- A positive Tinel sign which means that gentle tapping of the median nerve at the wrist elicits tingling in the distribution of the median nerve.[29] Three taps are considered positive if tingling results from each tap.
- A positive Phalen test, which means making a forceful flexion of the patient's wrist and holding it there for 1 minute can reproduce the paresthesia.[30,31] Phalen felt no need for electrodiagnostic testing if results of both the Tinel and Phalen tests were positive.[30] Careful studies[32] have refuted the value of a Tinel sign but continue to accept the Phalen test.

Weakness of the abductor pollicis brevis[33] and change in sensory testing by light palpation, vibration test or Semmes-Weinstein filament test are also indicators.

Nerve conduction is diagnostic and electromyographic (EMG) testing is necessary in the presence of significant motor weakness.

Occupational factors that need concern the examiner are:

- Repetitive activities[33]
- Computer keyboard activities
- Grip force[34]

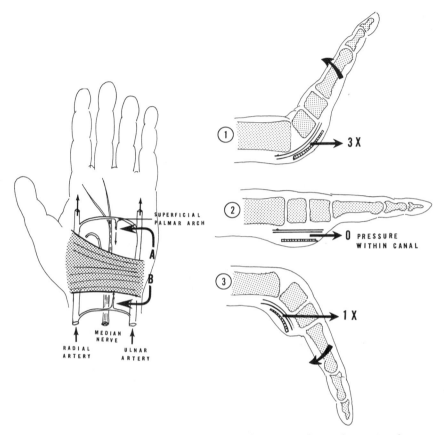

Figure 10–11. Postulated mechanism of paresthesia: carpal tunnel pressure changes. The large drawing shows arterial circulation of the median nerve, which is a small branch distal to the superficial palmar arch (*A*) and a proximal branch from the ulnar artery (*B*). Pressure on the arterial source varies with palmar position. (*1*) Wrist extension (dorsiflexion) increases the tunnel pressure three times that caused by wrist flexion (*3*). Normal pressure is shown in neutral wrist position (*2*).

- Pinch force
- Wrist flexion
- Palm pressure
- Vibration[35–37]
- Glove use
- Exposure to cold
- Intensity of work conditions

After the occupational situation and early delayed conduction times are confirmed, the following measures appear to be indicated:

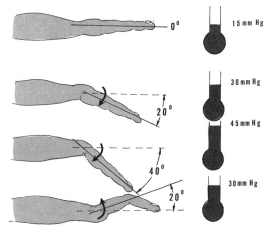

Figure 10–12. Variants of tunnel pressures from wrist positions. In neutral position the carpal tunnel pressure is 15 mm Hg, doubles with flexed wrist as 20°, and triples with wrist flexed to 40°. Wrist extension causes an increase of tunnel pressure to 30 mm Hg.

1. Night splinting and splinting during working hours (Fig. 10–14).[38,39]
2. Prework exercises
    Flexibility
    Strengthening (Fig. 10–15)
3. Job technique modification[40,41]

   Dynamic studies on repetitive *passive* flexion-extension motions *pumps up* carpal tunnel pressure in patients with CTS and remains higher than normal even after rest.[42] Active flexion-extension has additional effect. Flexion-extension isometric or isotonic exercises of the forearm muscles[43] increase carpal tunnel pressure, but because forearm muscles do not extend into the wrist, the reason for increased carpal tunnel pressure is not clear. Certain advocates suggest active flexion-extension exercises to provoke symptoms of CTS. These factors cast doubt on the advocacy of forearm exercises in the treatment of

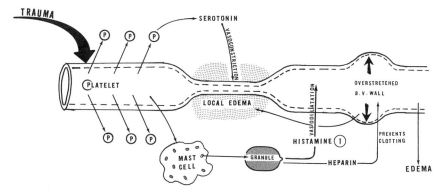

Figure 10–13. The effect of trauma: a vasochemical reaction.

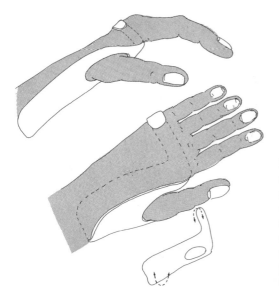

Figure 10–14. A cock up splint for carpal tunnel syndrome. One of numerous types of wrist splints used in treatment. It immobilizes the wrist at a neutral position. The thumb and fingers at their metacarpophalangeal joints are free to allow active motion.

CTS[19] even though they have proven effective. Exercises *may* mobilize the tendons within the tunnels, but this remains conjectural. Rest is apparently effective as is immobilization of the wrist during activities of daily living.

4. Local steroid injections[44]

A provocative paper[19] has asserted a relationship between cervical pressure and CTS. Hellenbrandt, Houtz, Partridge, and Waltos[45] demonstrated that repetitive, fatiguing upper extremity movement ex-

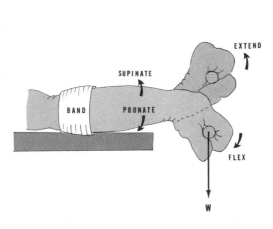

Figure 10–15. Exercises for the forearm flexors and extensors. With the forearm resting on a firm surface, a weighted (W) object with a rounded contour handle is lifted up (extended) and allowed to slowly descend. The forearm is then supinated and the same exercise strengthens the flexors. With varying degrees of pronation and supination, a combination of flexion-lateral flexion (extension-lateral flexion) is strengthened. Full range of motion is attempted to increase range of motion.

erted reciprocal reflex activities in the neck muscles. Changing neck and head postures affects the limb muscle activity and *vice versa*. Neck muscle fatigue significantly affects limb muscle activity.[46] Increased load on the tendons from increased forearm muscle tonus, resulting from cervical muscle asymmetry, increases the inflammatory response that leads to CTS.

The protocol is to evaluate muscle imbalance and asymmetry and then to strengthen the weaker side. Asymmetric weakness has been found in the sternocleidomastoid and neck extensors. After strengthening exercises, frequent rotation to one side with sustained contraction is followed by a return to midline. This procedure should be implemented in daily working activities.

Steroid Injection Technique. A mixture of 0.75 mL of a soluble steroid and 0.75 mL of 1% lidocaine without epinephrine is used. A 25-ga needle is inserted 1 cm proximal to the distal wrist flexion crease between the palmaris longus and flexor carpi radialis tendon (Fig. 10–16). The needle is angled at 45° to 60° distally and is inserted 1 cm to penetrate the flexor retinaculum, then inserted 1 cm further before solution is inserted. If the needle insertion elicits paresthesia, the needle should be withdrawn and reinserted slightly more superficially. Injection *into* the nerve should be assiduously avoided. After injection, the wrist should be splinted or casted at a neutral position for 3 weeks.

If objective nerve impairment is noted and conservative treatment fails,

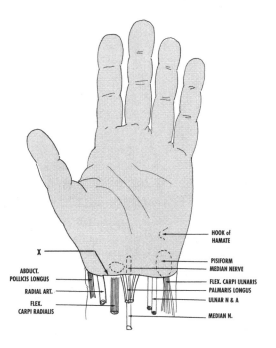

Figure 10–16. Superficial landmarks at the palmar surface of the wrist. X indicates the palmar crease. The median nerve lies directly under the palmaris longus tendon. All tendons are palpable and ascertained by having the involved muscle contracted during palpation.

surgical decompression should be considered (Fig. 10–17). Complete visualization should be assured and damage to the nerve and its branches avoided (Fig. 10–18). Both layers of the ligament should be addressed.

Numerous theories are evolving as to the probable causation of CTS. These suggestions alter the approach to its management. General agreement exists that CTS is a cumulative trauma disorder (CTD) or a repetitive strain injury (RSI) or both, they are identical in concept. The incidence of CTS has increased over the decades as more workers perform fine manual motor activities for increasingly longer periods.

Awkward hand and wrist positions and repetitive hand-finger activities are prominent in CTDs.[47–49] Flexion-extension acceleration studies that did not require the use of hand tools were found to be prominent in CTDs[50] and were supported by anatomic, physiologic, and biomechanical modeling studies.

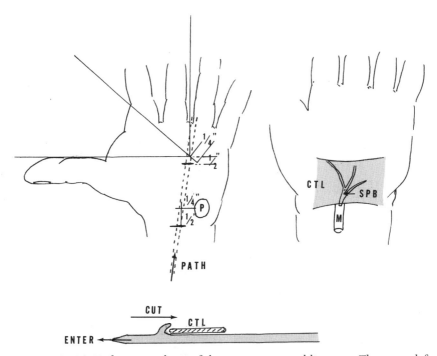

Figure 10–17. Endoscopic release of the transverse carpal ligament. The upper left drawing shows the pathway of the trocar entering $\frac{1}{4}$ inch medial to the pisiform bone (P) and $\frac{1}{2}$ inch proximal to the palmar crease. It exits distally between the third and fourth fingers. The upper right drawing shows the site of the median nerve (M) under the carpal transverse ligament (CTL). The sensory palmar branch (SPB) leaving the median nerve, which must be avoided is shown. The lower drawing shows the trochar with its cutting blade passing under the carpal tunnel ligament (CTL). Once the blade has passed the ligament, the blade is pulled back to cut the ligament.

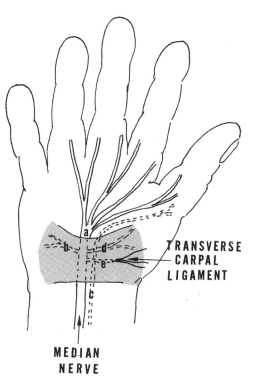

Figure 10–18. Anatomic variations of the median nerve at the wrist. (*a*) The usual distribution of the median nerve. (*b*) A transligamentous branch distribution going to the abductor digiti quinti. (*c*) A divided median nerve. (*d*) A transligamentous branch that remains under the ligament. (*e*) is a transligamentous branch that penetrates the ligament toward the thenar eminence.

Robbins[51] postulated that extreme flexion-extension of the wrist reduced the volume of the carpal tunnel by compressing the median nerve. Smith, Sontegard, and Armstrong[52] replaced the median nerve with a water-filled cylindrical balloon and found that pressure on the nerve (balloon) was increased when the wrist was flexed to an extreme angle and when the flexor tendons were tensed at various wrist flexion angles.

Biologic changes occur in the flexor tendons as they pass under the carpal tunnel ligament with resultant hyperplasia and increased density[53] from repeated exertions of the wrist, hand, and fingers. Repeated flexion-extension movements also increase the shear traction forces of the tendons from their pulley action at the transverse ligament.[54]

From these studies, the forces upon the tendons in their flexion-extension acceleration cause tenosynovitis of the tendons with resultant compression on the median nerve.

Compressive forces are also exerted by forearm muscles that generate forces for repetitive contraction. These muscles also exert torque forces and cocontraction of the muscles to stabilize the wrist while the fingers are flexing and extending thus increasing the compressive forces within the carpal tunnel.[55]

CTDs result, therefore, from repetitive flexion-extension activities with concurrent static wrist stabilizing forces (Fig. 10–19). Static muscle tension from inappropriate muscular activity and prolonged *isometric* contraction of the stabilizing muscles with cocontraction of the kinetic muscles performing the dexterity action has been asserted but, as yet, has not been fully confirmed.

Prolonged static contraction also probably impairs the agonist-antagonist reflex action with the kinetic muscles causing the agonists to function against the action of unreleasing antagonist muscles. This becomes *cocontraction*, rather than reciprocal agonist-antagonist action. Resultant improper tendon action is manifested at the carpal tunnel, producing CTS. This is being studied using intricate EMG testing, which may lead to precise pathonomonics of CTS. Other involved factors are evolving, such as posture, stress, and individual psychosocial considerations.

Some mechanisms *trigger* the pathophysiology of CTS in certain particularly susceptible individuals. One recent concept is the *double-crush theory* in which proximal nerve compressive syndromes cause or predispose to distal nerve entrapment. Such proximal factors include brachial plexus compression from scalene pressure (see Chap. 7) (Fig. 10–20).

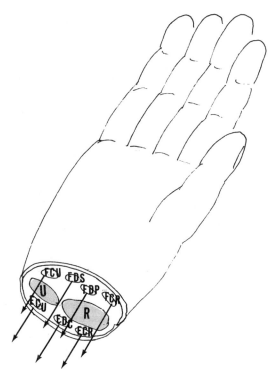

Figure 10–19. Cross section of the wrist. The seven tendons at the wrist transmit force exerted by the extrinsic muscles of the forearm. They achieve grip-and-pinch force as well as torque about the wrist. The cocontraction of extensors and flexors generates compressive forces at the wrist and in the carpal tunnel. The tendons are as follows: FCR = flexor carpi radialis; FDS = flexor digitorum superficialis; FDP = flexor digitorum profundus; FCU = flexor carpi ulnaris; ECR = extensor carpi radialis; ED = extensor digitorum; ECU = extensor carpi ulnaris; U = ulna; and R = radius bones of the forearm.

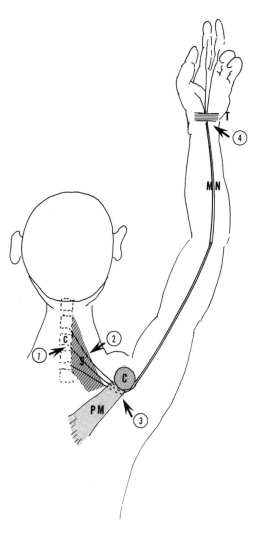

Figure 10–20. "Double crush": median nerve compression syndrome. The median nerve (MN) can be compressed at numerous sites causing it to be hypersensitive: (*1*) at the cervical (c) intervertebral foramen, (*2*) at the scalene muscles (S), (*3*) under the pectoralis minor (P) or under the corocoid process (C), and (*4*) at the transverse carpal tunnel (T).

The *crush* syndrome is one wherein neural compression allegedly alters the axoplasmic neural transport system.[56] The axoplasmic transport theory is illustrated in Figure 10–21. The crush occurs on a myelinated nerve with displacement of the nodes of Ranvier (Figs. 10–22 and 10–23). The resultant changes in the axonal transmission distally predispose to further impairment from a potential distal crush.

Why the proximal muscles cause the proximal aspect of the double-crush syndrome is being explored. These muscles fatigue and fail to recover in an appropriate time. Biomechanical stress of these muscles on contiguous nerves lead to entrapment. The fibers that fatigue first are the slow-twitch fibers[57]

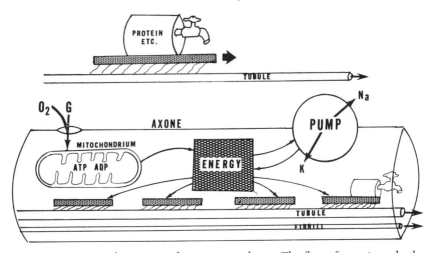

Figure 10–21. Axoplasmic neural transport: a theory. The flow of protein and other derivatives begins with entry of glucose (G) into the fiber. Glycolysis and phosphorylation occur (O_2) in the mitochondria through metabolism of adenosine-triphosphate (ATP), which creates the energy to the sodium pump. This pump regulates balance of sodium (Na) and potassium (K) and determines nerve activity. The transport filaments (F) move along the axon by oscillation and carry the nutritive protein elements along the nerve pathway. (Data from Ochs, S: Axoplasmic transport: A basis for neural pathology. In Dyck, PJ, Thomas, PK, and Lambert, EH: Peripheral Neuropathy, Vol 1. WB Saunders, Philadelphia, 1975, pp 213–230.)

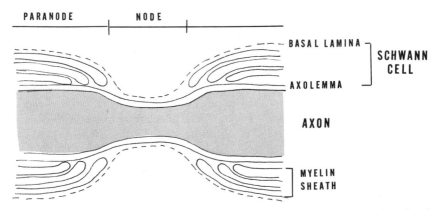

Figure 10–22. A node of Ranvier. The myelinated axon is narrowed at each node of Ranvier formed by Schwann cells that invaginate to form a node with the remaining portion comprising a paranode.

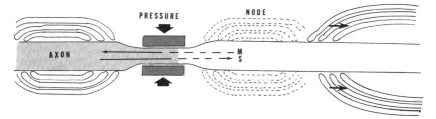

Figure 10–23. Effect of pressure (crush) on a myelinated nerve. Application of pressure on a myelinated peripheral nerve causes longitudinal displacement of the nodes of Ranvier especially at the proximal edge of the pressure site. The dotted drawing is the normal site of the node before application of pressure, and the node with arrows shows the migration. Pressure on an axon causes a deficit in nerve conduction both in sensory (S) and motor (M) fibers (*arrows*).

which, if not periodically rested, *shut off*. Areas of local ischemia that develop become sites of fibromyalgia (see Chap. 3).

Stages of dysfunction follow with the proximal muscles initiating the process. The muscles involved are the trapezius muscles that support the scapula and normally maintain the supraclavicular space through which the plexus emerges. With a postural forward head position necessary for the task, a scalene syndrome results with neurovascular compression as the scalene muscles assume the function of other scapular muscles. These muscles cause a proximal neurovascular compression that ultimately result in neurovascular distal compression within the carpal tunnel.

The initial symptoms are numbness and tingling with no discernible edema or delayed nerve conduction. The initial microscopic edema is in the forearm compartment. The intrinsic muscles of the hand undertake the function of the proximal forearm (flexor) muscles.[58]

The slow-twitch muscles that are fatigued become unable to sustain prolonged activities. This is initially in the capsular, and then possibly the cervical, muscles.

Treatment protocols of incipient CTS thus treat the proximal component early. Work-rest cycles are mandatory and must be frequent. Strengthening of scapular muscles found to be weak must be undertaken. Treatment of the *distal* aspect of the syndrome must be initiated as well, but this therapy will fail if the proximal component is ignored.

PRONATOR TERES MEDIAN NERVE COMPRESSION

The median nerve leaves the cubital fossa passing between the heads of the pronator teres muscle then passes under the tendinous edge of the flexor digitorum sublimis muscle (Fig. 10–24). The course of the median nerve

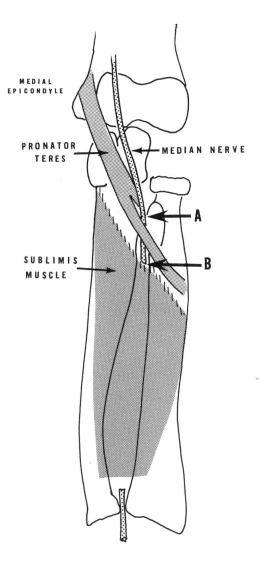

MEDIAL EPICONDYLE

PRONATOR TERES

MEDIAN NERVE

A

SUBLIMIS MUSCLE

B

Figure 10–24. Pronator teres median nerve compression. (*A*) The median nerve leaves the cubital fossa (*upper portion of drawing*) to pass between the heads of the pronator teres muscle, then (*B*) passes under the tendinous edge of the flexor digitorum sublimis muscle. On leaving the pronator teres, the median nerve gives rise to the anterior interosseous nerve.

through the pronator teres muscle varies[58] between the heads (56%), behind the heads (11%), through the humeral head (3%), and through the ulnar head (2%). In some patients, the ulnar head of the pronator teres is missing. After leaving the pronator teres, the median nerve gives rise to the anterior interosseous nerve.

After traversing the teres muscle, the median nerve divides under the tendinous arch of the flexor digitorum sublimis and into the layer between the flexor digitorum sublimis and the flexor digitorum profundus. The median nerve runs between the flexor digitorum sublimis and the flexor digitorum profundus, ultimately between the flexor carpi radialis and the palmaris longus to reach the carpal tunnel.

In the forearm, the median nerve supplies the pronator teres, flexor carpi radialis, palmaris longus, and digitorum superficialis. Just distal to the pronator muscle, the median nerve sends branches to the ulnar half of the flexor digitorum profundus, flexor pollicis longus, and pronator quadratus. This anatomic knowledge is vital in diagnostically exploring the muscle involved in this syndrome.

The pronator teres pronates the forearm with the elbow preventing rotation by elimination of pronation from the brachioradialis and the long flexors of the forearm.

The numerous causes of nerve compression vary from direct trauma,[59] to static compression from a fibrous band and to prolonged external compression as seen in *honeymoon paralysis*.[60]

Symptoms and Signs

Subjective symptoms and objective signs of median nerve involvement found in that upper extremity are similar to CTS. The pronator teres syndrome, however, involves not only the muscles of the thenar eminence but also the flexors of the wrist and the finger flexors. The patient's complaints are related to thumb, index finger, and middle finger flexion. Sensory disturbances involve the volar and dorsal surfaces of the hand, palm, and several fingers.[61]

Sensory disturbances of the palm indicate compression *proximal* to the tunnel because the median nerve normally gives over to the palmaris branch before entering the tunnel. This is probably the most important sign diagnostic for differentiating the pronator teres syndrome from carpal tunnel median nerve compression.

A stress test[62] that suggests pronator teres compression is the evoking of pain and paresthesia by *resisted pronation of the forearm with the elbow extended*. Further aggravation of the symptoms occur by resistance of flexion of the elbow and simultaneous supination of the forearm, implicating the lacertus fibrosus. Resistance of flexion of the proximal interphalangeal joint of the middle finger implicates the FDS muscle belly.

A positive Tinel sign can be elicited by tapping or exerting direct pressure in the region of the two heads of the pronator teres muscle below the cubital space.

Use of EMG studies can assist by demonstrating abnormalities and delayed conduction velocity of the flexor carpi radialis, flexor digitorum sublimis, and flexor palmaris longus. In contrast to carpal tunnel median nerve compression, which usually involves the muscles of the thenar eminence, compression at the pronator teres site involves not only the thenar muscles but also

those of the wrist and finger flexors. Because the median nerve gives off a palmar branch before entering the carpal tunnel, a sensory deficit of the palm implies median nerve compression proximal to the carpal tunnel.

Treatment of the PTS

Most pronator teres syndromes are mild and self-limited, thus merely reducing provocative movement of the forearm, wrist, and finger flexors for several weeks will be beneficial. This process can be assisted by splinting the forearm in a neutral position between pronation and supination. Local injections
of steroids into the region of compression is also valuable.[63]

Persistent symptoms and objective evidence of insidious paresis and anas-
thesia justify surgical decompression, which will allow identification of the involved structures, release of the origin of the humeral head of the pronator,
and even neurolysis of the median nerve, if indicated.[65]

ANTERIOR INTEROSSEOUS SYNDROME

The motor branch of the median nerve, the anterior interosseous nerve,
in the cubital region can undergo compression, impairing function of the distal
phalanx of the thumb and index finger.

The anterior interosseous nerve originates from the division of the median nerve progressing under the deep fascial layer of the flexor digitorum superficialis running along the interosseous membrane. It ultimately innervates
the flexor pollicies longus and the flexor digitorum profundus to the second
finger. Many variations occur in the course of this nerve, which has prompted
authors to consider this syndrome as being identical to the pronator teres syndrome.[64,65]

Because numerous fascial tunnels possibly exist in the forearm, the exact
tunnel involved remains in question.

Clinically the patient develops an inability to pinch between the thumb
and index finger because of paresis of the distal phalanges of both fingers.
Pinching is then attempted with both joints in extended position. In addition,
the patient is unable to clench the fist or write (Fig. 10–25).

Treatment consists of immobilization and avoidance of causative factors
determined, but with persistent symptoms and EMG confirmation, surgical
decompression is indicated.

ULNAR NERVE COMPRESSION

The ulnar nerve is subjected to compression at numerous sites along its
course, causing characteristic sensory and motor symptoms (Fig. 10–26). At
the wrist the ulnar nerve enters the hand in a shallow trough between the

Figure 10–25. Anterior interosseous syndrome. The motor deficit of the anterior interosseous nerve syndrome causes inability to flex the distal phalanges (DP) of the index finger and thumb. The normal pinch (*upper A*) with tip-to-tip opposition is not possible (*upper B*) with the distal phalanges extended. In making a fist (*lower A*) the normally flexed fingers cannot flex at the index and thumb distal phalanges (*lower B*).

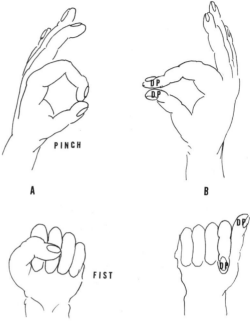

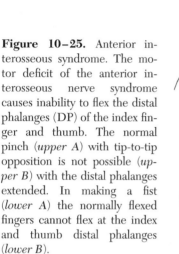

pisiform bone and the hook of the hamate bone (Guyon's canal)[66] (Fig. 10–27).

The floor of this tunnel is a thin layer of ligament and muscle. Its roof is composed of the volar carpal ligament and the palmaris longus muscle (Fig. 10–28). Proximal to its entry the nerve divides into dorsal and palmar branches that further divide into superficial and deep palmar branches that run into the tunnel. Only these two terminal branches run into the tunnel, therefore compression *from* tunnel entrapment spares the dorsal branch.

The superficial branch of the palmar branch innervates the palmaris brevis muscle, the palmar skin of the fifth finger, and the ulnar skin of the fourth finger. The deep branch innervates the hypothenar muscles, the two lateral lumbricals, all the interosseus muscles, the adductor pollicis, and the deep head of the flexor pollicis brevis muscles. Compression of the superficial branch causes motor and sensory symptoms (Fig. 10–29) whereas compression of the deep branch causes only motor symptoms (Figs. 10–30 and 10–31).[66]

Numerous etiologies are proposed to explain ulnar nerve compression at Guyon's canal, but most are traumatic, such as bicycle or motorcycle riding, operating a pneumatic drill, among others.

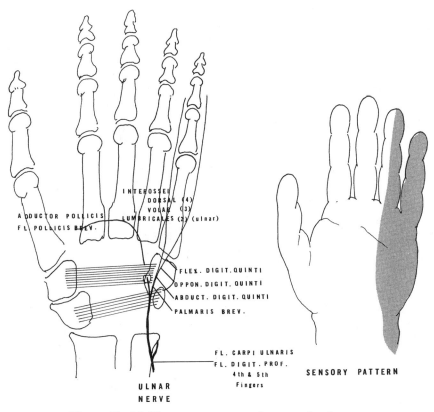

Figure 10-26. Ulnar nerve: motor and sensory distribution.

Symptoms may describe *difficulty* in hand grasping activities and paresthesiae of the dermatomal regions of the ulnar nerve. Motor weakness may be described as *clumsiness* in performing fine movements; reduced *pinch strength* of the thumb is also apparent. Atrophy of the interossei gradually becomes evident with deepening of the interosseus grooves on the dorsum of the hand. A positive Tinel sign over the ulnar nerve may be elicited. Confirmation using EMG is diagnostic.

Treatment should be conservative avoiding activities found to be responsible, and therapy with oral anti-inflammatory medication, steroid injections, and splinting. Without significant relief, waiting longer than 6 months is not advocated.[67] If both Guyon's syndrome and CTS are present surgical release of the median nerve should also be contemplated.[68]

Figure 10–27. Guyon's canal: the ulnar nerve tunnel. Guyon's canal is adjacent to the carpal tunnel (CT). The canal is within the flexor retinaculum, which contains the ulnar nerve, flexor carpi ulnaris tendon (FCU), blood vessels (BV) (the ulnar artery and vein), and the flexor carpi radialis (FCR) muscle. The base of the tunnel is the scaphoid (S) (navicular), capitate (C), hamate (H), triquetrum (Tq), and the pisiform (P) bones. The canal's pressure is different than that within the carpal tunnel.

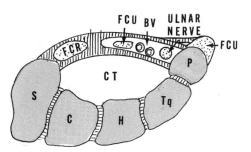

CUBITAL TUNNEL SYNDROME

Compression of the ulnar nerve at the elbow is commonly called **cubital tunnel syndrome,** which is considered the second most common nerve entrapment of the upper extremity, second only to CTS.

Cubital tunnel syndrome, recognized for over 100 years[69] is apparently becoming increasingly more common due to the increasing use of computers whose operators repetitively use the upper extremity held in a elbow-flexed

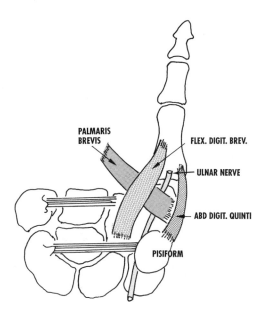

Figure 10–28. Guyon's canal: entry into the hand.

ULNAR NERVE
(SENSORY)

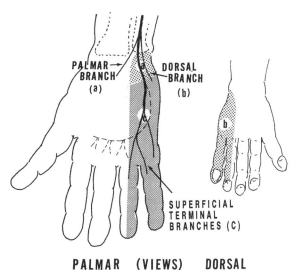

Figure 10–29. Ulnar nerve: sensory pattern.

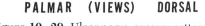
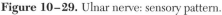
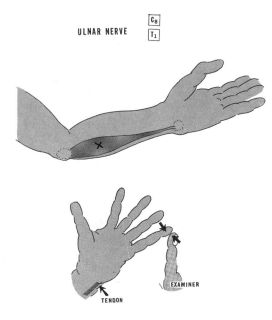

Figure 10–30. Flexor carpi ulnaris. The flexor carpi ulnaris originates from the medial epicondyle of the humerous medial to the olecranon and the dorsal border of the ulna. It inserts into the piriformis and flexes the wrist in an ulnar direction. The examiner resists abduction and flexion of the fifth finger, which tenses the flexor carpi ulnaris at the pisiform.

ULNAR NERVE $\boxed{C_8}$ $\boxed{T_1}$

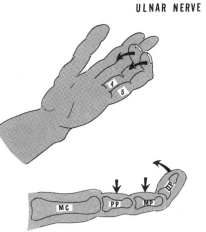

Figure 10–31. Flexor digitorum profundus. The flexor digitorum profundus flexes the distal phalanx and is tested by fixing the middle and proximal phalanges. This muscle originates from the midulnar bone and interosseous membrane. It inserts into the base of the distal phalanx.

position and put direct pressure on the nerve at the cubital tunnel (Fig. 10–32). The ulnar nerve is very superficial at this site.

At the elbow the ulnar nerve enters the cubital groove on the posterior aspect of the medial epicondyle with its roof being formed from an aponeurotic band at an angle transverse to the nerve. As the nerve leaves the tunnel, it passes between the two heads of the flexor carpi ulnaris muscle.

The aponeurotic band stabilizes the ulnar nerve behind the medial epicondyle, thus preventing subluxation of the nerve during elbow actions. Hypermobility of the nerve exists,[57] however, making compression *outside* the

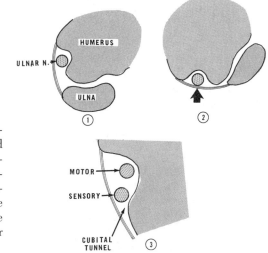

Figure 10–32. Cubital tunnel-ulnar nerve. In the supinated elbow (1), the ulnar nerve is removed from possible compression, whereas pronation (2) encourages compression. (3) The sensory fibers are closer to the surface than are the motor nerve fibers.

canal more possible. The retinaculum is lax in elbow extension and taut only in full flexion.[70] With flexion the volume of the cubital tunnel decreases and causes greater pressure upon the nerve.[71] Cubital pressure also increases with the wrist extended and with the shoulder forward, flexed, and abducted, which replicates many postures used in the workplace.[72]

Within the tunnel, the motor fibers supplying the intrinsics of the hand are superficial, whereas those supplying the flexor carpi ulnaris and the digitorum profundus are deeper.[73] The superficial location of the sensory nerves also explains the impaired sensation found early in this process.

More proximally to the cubital tunnel, the ulnar nerve passes under the *arcade of Struthers*, which is a thick fascial band running from the medial head of the triceps muscle to the medial intermuscular septum.[74] This septum may also be a site of entrapment.

Because symptoms from entrapment at the site are often delayed, the term **tardy ulnar palsy** has evolved.[75] Surgical findings of this syndrome revealed a "markedly swollen and adherent ulnar nerve within the groove with no significant elbow deformity." All patients who had operations to release the arch 'without nerve transposition' had relief of symptoms.[76]

Symptoms of Cubital Tunnel Ulnar Nerve Compression

Aching pain on the medial site of the elbow near the medial epicondyle is frequently associated with shooting pains in the ulnar aspect of the hand and little finger. This hypasthesia is activity related and is provoked by elbow flexion and occasionally relieved from elbow extension. Unlike the carpal tunnel syndrome, the paresthesiae are *not* nocturnal. Clumsiness of hand activities may be an associated complaint depending on the degree of motor involvement.

A positive Tinel sign may be elicited, but care must be exercised in this sign's being elicited because normal ulnar nerves at the elbow respond to excessive tapping. The sensory modality tests previously described (light palpation, vibration, Semmes-Weinstein monofilament, and two-point discrimination) are diagnostic of nerve involvement.

A provocative test is made by flexing the elbow fully and extending the wrist for 3 minutes.[77] Motor evaluation begins with weakness of the first dorsal interosseous (resisting index finger abduction) and abductor digiti minimi (testing little finger abduction). Ultimately the presence of atrophy in the hypothenar region and the first web with clawing of the ring finger and little finger becomes apparent. A positive Froment sign (pinching a piece of paper between thumb and side of the index finger) is apparent. In this sign the distal thumb joint is flexed.

The major muscles to test are the flexor carpi ulnaris (testing wrist flexion in an ulnar direction) and the ulnar portion of the flexor digitorum profundus (testing flexion of the distal interphalangeal joint).[78] The normality of the bony aspect of the tunnel can be evaluated radiologically by special views.[79]

Treatment

Prevention is obviously desirable, that is, avoidance of direct pressure on the flexed elbow. Moderate flexion with a cushioning is desirable if possible. Sleep position-induced compression must be identified and modified using a small pillow to maintain elbow extension and to avoid flexion. Modification of vocational activities must also be addressed. Frequent and forceful elbow flexion may also be incriminated and when identified, must be eliminated.

Oral anti-inflammatory nonsteroidal drugs (NSAIDs) have value; perineural steroid injection has also been proposed.[80] Disadvantages with the latter include subcutaneous atrophy and cosmetic skin depigmentation. A physician attempting an injection in the cubital tunnel must warn the patient of these possibilities.

Surgical Intervention

Controversy exists of the surgical approach that affords the greatest benefit. The degree of preoperative compression strongly influences prognosis of success with those patients who exhibit intrinsic muscle weakness and atrophy having the poorest prognosis.[81]

Procedures vary from simple decompression to anterior transposition and medial epicondylectomy. These procedures are beyond the scope of this textbook—moreover, the choice resides in the expertise of the individual surgeon.

TENDON PROBLEMS

Common Tendinitis

Trauma to the tendons of the hand is a frequent cause of pain and impairment, yet symptomatic inflammation of the tendons and peritendinous tissues of the body remain poorly understood. The gross and histopathologic changes in these tissues are nonspecific. They include fibrocytic proliferation, thickening, destruction of synovial tissue, and often adhesion to adjacent soft tissues. Tendinitis implies inflammation that causes abnormal function of a tendon with impairment and often pain.

Tendons normally connect muscle to bone for extremity articular function; muscle tonus generally determines the tension within the tendon fibers. The collagen fibers (Fig. 10–33) that form the tendons normally have a curled

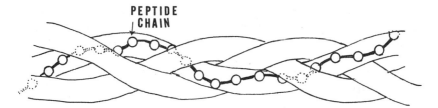

Figure 10–33. Trophocollagen trihelix fiber (schematic). Type I collagen fiber molecule is composed of peptide chains composed of two α_1 and one α_2 peptide chains in which every third molecule is a glycine amino acid. The three intertwining peptide chains form a trihelix collagen fiber. (Modified from Alberts, B, Bray, D, Lewis, J, et al: Molecular Biology of the Cell. Garland, New York, 1983, p 694.)

configuration. The collagen fibril is a trophocollagen crystalline molecule formed by chemically bonded atoms. These fibrils are imbedded within a ground substance containing glycosaminoglycans, proteoglycans, and glycoproteins. In a tendon the collagen fibers lie parallel to each other (Fig. 10–34). In the resting stage of physiologic curl, they maintain tone. The tone of the muscle tendon complex mechanism[82] determining the tone within the tendon is set by the tone of the extrafusal fibers of the muscle (Fig. 10–35). Muscle tone is determined by intrinsic neurologic mechanisms in which the spindle system feedback, in conjunction with Golgi apparatus feedback within the tendon itself. The spindle system determines the rate of elongation, whereas the Golgi apparatus determines the strength (i.e., force) of the contraction.

The extrafusal muscles contract concentrically and eccentrically, thus causing the tendon fibers also to undergo commensurate tension and elongation. Deceleration of a musculotendinous unit occurs frequently in daily neuromuscular actions and places even greater newtonian forces than concentric forces[83]—a fact frequently overlooked in the clinical setting.

Relaxation after a muscular contraction allows the tendon fibrils to recoil. If the contraction is excessive or prolonged without an interim test period, the fibrils undergo excessive elongation with some structural internal disruption.

The mechanical tendency of tendons to elongate until there is a specific degree of rupture has been a subject for study. Rupture is a break in the peptide chain after a nonphysiologic force of elongation. These forces are plotted in a *stress* and *strain curve* in which stress is the amount of load per unit of cross-sectional area and *strain* is the resultant proportional elongation resulting.

It has been postulated that different regions of the tendon react to elongation forces within the stress-strain curve:

- Toe region[84]—*physiologic* loading occurs for 1 hour.

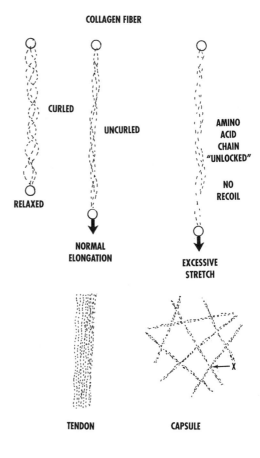

Figure 10–34. Collagen fibers. Each fiber is a trihelix chain of amino acids bound together chemically (electrically) (see Fig. 10–33). These chains uncurl to their maximum physiologic elongation, then recoil when the elongation force is removed. If the force exceeds physiologic limits, the fiber uncoils, thus essentially disrupting the amino acid chains. The fiber remains extended. In a tendon, the collagen fibers are in a parallel relationship. Within a capsule they crisscross, gliding over each other at their intersections (X).

- Linear region—stress increases rapidly causing prolonged elongation. Microfailure results.
- Progressive failure region—the tendon remains intact to the naked eye but microscopically will demonstrate significant failure.
- Major failure region—the tendon still remains *intact*, but frank ruptures exist.
- Complete rupture region—a gross tendon disruption.[85]

These *regions* are arbitrary, microscopic, and their true value lies in *recovery*, that is, the return to their original length. The recovery of a tendon after stretch can be beneficially modified by conditioning the tendon using gentle stretching prior to testing.[86] The term **recovery** has unfortunately been used to imply that no permanent damage or permanent elongation remains after stretching. Microfailure apparently remains.[87]

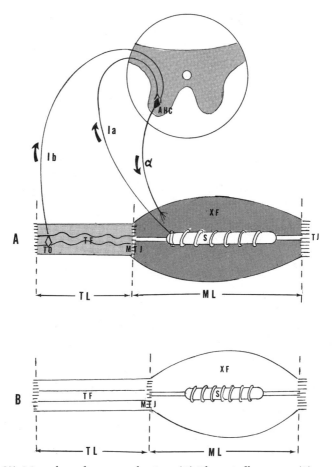

Figure 10–35. Musculotendinous mechanism. (A) The spindle system (S) measures the length of the muscle (ML) and the tendon organs (TO) (Golgi) monitor the tension. Stretching of the spindle system activates the Ia fiber, whereas stretching the TO activates the Ib fibers. These influence the anterior horn cell (AHC), which sends motor fiber activity via the α fibers to the extrafusal fibers (XF). With the muscle at resting level (A) the tendon fibers (TF) are slightly coiled. When the extrafusal fibers contract (B), the muscle shortens (ML), the tendon elongates (TL) to the degree that the tendon fibers can elongate. The tendon fibrils (TF) uncoil. Excessive muscle contraction can tear the muscle-tendon juncture (MTJ).

The stress and strain curve relates to many factors besides prestretch *conditioning*. The rate of stretch influences ultimate recovery.[88] The ideal *spring* elongation depends on the speed of stretch with the tension remaining constant at any given length. Collagen does not perform as an ideal spring. A tendon gradually lengthens from a constant or repeated load. This slow elongation is termed **creep**—it is transient if the force is within physiologic limits.

The viscoelastic properties of collagen vary with temperature. Temperature below 37°C can be considered physiologic with good chances for recovery, whereas temperatures between 37° and 40°C increase creep and temperatures above 40°C enhance permanent damage by *melting* the bonds between tropocollagen molecules. These factors have clinical significance, because damage and recovery depend on stress and ambient temperature.

There are some nontraumatic factors that affect tendons. Immobilization cause significant loss of strength. The dense connective tissue of muscle loses 80% of its strength within 4 weeks, 50% in ligaments after 8 weeks. Length and flexibility diminish rather than strength.

In their daily functions, tendons are subjected to tensile forces, compressive stresses, and shear stresses.[89] Microfailure occurs if the tendon load is excessive or if the rest between loads is inadequate to allow the tendon fibrils to recover their resting length.[90] Repetitive loading stress accelerates the microtrauma by exceeding the reparative capacity of the tendon.[91]

Pathologic changes within the tendon include swelling and thickening of the sheaths that cause vascular impairment within the mesotendon and failure of normal diffusion of nutritive elements.[92]

Tendons glide upon their contiguous tissues. This action is facilitated by the thin fibrous and cellular layers of the tendon termed **epitenon,** which adheres to tendon surfaces. The tendons contained within sheaths contain synovial fluid for lubrication of the tendon within the sheath. The sheath itself has external lubricant against peritendinous tissues.

Systemic factors affect the viability and integrity of tendons such as rheumatoid arthritis, hypothyroid, diabetes mellitus, gout, calcium pyrophosphate, collagen vascular disease, and infections.[93]

Occupational stress factors frequently cause tendinitis. These CTS[94] include repetitive tasks requiring forceful motions, unusual postures, exposure to temperature extremes, and exposure to vibration. These factors were recognized as early as 1717.[95]

Diagnosis reveals swelling, tenderness, warmth, crepitus, snapping, and occasional numbness. Direct identification of the involved tendon is mandated; placing that specific tendon under stress (resisted movement) or passive elongation reveals the precise tendon.

Every tendon in the hand is a potential site of tendinitis. Most such sites can be identified by evaluating the specific functional impairment of that precise tendon. Generalities of tendon injuries apply to the more specific sites.

Tendon Rupture

A tendon may be ruptured by an acute stretch injury when the fibrils are elongated beyond the limit of their physiologic recoil. The tendon is normally strongest at its musculotendinous link where it seldom tears. Tearing occurs at its insertion site with and without avulsion of the bone or periosteum. A tendon damaged by a systemic disease or a tendon which has sustained numerous micro-traumata will tear more frequently from a lesser stress.

Extensor Tendons. Injury to extensor tendons of the fingers and thumb is common because they are superficially prominent and have little overlying skin and subcutaneous tissue to protect them. They are also subject to direct injury when the hand and other fingers are extended. A thorough knowledge of functional anatomy is necessary to diagnose and treat these injuries accurately.

Extensor tendons tend **not** to retract after being severed and thus can be sutured soon after injury, when they will require 3 to 4 weeks before they regain integrity. The suture material used should not be absorbable because integrity, usually gained at 3 weeks, may not be attained before the absorption of the suture material.

After approximation and suture, during the first 2 to 3 days, an outpouring of fibrin is invaded by fibroblasts within 5 days. These fibrin fibrils fuse into long threads that bridge the gap between the two severed ends. By the third week, edema has usually subsided and excessive vascularity is decreased. The union is, at this time, sufficiently strong to allow some traction upon the tendon.

Tendons contained *within* a sheath when severed show greater deterioration and heal more slowly than those not contained within a sheath. The reason is that the swelling of the injury tendon within the sheath obstructs venous and lymphatic return, which impairs tendon nutrition and subsequent healing. Adhesions may form about the tendon which may also impair nutrition and ultimate function.

The exact technique of tendon suturing is beyond the scope of this book, but postsuture management needs discussion. Once sutured, the wrist must be immobilized for 3 to 4 weeks with 30° to 40° extension of the fingers. This violates the principle of immobilization in a *position of function* with the wrist slightly extended and the fingers flexed. Sutured extensor tendons fortunately usually result in good function despite postoperative immobilization.

The extensor pollicis longus tendon usually retracts a considerable distance and it may be difficult to locate the proximal end. Search of this portion of the tendon is best achieved through an incision above the wrist and approximating the ends using a probe.

Due to varying characteristics of extensor tendon anatomy, injuries must be oriented by area. Anatomic zones have been delineated (Fig. 10–36).

Flexor Tendon Injury

Suturing a flexor tendon in "no man's land" (Fig. 10–37) has an unfavorable prognosis. The anatomic structure and relationship of the tendons in the area indicate the reason for this poor prognosis. A sutured tendon usually

Figure 10–36. Anatomic zones of tendon injuries. Zone I is at the distal interphalangeal joint level and zone 8 (not shown) is at the distal forearm level. Muscular injuries occur proximal to zone 8 and tendons at zone 7 and 8 are beneath subcutaneous, reticulum, and fascial levels. The tendons at zone 6 are very superficial, rounded or ovoid. Lacerations at zone 5 are at the MP joint level. Tendons at this level usually do not retract. Zones 4 and 3 are at the interphalangeal joint level and rarely include complete lacerations of the dorsal apparatus. Lacerations at zones 2 and 1 are conceptually simple: thin and oriented on the dorsal aspect of the middle phalanx. The thumb zones (TI-V) are discussed in the text. (From Cailliet, R: Hand Pain and Impairment, ed 4. FA Davis, Philadelphia, 1994, p 167, with permission.)

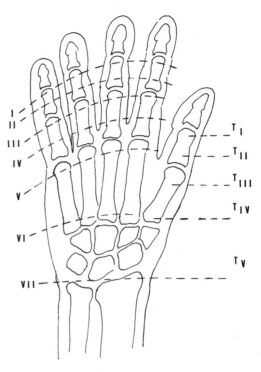

swells—in this area of the fingers no room is available for expansion of the tendon. Ischemic necrosis can result.

"Primary suturing of a flexor tendon within no man's land should be avoided." Primary care should be concerned with the wound and a tendon transplant should be considered only 4 to 5 weeks later. Tendons severed *distal* to no man's land, for example, profundus tendons, may be primarily sutured. In these severed tendons, the distal portion of the profundus tendon can be surgically removed and the proximal end reattached. The resultant shortened tendon does not interfere with the uninjured superficialis function.

Severed flexor tendons proximal to no man's land, especially at the wrist level, can be primarily sutured with good functional results. Attempting to resuture "individual" tendons, that is, profundus to profundus or superficialis to superficialis, will usually result in functional failure. Only the profundus tendon can be repaired in this manner. Because this tendon flexes the distal interphalangeal joint, good return of finger function results.

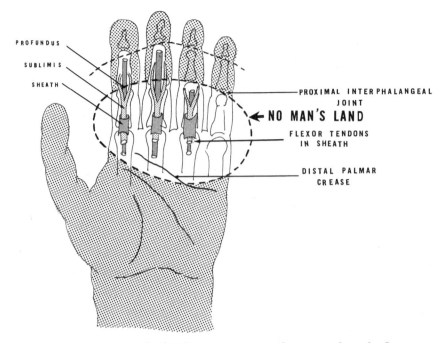

PROFUNDUS

SUBLIMIS

SHEATH

PROXIMAL INTERPHALANGEAL
JOINT

←NO MAN'S LAND

FLEXOR TENDONS
IN SHEATH

DISTAL PALMAR
CREASE

Figure 10–37. "No man's land." This area represents the region where the flexor tendons (profundus and sublimis) are tightly enclosed within a sheath. Primary repair of the tendons in this region is *contraindicated*. Only suture of the skin should be contemplated. Primary suture between the two interphalangeal joints should be avoided because of the tendons' relationship in this region.

Specific Tendinitis Problems of the Hand

Extensor Tendon Tears

Mallet Finger. Tear of the extensor tendon from its attachment on the distal phalanx (Fig. 10–38) usually occurs during an acute flexion injury to the finger, that is, when the extensor tendon is taut. Most patients have the tendon torn at its point of insertion on the phalanx, although 25% also sustain a bone avulsion from the injury.

Conservative treatment includes immobilization of the distal phalanx in hyperextension (Fig. 10–39) for 5 weeks; this usually results in functional recovery. By flexing the middle phalanx and by extending the distal phalanx, the central extensor slip pulls the extensor mechanism distally and allows the torn tendon to reunite (Fig. 10–40). In this finger position the lateral bands are relaxed. If treatment is begun within 10 days of injury, a cast (Fig. 10–41) for 5 weeks followed by splinting the distal phalanx for another 4 weeks usually suf-

Figure 10-38. Distal phalanx extensor tendon tear (mechanism). The mechanism of the mallet finger is described. The arrow depicts flexion of the distal phalanx: (*1*) Tear of the extensor tendon on the distal phalanx. (2) Landsmeer ligament that connects the extensor and flexor tendons. (3) Extensor tendon pull. (4) Lumbical muscle pull. (5) Profundus flexor muscle pull.

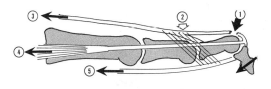

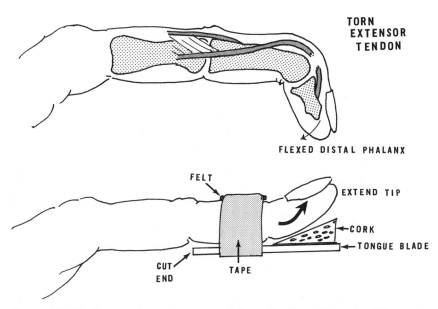

Figure 10-39. Conservative management of the mallet finger. Rupture of the extensor tendon to the distal phalanx results in an acute flexion of the finger tip with inability to extend this joint actively. Immobilization of the distal phalanx in *hyperextension* for 4 to 5 weeks usually allows functional healing. The splint is a wooden tongue blade reaching only to the middle phalangeal joint, which extends past the finger tip to protect the digit. The shaped cork is glued to the blade. A small layer of felt is placed under the tape that protects the dorsum of the finger.

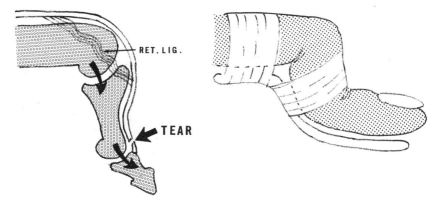

Figure 10–40. Rationale of treatment for mallet finger. Flexing the middle phalanx and extending the distal digit permits the extensor tendon to reunite. This position pulls the extensor mechanism distally and relaxes the lateral bands.

fices to allow functional recovery. If contracture of the flexors has occurred, passive stretch may be needed, as well as gentle active extensor exercises. Surgical intervention is indicated when functional restoration has not been achieved or is not accepted by the patient.

Extensor Tendon Rupture at the Middle Phalanx. Rupture of the insertion of the extensor tendon into the middle phalanx, with or without bony avulsion, may be caused by a direct blow or by a crushing injury. Earlier injuries may have permitted attenuation of the tendon that has not been ruptured by a lesser force.

Rupture of the extensor tendon at that site causes the proximal phalanx to extend and the middle phalanx to flex (Fig. 10–42). This deformity is termed boutonniere deformity; it may result from rheumatoid disease or trauma. Because of inadequate extensor slip function, the lateral bands dislocate to the flexor side of the joint fulcrum, thus causing a flexion deformity of the proximal interphalangeal joint and hyperextension of the distal joint.

Treatment of this deformity is difficult because a functional splint (Fig.

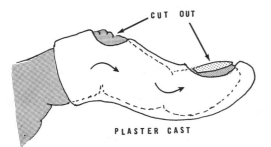

Figure 10–41. Plaster cast treatment of mallet finger. The cast is molded to hold the distal phalanx hyperextended and middle joint flexed. The dorsum of the middle joint and the nail are exposed to prevent friction and pressure.

Figure 10–42. Mechanism of extensor tendon rupture at the middle phalangeal joint. This is termed a **boutonniere.** The tear in the extensor tendon (*1*) allows the lateral bands (*2*) to migrate volarly from contraction of the extensor mechanisms (*6*). The intrinsics (*5*) contract and flex the proximal interphalangeal joint (*3*). The distal phalanx extends (*4*).

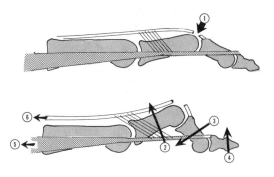

10–43) is often ineffective and a rigid splint may maintain the manually corrected deformity (Fig. 10–44).

Extensor Pollicis Longus Rupture. The extensor pollicis longus tendon curve around the dorsal radial tubercle of Lister (Fig. 10–45) passes over the radial wrist extensors and continues to the thumb. At the point where the tendon angulates wear and tear can occur. Rupture of this tendon results in an inability to extend the distal joint of the thumb and weakness extending to the proximal joint. Normally the tendon can be palpated when the wrist is actively extended and the thumb abducted.

After primary rupture, suturing the two fragmented ends of the tendon is *not possible*, because such repairs neither hold nor function. Repair requires a graft from a site extending proximal to the dorsal retinaculum to the end located at the metacarpal. Repair may necessitate the transfer of the tendon of the extensor indicis. Once grafted the thumb must be splinted for at least 1 month before use.

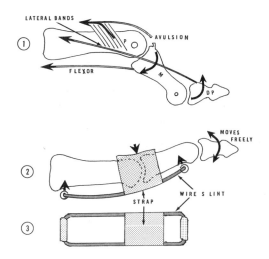

Figure 10–43. Treatment of a boutonniere deformity. The deformity occurs (*1*) (as stated in Fig. 10–37). PP = proximal phalanx; M = middle; and DP = distal phalanx. (*2*) Shows the positioning of the splint (*3*) with the *arrows* depicting the applied forces.

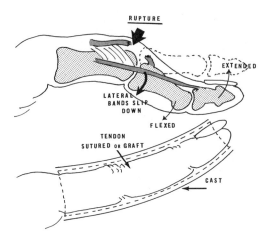
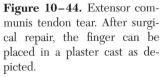

Figure 10–44. Extensor communis tendon tear. After surgical repair, the finger can be placed in a plaster cast as depicted.

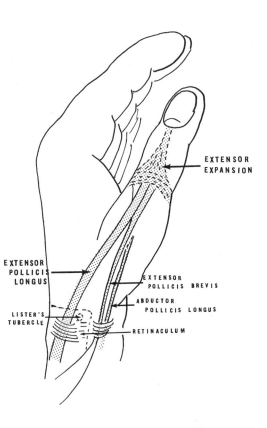

Figure 10–45. Rupture of the extensor pollicis longus. The extensor pollicis longus tendon extends to the distal phalanx. Its rupture results in the inability to extend the distal digit of the thumb. This tendon retracts considerably, thus making end-to-end suturing difficult. A graft is usually required.

Tendinitis of the Extensor Compartments

De Quervain's Disease. Tenosynovitis of the thumb abductors at their radiostyloid process and subsequent stenosis is very common. The condition was named after the Swiss surgeon de Quervain.[91] The first dorsal compartment contains the abductor pollicis longus and the extensor pollicis brevis confined by the radial styloid and covered by a synovially lined ligament 1.5 inches long.[92,93]

Symptoms include edema and pain over the radial styloid with the pain initiated and aggravated by forcing the wrist into an ulnar-deviated position and the thumb flexed and adducted: it is known as Finkelstein's test.[94] Tenderness over the extensor sheath is often accompanied by swelling and thickness (Fig. 10–46).

The pathology is increased vascularity of the outer sheath combined with edema that thickens the sheath and constricts the enclosed tendon. The synovial fluid tends to increase and thicken with formation of fine hair-like fibers that adhere the adjacent tissues.

Treatment. For de Quervain's disease, splinting of the thumb and oral anti-inflammatory medication can be tried but local injection of steroids is preferable because one injection often suffices. Accuracy of technique is mandated. The needle is inserted into the distal end of the compartment where the gradual swelling from the anesthetic agent confirms its entry into the compartment.

In refractory patients, surgical release may be required although results have been disappointing. Techniques are beyond the scope of this text but it may be stated that incisions must not be longitudinal along the tendon sheath because this type of incision tends to scar or even to form keloid.

Tendinitis in the Flexor Compartments

Trigger Fingers. The parallel collagen fibers that form a tendon undergo attritional changes from overuse, trauma, and occasionally disease. As a result of trauma, the ligamentous sheath thickens impairing repeated gliding. Thickening results from microscopic tearing of the collagen fibers and thickening of the sheath.[95] After being torn, a collagen fiber has the tendency to retract and form a nodule (Fig. 10–47).

Snapping of the flexor tendons during active finger flexion is termed "trigger finger" and is palpable and audible during flexion and re-extension. Flexion is restricted but if flexion is further attempted it occurs suddenly. Once flexed the nodule within the finger has passed annular ligament remains *locked* in the flexed position, and cannot be reextended.

This trigger action occurs most frequently in the middle or ring finger and is related to direct, repetitive trauma to the flexor tendons of the fingers (Fig. 10–48).

Treatment consists of injecting a steroid into the sheath to lessen its constriction.[96] Although the nodule remains, it now may be able to pass the previous obstruction. Failure of this procedure necessitates surgical intervention in

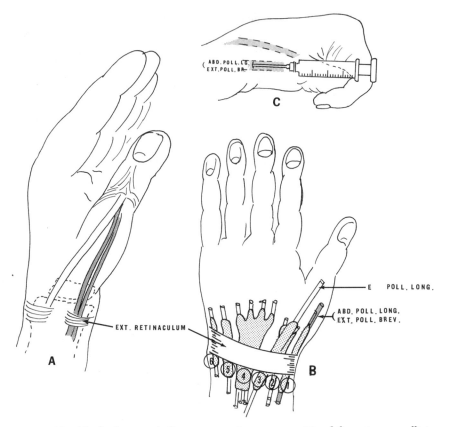

Figure 10–46. de Quervain's disease: stenosing tenosynovitis of the extensor pollicis brevis and abductor pollicis longus. (*A*) The tendons pass over the prominence of the radial styloid process and form the ulnar border of the "snuff box." (*B*) Six tendon sheaths pass under the extensor retinaculum. 1 = abductor pollicis longus; 2 = extensor carpi radialis; 3 = extensor pollicis longus; 4 = extensor digitorum communis; 5 = extensor digiti minimi; 6 = extensor carpi ulnaris. Tenosynovitis usually occurs at 1. (*C*) Method of treatment and site of injection of steroidal solution.

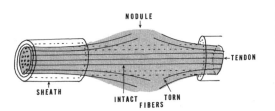

Figure 10–47. Formation of a tendon nodule. The parallel arrangement of collagen fibers in a tendon becomes disrupted by friction, attrition, and direct trauma. The fibers tear and undergo retraction, thus forming a nodule. The sheath enlarges and thickens.

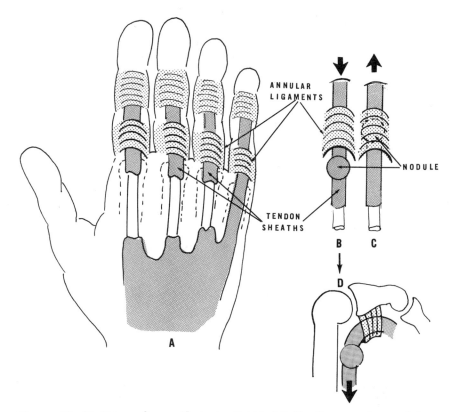

Figure 10–48. Trigger fingers (flexor tendinitis). (*A*) The flexor tendons and their sheaths as they pass under the annular ligaments. (*B*) The fusiform swelling of a tendon proximal to the ligament. (*C*) The nodule is now under the ligament. (*D*) The nodule has passed proximal to the ligament and has *locked* the finger in flexion preventing extension.

which a transverse incision of the sheath proximal to the nodule exposes the annular band which has been slit. Excision of the nodule invariably causes formation of a new and often larger nodule.[101]

Flexor Carpi Ulnaris Tendinitis. Tendinitis of this tendon (FCU) is common and results from repetitive trauma. It is especially common in tennis players and carpenters.

Clinically pain and swelling exist, proximal to the pisiform and exacerbated by wrist flexion in a radial direction. Because of its proximity, concurrent compression of the ulnar nerve within Guyon's canal may be present. Differentiation of pain located in this region from that of a pisiform fracture or arthritis of that bone is made by reproducing the pain with a side-to-side motion of the bone.

Treatment requires splinting in a mild wrist flexion and oral steroid or NSAID medication, or direct injection of steroids into the area. In resistant patients, the ligament can be lengthened or the pisiform bone excised.

Other sites of tendinitis with nodularity can be ascertained by clinical examination but are not discussed here. They are, however, similar in symptoms and treatment.

FRACTURES AND DISLOCATIONS

With all hand and wrist fractures, knowledge of normal anatomy of the part is mandatory to ensure proper management.[98] The metacarpals inform three arches: the proximal, distal transverse, and the longitudinal. The proximal carpal arch is formed by the carpal bones. The distal transverse arch is composed of the distal portions of the metatarsal heads (Fig. 10–49).

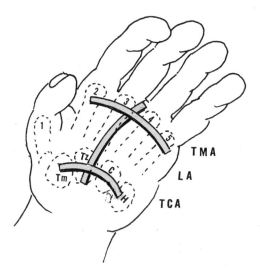

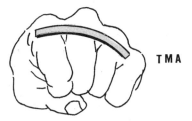

Figure 10–49. Arches of the hand. The metacarpals are numbered and the carpal bones are designated. Tm = trapezium; Tz = trapezoid; H = hamate; C = capitate: TMA = transverse metatarsal arch; TCA = transverse carpal arch; LA = longitudinal arch.

Principles of Treatment

Fractures and dislocations of the fingers have frequently been ignored or treated only cursorily with resulting severe disability. Loss of finger function interferes markedly with use of the upper extremity and poses significant workplace difficulties.

The following principles in the care of injured phalanges and interphalangeal joints must not be violated:

1. Immobilization must be instituted to relieve pain and permit primary healing. Too early or inappropriate active or passive motion exercise may result in more pain and contracture. Usually immobilization must be maintained for at least 10 to 14 days.
2. Immobilization must be maintained in degrees of physiologic flexion (Fig. 10–50). No fracture must be immobilized by using extension of all three joints.
3. All digits that do not require immobilization must be actively, not passively, mobilized.
4. The uninvolved digits of the hand, wrist, elbow, and shoulder must be actively placed through their normal range of motion with emphasis on frequent elevation of the hand above the level of the heart.

Duration of immobilization is "not equated with the time of healing:[103] it is shorter than this time factor" (Fig. 10–51). Active range-of-motion exercises must be started before radiographs show evidence of healing: usually within 1 to 2 weeks.

The specific fractures of the hand, albeit soft tissues, are well documented in the literature[100] and will not be further discussed in this text. Diagnosis of a fracture of the forearm or hand mandates immediate referral to an orthopedist to ensure the patient's return to normal function.

The prevalence of work-related upper extremity disorders has significantly increased in past decades.[101] Data from the National Ambulatory Med-

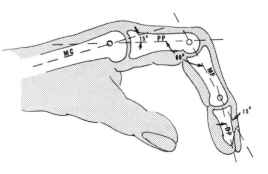

Figure 10–50. Physiologic position of the hand for immobilization. MC = metacarpal; PP = proximal phalanx; MP = middle phalanx; DP = distal phalanx. The MC-PP angle is 15°, the PP-MP angle is 60°, and the MP-DP is 15°. (From Cailliet, R: Hand Pain and Impairment, ed 4. FA Davis, Philadelphia, 1994, p 194, with permission.)

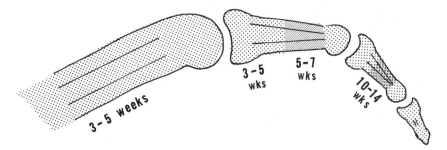

Figure 10–51. Fracture healing time. (Modified from Moberg, E: Emergency Surgery of the Hand. Livingstone, London, 1969.)

ical Care Survey[102] on the use of medical services for new and chronic conditions related to hand and wrist problems indicated that 1.8% of 1,264,662 visits in 1980 were related to hand and fingers and 1%[99] were related to wrist problems. Medical visits for chronic pain of the hands, fingers, and wrists were approximately 800,000 per year for 1980 to 1981. In 1988[103] 28.6% of total closed cases (31,756 out of 110,975) involved upper extremity disorders.

Persistent pain, loss of function, and work-related disability involving an upper extremity are affected by multiple factors.[104] These include physical capabilities as related to work demands, ergonomic risk factors in the workplace, psychologic factors related to the worker in terms of work, and the ability to manage symptoms as required by the patient's desire to return to work.

Long-term vocational outcome involves multicomponent rehabilitative efforts:

1. Physical reconditioning
2. Modification of workplace ergonomics
3. Stress management
4. Vocational counseling and placement

With so many factors involved in upper extremity disability, a multidisciplinary program must be instituted to address all factors. Despite widespread growth of programs and services providing multidisciplinary rehabilitation, little or no outcomes assessment statistics have evolved.

Because many, if not most, are soft tissue injuries, it is apparent that these injuries must be recognized, and then understood in a meaningful way, so that the components of disability can provide the basis of therapy and functional restoration.

Not all upper extremity disabilities need a multidisciplinary approach but when the condition is not recognized and does not respond to meaningful therapeutic approach before onset of chronic pain and persistent disability, the multidiscipline approach must be considered.

Simplistically, the patient's return to work has become the standard for judging the benefit of therapy. Return to work before therapy is complete or before even pain is now significantly lessened mandated by employers and insurers. This edict implies reassuring the patient of performance of function "in spite of pain" is not only not harmful but may even be beneficial. "Fear of reinjury" is, however, a prominent concern that only a meaningful, thorough, accurate examination and related treatment will be able to overcome.

Return to work must also address the workplace ergonomics in a meaningful and realistic manner. Prevention here, as in all other injuries, is as mandatory as recover from injury and its sequelae.

REFERENCES

1. Blecker, ML: Medical surveillance for carpal tunnel syndrome in workers. J Hand Surg 12A:845–848, 1987.
2. Scelsi, R, Zandungo, M, and Tenti, P: Carpal tunnel syndrome: Anatomical and clinical correlations and morphological and ultrastructural aspects of tenosynovial sheath. J Orthop Trauma 15:75–80, 1989.
3. Armstrong, T, Castelli, W, Evans, F, and Diaz-Perez, R: Some histological changes in carpal tunnel contents and their biomechanical irregularities. J Occup Med 26:197–201, 1984.
4. Armstrong, T and Chaffin, D: Some biomechanical aspects of the carpal tunnel. J Biomech 12:567–569, 1979.
5. Kline, SC, Beach, V, and Moore, R: The transverse carpal ligament. J Bone Joint Surg 74A:1478–1485, 1992.
6. Doyle, JR: Dynamics of the flexor tendon sheath and pulley system. In Hunter, JM, Schneider, LH, and Mackin EJ (eds.): Tendon Surgery in the Hand. CV Mosby, St. Louis, 1987, pp 20–23.
7. Blix, M: Die Lange und die Sannung des Muskels. Scand Arch Physiol 3:295–318, 1891.
8. Elftman, H: Biomechanics of muscle. With particular application to studies of gait. J Bone Joint Surg 48A:363–377, 1966.
9. Freehafer, AA, Peckman, PM, and Keith, MW: Determination of muscle-tendon unit properties during tendon transfer. J Hand Surg 4:331–339, 1979.
10. Idler, RS: Anatomy and biomechanics of the digital flexor tendons. Hand Clin 1:3–111, 1985.
11. Cailliet, R: Hand Pain and Impairment, ed 4. FA Davis, Philadelphia, 1994.
12. Doyle, JR and Blythe, W: The finger flexor tendon sheath and pulleys: anatomy and reconstruction. In The American Academy of Orthopaedic Surgeons: Symposium on Tendon Surgery of the Hand. CV Mosby, St. Louis, 1975, pp 81–87.
13. Das, SK and Brown, HG: In search of complications in carpal tunnel decompression. Hand 8:243–249, 1976.
14. Gelberman, RH, Rydevik, BL, Pess, GM, et al: Carpal tunnel syndrome: A scientific basis for clinical care. Orthop Clin North Am 19:115–124, 1988.
15. Kulick, MI, Gordillo, G, Javidi T, et al: Long-term analysis of patients having surgical treatment for carpal tunnel syndrome. J Hand Surg 11A:59–66, 1986.
16. Manske, PR and Lesker, PA: Strength of human pulleys. Hand 9:147–152, 1977.
17. Rydevik, B and Lundborg, GN: Permeability of intraneural microvessels and perineurium following acute graded experimental nerve compression. Scand J Plast Reconstr Surg 11:179, 1977.

18. Gelberman, RH, Szabo, RM, Williamson, RV, et al: Tissue pressure threshold for peripheral nerve viability. Clin Orthop 178:285, 1983.
19. Skubick, DL, Clasby, R, and Donaldson, CCS: Carpal tunnel syndrome as an expression of muscular dysfunction in the neck. J Occup Rehabil 3:31–43, 1993.
20. Phalen, GS: Spontaneous compression of the median nerve at the wrist. JAMA 145:1128–1132, 1951.
21. Hybbinette, C and Mannerfelt, L: The carpal tunnel syndrome. A retrospective study of 400 operated patients. Acta Orthop Scand 46:610–620, 1975.
22. Proceedings and Reports of Councils and Associations: etiology of carpal tunnel compression of the median nerve. J Bone Joint Surg 34B:515, 1952.
23. Nissen, KI: Etiology of carpal compression of median nerve. J Bone Joint Surg. 34B:514, 1952.
24. Fuchs, PC, Nathan, PA, and Myers, LD: Synovial histology in carpal tunnel syndrome J Hand Surg 16A:753–758, 1991.
25. Faithfull, DK, Moir, DH, and Ireland, J: The micropathology of the typical carpal tunnel syndrome. J Hand Surg 11B:131–132, 1986.
26. Sunderland, S: The nerve lesion in the carpal tunnel syndrome. J Neurol Neurosurg Psychiatry 39:615–626, 1976.
27. Brain, WR, Wright, AD, and Wilkinson, M: Spontaneous compression of both median nerves in the carpal tunnel. Six cases treated surgically. Lancet 1:277–282, 1947.
28. Jaeger, SH, Spitz, LK, Powell, M, and Trans, ZV: The prevention of occupational carpal tunnel syndrome: An experience in a high risk population. Personal correspondence. Publication pending.
29. Gellman, H, Gelberman, RM, Tan, AM, and Botte, MJ: Carpal tunnel syndrome: An evaluation of the provocative diagnostic tests. J Bone Joint Surg 68A:735–737, 1986.
30. Phalen, GS: Refections on 21 years experience with carpal tunnel syndrome JAMA 212:1365–1367, 1970.
31. Phalen, GS: Spontaneous compression of the median nerve at the wrist. JAMA 145:1128–1132, 1951.
32. Kuschner, SH, Ebramzadeh, E, Johnson, D, et al: Tinel's sign and Phalen's test in carpal tunnel syndrome. Orthopedics 15:1297–1302, 1992.
33. Carragee, EJ and Hentz, VR: Repetitive trauma and nerve compression. Orthop Clin North Am 19:157–164, 1988.
34. Wieslander, G, Norback, D, Gothe, CJ, and Juhlin, L: Carpal tunnel syndrome (CTS) and exposure to vibration, repetitive wrist, movements, and heavy manual work: a case referent study. Br J Ind Med 46:43–47, 1989.
35. Bostrom, L, Gothe, CJ, Hansson, S, et al: Vibration-induced carpal-tunnel syndrome (letter): Lancet. 337:744–745, 1991.
36. Conner, DE and Kolisek, FR: Vibration-induced carpal tunnel syndrome. Orthop Rev 15:447–452, 1986.
37. Koskimies, F, Farkila, M, Pyykko, I, et al: Carpal tunnel syndrome in vibration disease. Br J Ind Med 47:411–416, 1990.
38. Falkenburg, SA: Choosing hand splints to aid carpal tunnel syndrome recovery. Occup Health Saf 56:60–64, 1987.
39. Kruger, VL, Kraft, GH, Deitz, JC, et al: Carpal tunnel syndrome: Objective measures and splint use. Arch Phys Med Rehabil 72:738–742, 1991.
40. McGraph, MH: Local steroid therapy in the hand. J Hand Surg 9A:915–921, 1984.
41. Pinkham, J: Carpal tunnel syndrome sufferers find relief with ergonomic designs. Occ Health Saf 57:49–53, 1988.
42. Szabo, RM and Chidgey, LK: Stress carpal tunnel pressure in patients with carpal tunnel syndrome and normal patients. J Hand Surg 14A:624–627, 1989.
43. Rydholm, U, Werner, C, and Ohlin, P: Intracompartmental forearm pressure during rest and exercise. Clin Orthop 175:213–215, 1983.

44. Eisma, TL: Ergonomic design protects hands from repetitive motion stress, vibration. Occup Health Saf 59:75–77, 80–82, 1990.
45. Hellenbrandt, FA, Houtz, SJ, Partridge, MJ, and Waltos, CE: Tonic neck reflexes in exercises of stress in man. Am J Phys Med 35:144–159, 1956.
46. Aiello, I, Rosati, G, Sau, GF, et al: Tonic neck reflexes on upper limb flexor tone in man. Exp Neurol 101:41–49, 1988.
47. Marras, WS and Schoenmarklin, RW: Wrist motions in industry. Ergonomics 36:341–351, 1993.
48. Schoenmarklin, RW and Marras, WS: Dynamic capabilities of the wrist joint in industrial workers. Int J Ind Ergonomics 11:207–224, 1993.
49. Ochs, S: Axoplasmic transport: A basis for neural pathology. In Dyck, PJ, Thomas, PK, and Lambert, EH (eds): Peripheral Neuropathy, vol 1. WB Saunders, Philadelphia, 1975, pp 213–230.
50. Schoenmarklin, RW, Marras, WS, and Leurgans, SE: Industrial wrist motions and incidence of hand/wrist cumulative trauma disorders. Ergonomics. Publication pending.
51. Robbins, H: Anatomical study of the median nerve in the carpal tunnel syndrome. J Bone Joint Surg 45A:953–966, 1963.
52. Smith, EM, Sontegard, DA, and Armstrong, TJ: Contribution of flexor tendons to the carpal tunnel syndrome. Arch Phys Med Rehabil 58:379–385, 1977.
53. Armstrong, TJ and Chaffin, DB: Some biomechanical aspects of the carpal tunnel. J Biomechanics 12:567–570, 1979.
54. Goldstein, SA, Armstring, TJ, Chaffin, DB, and Mathews, LS: Analysis of cumulative strain in tendons and tendon sheaths. J Biomechanics 20:1–6, 1987.
55. Schoenmarklin, RW and Marras, WS: An EMG-Assisted Biomechanical Model of the Wrist Joint. In Kumar, S (ed): Advances in Industrial Ergonomics and Safety IV. Taylor & Francis, Philadelphia, 1992.
56. Stokes, M, Edwards, R, and Cooper, R: Effect of low frequency fatigue on human muscle strength and fatigability during subsequent stimulated activity. Eur J Appl Physiol 57:312–321, 1989.
57. Jorgensen, K, Fallentin, N, Krough-Lund, C, and Jensen, B: Electromyography and fatigue during prolonged, low-level static contractions. Eur J Appl Physiol 57:316–312, 1988.
58. Kopell, HP and Thompson, WA: Peripheral Entrapment Neuropathies. William & Wilkins, Baltimore, 1963.
59. Pecina, MM, Krmpotic-Nemanic, J, and Markiewitz, AD: Tunnel Syndromes. CRC Press, Boca Raton, 1991, pp 31–34.
60. McCue, FC III and Miller, GA: Soft-tissue injuries of the hand. In Pettrone, FA (ed): Symposium of Upper Extremity Injuries in Athletes. CV Mosby, St. Louis, 1986, pp 79–94.
61. Spinner, M: Injuries to the Major Branches of Peripheral Nerves of the Forearm, ed 2. WB Saunders, Philadelphia, 1978.
62. Commandre, F: Pathologie Abarticulaire. Laboratoire Cetrane, Paris, 1977.
63. Mosher, JF: Peripheral nerve injuries and entrapment of the forearm and wrist. In Pettrone, F (ed): Symposium on Upper Extremity Injuries in Athletes. CV Mosby, St. Louis, 1986, pp 174–181.
64. Howard, FM: Controversies in nerve entrapment syndromes in the forearm and wrist. Orthop Clin North Am 17:375, 1986.
65. Pecina, M, Krmpotic-Nemanic, J, and Markiewitz, AD: Ulnar Tunnel Syndrome. In Pecina, MM, Krmpotic-Nemanic, J, and Markiewitz, AD (eds): Tunnel Syndromes. CRC Press, Boca Raton, 1991, pp 69–73.
66. Yocum, LA: The diagnosis and nonoperative treatment of elbow problems in the athlete. Clin Sports Med 8:439, 1989.
67. DelPizzo, W, Jobe, FW, and Norwood, L.: Ulnar nerve entrapment syndrome in baseball players. Am J Sports Med 8:439, 1989.

68. Silverstein, BA, Fine, LJ, and Armstrong, TJ: Hand wrist cumulative trauma disorders in industry. Br J Industrial Med 43:779–784, 1986.
69. Childress, HM: Recurrent ulnar-nerve dislocation at the elbow. J Bone Joint Surg 38A:978, 1956.
70. O'Driscoll, SW, Horii E, Carmichael, SW, et al: The anatomy of the cubital tunnel and its relationship to ulnar neuropathies (abstract SS-03). Abstracts of the American Society for Surgery of the Hand 45th Annual Meeting, Toronto, 1990, pp 3–11.
71. Kumar, K, Deshpande, S, Jain, M, et al: Evaluation of various fibro-osseous tunnel pressures (carpal, cubital and tarsal) in normal human subjects. Ind J Physiol Pharmacol 32:139, 1988.
72. Macnicol, MF: Extraneural pressures affecting the ulnar nerve at the elbow. Hand 14:5, 1982.
73. Sunderland, S: The intraneural topography of the radial, median and ulnar nerves. Brain 68:243, 1945.
74. Kane, E, Kaplan, EBN, and Spinner, M: Observations of the course of the ulnar nerve in the arm. Ann Chir 27:487, 1973.
75. Feindel, W and Stratford, J: The role of the cubital tunnel in tardy ulnar palsy. Can J Surg 1:287, 1958.
76. Buerhler, MJ and Thayer DT: The elbow flexion test. A clinical test for the cubital tunnel syndrome. Clin Orthop 233:213, 1988.
77. Vanderpool, DW: Peripheral compression lesions of the ulnar nerve. J Bone Joint Surg 50B:792, 1968.
78. St. John, JN and Palmaz, JC: The cubital tunnel in ulnar entrapment neuropathy. Radiology 158:119, 1986.
79. Pechan, J and Kredba, J: Treatment of cubital tunnel syndrome by means of local administration of cortisonoids. Acta Univ Carol [Med] (Praha) 26:125, 1980.
80. Foster, RJ and Edshage, S: Factors related to the outcome of surgically managed compressive ulnar neuropathy at the elbow level. J Hand Surg 6:181, 1981.
81. McPherson, SA and Meals, RA: Cubital tunnel syndrome. In Szabo, RM (ed): Common Hand Problems Orthop Clin North Am 23:111–123, 1992.
82. Seliger, V, Dolejs, L, and Karas, V: A dynamic comparison of maximum eccentric, concentric and isometric contractions using EMG and energy expenditure measurements. Eur J Appl Physiol 45:235–244, 1980.
83. Rigby, BJ, Horai, N, and Spikes, JD: The mechanical behavior of rat tail tendon. J Gen Physiol 43:265–283, 1959.
84. Lehman, JF, Masock, AJ, Warren, CG, et al: Effect of therapeutic temperatures on tendon extensibility. Arch Phys Med Rehabil 50:481–487, 1970.
85. Warren, CG, Lehman, JF, and Koblanski, JN: Elongation of rat tail tendon: Effect of load and temperature. Arch Phys Med Rehabil 52:465–484, 1971.
86. Van Brocklin, JD and Ellis, DG: A study of the mechanical behavior of toe extensor tendons under applied stress Arch Phys Med Rehabil 46:369–370, 1965.
87. Tillman, LJ and Cummings, GS: Biologic mechanisms of connective tissue mutability. In Dean, P, Currier, and Nelson, RM (eds.): Dynamics of Human Biologic Tissues. FA Davis, Philadelphia, 1992, pp 1–44.
88. Armstrong, TJ: Ergonomics and cumulative trauma disorders. Hand Clin 2:553, 1986.
89. Goldstein, SA, Armstrong, TJ, and Chaffin, DB: Analysis of cumulative strain in tendons and tendon sheaths. J Biomech 20:1, 1987.
90. Manske, PR, Ogata, K, and Lesker, PA: Nutrient pathways to extensor tendons of primates J Hand Surg 10B:8, 1985.
91. Cohen, BK: DeQuervain's disease. J Bone Joint Surg 33B:96–99, 1951.
92. Lipscomb, PR: Tenosynovitis of the hand and wrist: Carpal tunnel syndrome, deQuervain's disease, trigger digit. Clin Orthop 13:164, 1959.
93. Lipscomb, PR: Stenosing tenosynovitis at the radial styloid process. Ann Surg 134:110, 1951.

94. Finkelstein, H: Stenosing tenosynovaginitis at the radial styloid process. J Bone Joint Surg 12A:509, 1930.

95. Hueston, JT and Wilson, WF: The etiology of trigger finger. Hand 4:257, 1972.

96. Kolin-Sorensen, V: Treatment of trigger fingers. Acta Orthop Scand 41:428, 1970.

97. Newport, ML, Lane, LB and Stuchin, SA: Treatment of the trigger finger by steroid injection. J Hand Surg 15A:748, 1990.

98. American Society for Surgery of the Hand: Regional Review. Course in Hand Surgery Syllabus, ed 10. ASSH, Aurora, Colo., 1990 pp 9–12.

99. Moberg, E.: Emergency Surgery of the Hand. E & S Livingstone, London, 1967.

100. Cailliet, R: Fractures and dislocations of the wrist, hand and fingers. In Cailliet, R: Hand Pain and Impairment. FA Davis, Philadelphia, 1994 pp 193–215.

101. Bureau of Labor Statistics. Occupational Injuries and Illnesses in the United States by Industry, 1989. Bulletin 2379. US Department of Labor, Washington, 1991.

102. Koch, H: The management of chronic pain in office-based ambulatory care: National ambulatory medical care survey. US Department of Health and Human Services, Washington, 1986.

103. New York State Worker's Compensation Board. Compensated Cases Closed. 1981. Research and Statistics Bulletin, No. 42. State of New York, Albany, 1984.

104. Feuerstein M, Callan-Harris S, Hickey P, et al: Multidisciplinary rehabilitation of chronic work-related upper extremity disorders. J Occup Med 35:396–403, 1993.

CHAPTER 11

Hip Pain and Impairment

The hip joint in humans is, for the most part intended for weight bearing and walking. It is well constructed for these functions and despite the trauma possible in everyday activities, is only infrequently impaired. The current emphasis on athletic activities, an increase in vehicular accidents, and cumulative trauma disorders have not significantly increased hip joint problems. Actually hip pathology has only impaired participation in nonprofessional athletic activities. The medical literature is relatively sparse except for an increase in surgical intervention procedures for treating the pathology.

FUNCTIONAL ANATOMY

The hip joint is the outstanding example of a congruous joint (Fig. 11–1). The precise convex surface of the femoral head articulates symmetrically with the precise concavity of the acetabulum. All joint motions are possible and rotation moves about a consistent point of contact (Fig. 11–2).

The head of the femur is spherical and points upward and forward on its neck as the angle of inclination dictates (Fig. 11–3). The angle of anteversion follows a similar position (Fig. 11–4).

These angles are important because the articular contacts are influenced by them in affording normal lubrication (Fig. 11–5) and are also involved in the degenerative changes that occur when these contacts are violated.

The femoral head articulates with the acetabulum, which is horseshoe-shaped and coated with cartilage (Fig. 11–6). The center of the horseshoe is not so covered. The open lower portion of the acetabulum is filled in as a com-

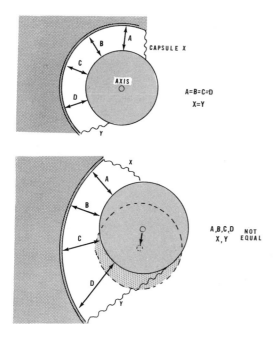

Figure 11–1. Congruous versus incongruous joints. The upper drawing depicts a congruous joint wherein the convex-concave articulating joint surfaces are symmetric throughout their arcs. Joint space is equal throughout the contact points $A = B = C = D$. The capsule (X and Y) is symmetric. The lower drawing shows an incongruous joint wherein the concave curves are different than the convex curves and motion requires gliding rather than mere rotation. At a given point, the distances (A, B, C, D, X) of the articulating surfaces are unequal. The capsule containing the joint is asymmetric (X and Y).

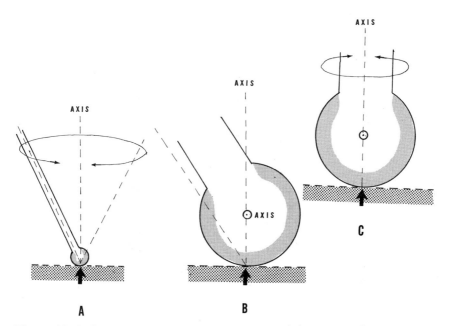

Figure 11–2. Joint motion: spin or rotation. True spin (C) is rotation about one point. If there is a change in the axis perpendicular (A) to the surface during spin, a spin rotation occurs (B). Spin rotation is movement in the hip joint as the axis of rotation remains relatively constant.

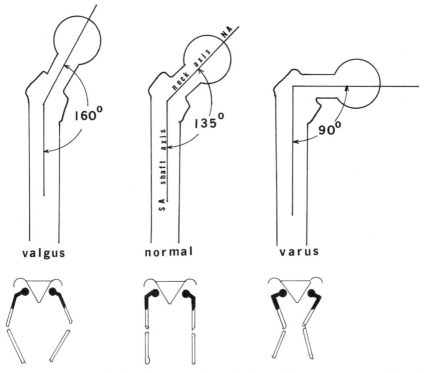

Figure 11–3. Angle of inclination. The angle formed by intersecting the femoral neck angle (NA) with an axis drawn through the shaft of the femur (SA) is termed the **angle of inclination.** This angle normally varies between 116° and 140° with an average of 135°.

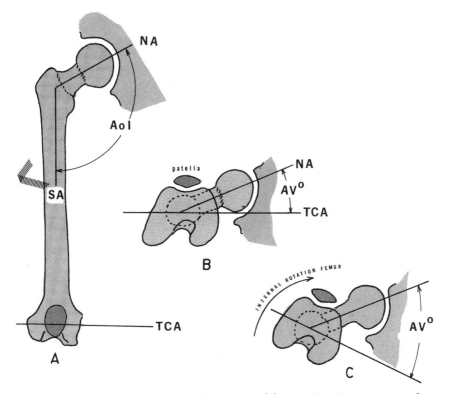

Figure 11–4. Angle of anteversion. The transcondylar axis (TCA) is a transverse line passing through the femoral condyles. An axis placed through the femoral neck (NA) forms an angle with TCA, which is termed **the angle of anteversion.** (B) is angle AV° with the femoral head viewed from above. A 15 to 25° of angle is considered normal. (C) The angle is increased due to internal rotation of the femur in relationship to the femoral neck. This is increased anteversion. Viewing the femur from anterior-posterior direction, (A) depicts the angle of inclination (see Fig. 11–3).

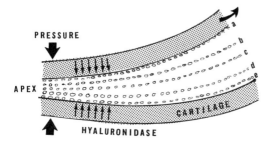

Figure 11–5. Hydrodynamic lubrication. Nonparallel joint surfaces, as they exist in incongruous joints, form a wedge-shaped lubricating fluid some of which stays at the apex. The lubricating fluid moves in layers *a, b, c, d,* and *e* at the same speed as the articulating bones. A layer, however, adheres to both surfaces. A shearing force between layers deforms fluid. The lubricant is both adhesive and viscous and is coated by hyaluronic acid, which is created by the synovium and cartilage. Even without movement, the layer(s) remain between the two opposing bony surfaces. It is apparent that there can be *no* congruity in any moving joint, only a degree of congruity. Constant pressure without movement diminishes the lubricant between surfaces.

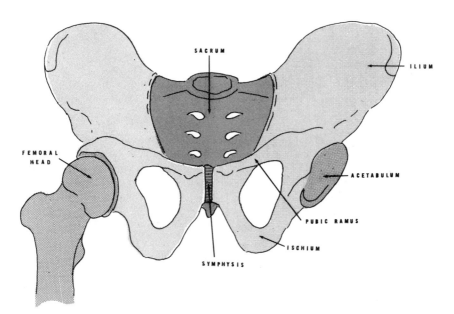

Figure 11–6. Anterior view of the bony pelvis. The left hip is removed to reveal the site of the acetabulum.

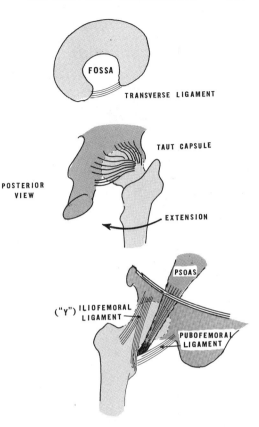

Figure 11–7. Hip joint. *Top view* depicts the acetabulum ring completed by the transverse acetabular ligament. *Center view* shows the capsule tightening as hip extends or internally rotates. *Lower view* shows the anterior capsule is reinforced by the iliofemoral, pubofemoral, and ischiofemoral ligaments and also the psoas tendon.

plete ring by the transverse acetabular ligament. The acetabulum is deepened by the cartilage-covered ring of fibrocartilage termed the **labrum.** The head of the femur is held firmly into the acetabulum by a thick capsule (Fig. 11–7), which tightens when the hip is rotated (Fig. 11–8).

Portions of the capsule are thickened forming ligaments, which are termed, according to their specific site of origin: the **iliofemoral, pubofemoral,** and the **ischiofemoral ligaments.**

In the erect stance, the center of gravity passes behind the center of rotation of the hip joint. The pelvis is angled so that the femoral head is seated directly into the acetabulum. The anterior portion of the capsule is thickened to form the iliofemoral ligament, which permits static stance to exist on a ligamentous support without supporting muscular activity.

In a toe-out stance, the head of the femur is directed forward (outward) out of the socket. To prevent subluxation of the joint the iliofemoral ligament is placed too far laterally, thus support derives from the iliopsoas tendon. Also involved is the *ligament of the head,* which is a hollow cone of synovial mem-

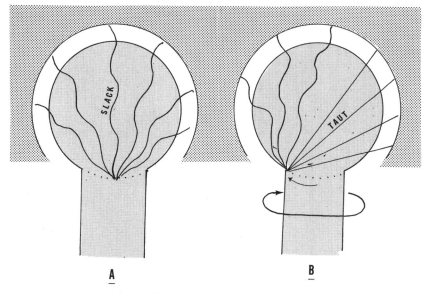

Figure 11–8. Femoral capsule. (A) The capsule, which is slack in the neutral hip position, becomes taut (B) on any rotation, internal or external.

brane which attaches to the acetabular fossa, which transmits blood vessels to the head of the femur and is not considered to be a strong support.[1]

The femoral head is covered with cartilage which, as is true with all cartilage, compresses to exude synovial fluid and recovers to imbibe nutritional fluid when nonweight bearing (Fig. 11–9).

HIP JOINT MOTIONS

Hip joint motions include flexion, extension, abduction, adduction, and rotation—all have physiologic limitations. Flexion is limited by the hamstring muscle group. Extension is limited by ligamentous thickening of the fibrous capsule. Abduction is limited by the adductor muscle group and adduction by the tensor muscle and fascia and abductor muscles. Rotation is limited by the fibrous capsule (Figs. 11–10 and 11–11).

In a clinical setting, the possible range of motion may indicate articular pathology or periarticular impairment which subsequent studies confirm. Tests for range are similar to the stretch exercises (Fig. 11–12) is the latter is the cause of impairment. If there is structural articular limitation, the test will also be valuable (Fig. 11–13).

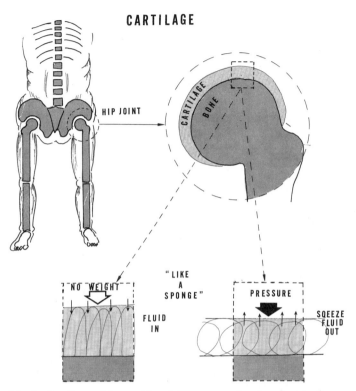

Figure 11–9. Cartilage of femoral head. The upper drawing depicts the covering of the femoral head by cartilage. In non–weight-bearing cartilage the cartilage expands by *imbibing* synovial fluid. During weight bearing or other pressure, the cartilage *flattens* and squeezes fluid into the joint to become lubricating synovial fluid.

Walking

Walking, besides applying pressure on the joint from gravity, repeatedly stretches the hip capsule, ligaments, and the fascia of the involved muscles. Discussion of normal determinants of gait could consume an entire test,[2,3] but salient points need emphasis for understanding of the effect upon the hip joint.

In normal gait, the femur rotates on the pelvis as the tibia rotates on the femur (Fig. 11–14). These motions require normal range of motion of the hip joint. Normal gait requires 60% of its timing in the stance phase and 40% in the swing phase (Fig. 11–15). The stance phase is weight bearing, thus adding compressive forces to the cartilage, whereas the swing phase requires greater flexibility to the capsular tissues. Patients with hip disease spend a dispropor-

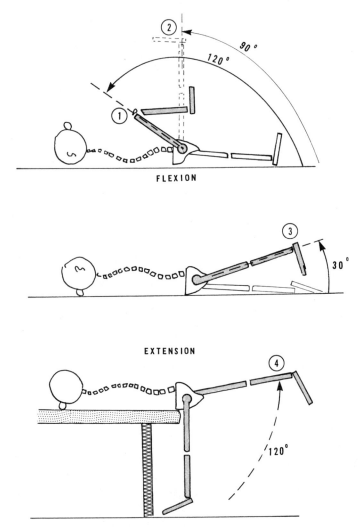

Figure 11–10. Hip range of motion. In clinical evaluation of hip range of motion, the following tests are initiated: (*1*) Hip flexion with knee flexed from 0° to 120° limited by contact of the thigh with the abdominal wall (*2*), (*3*) hip extension to 30° with patient prone; (*4*) with patient's other leg flexed the involved leg is extended to 90° to 120° as compared with the contralateral leg.

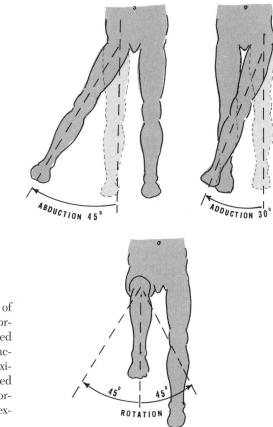

Figure 11–11. Hip range of motion. Hip abduction is normally 45° from 0° measured with leg fully extended. Adduction from neutral is approximately 30°. Rotation measured with flexed knee and hip is normally 45° of internal and 45° external rotation.

tionate amount of time in the stance phase with excessive rotation and lateral motion.

These variations change the gait velocity, stride length, and cadence of walking to minimize pain and to improve stability. Observation and evaluation of abnormal gait reveal these factors.

Standing

Weight distribution on the hip joint during standing has been calculated using a lever arm system (Fig. 11–16). The distance from the center of gravity of the body is approximately 4″ from the fulcrum of the hip joint. The abductor muscles exert the balancing force through a lever arm of 2″. This finding implies that an individual weighing 150 lbs imposes 450 lbs on the femoral head, thus indicating the biomechanical need for studying forces from activi-

HIP STRETCH

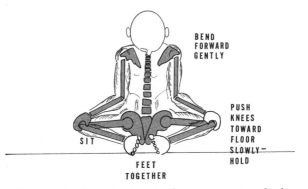

Figure 11–12. Hip stretch. Placing patient in the yoga position, the hip adductors and rotators can be stretched. Placing patient in this position can also test range of motion of each hip.

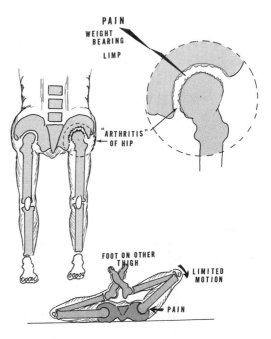

Figure 11–13. Limited motion from degenerative joint disease. In a patient with a damaged articular femoral head surface, there usually is pain on weight bearing. Examination reveals limited range of motion.

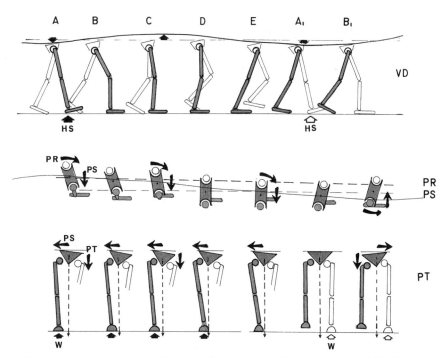

Figure 11–14. Composite schematic determinants of gait. VD, vertical displacement of the pelvis from a side view. PR, pelvic rotation viewed from above as the left leg swings through. PT, pelvic tilting. The bottom drawing shows the weight-bearing leg (W) going into a Trendelenberg position as the hip adducts. PS, the pelvic shift. All these determinants require normal hip motion.

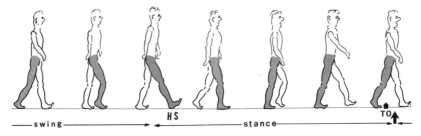

Figure 11–15. Gait. The shaded leg depicts the swing phase ending at heel strike (HS) and the stance phase continuing until toe off (TO). The hip extends at the beginning of swing and continues through midstance phase.

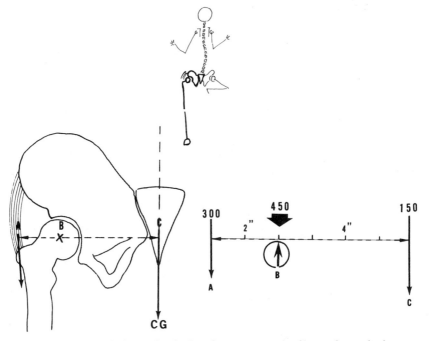

Figure 11–16. Weight borne by the hip during stance. (*Left*) Weight on the hip joint (*B*) combined from body weight (*C*) and balanced by pull of the abductor muscles (*A*) (*CG*-center of gravity). (*Right*) A 150-lbs adult with a 4-in distance from the center of gravity to the hip joint fulcrum is balanced by gluteal muscular action 2'' from the fulcrum. The glutei exert 300 lbs to balance, thus total pressure on the hip joint is 450 lbs.

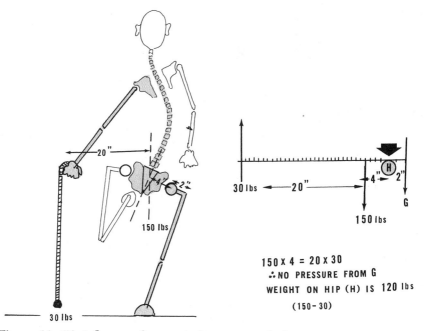

Figure 11–17. Influence of a cane in hip joint weight bearing. Assuming that the cane is held 20″ from the center of gravity with 30 lbs of pressure on the floor, the force on the hip is balanced by decreasing the dependence on the gluteal muscles. A decrease of 30 lbs is estimated.

ties and methods for relieving these forces. The use of a cane has been confirmed by studies (Fig. 11–17) to diminish weight bearing on the affected hip when used in the *opposite* hand.[4]

PAIN MECHANISMS OF THE HIP

Four major specific structures in the hip contain nociceptive nerves capable of evoking pain: the fibrous capsule and its ligaments, surrounding muscles, bony periosteum, and the synovial lining of the joint capsule. Cartilage itself is insensitive, but the subchondral bone is sensitive because of its blood supply and accompanying vasomotor innervation.

The nerves that supply the hip joint are the femoral, obturator, superior gluteal, accessory obturator. The femoral nerve supplies the iliofemoral ligament, the obturator the medial portion of the capsule, and the superior gluteal nerve the superolateral region. The sciatic nerve is thought to supply the posterior aspect of the hip joint capsule. The muscles of the hip joint are amply supplied both motor and sensory nerves.

The skin about the joint is supplied by the lateral femoral cutaneous nerve (Fig. 11–18) and the anterior thigh area is served by the femoral nerve. The abundant innervation of the hip justifies the statement "disorders of the hip region, including buttocks, are among the most important and frequent causes of prolonged pain, suffering, and serious disability."[5] A 1977 survey by the National Center for Health Statistics revealed that impairment related to the hips and lower extremities accounts for nearly a third of the total impairments affecting the entire musculoskeletal system.[6]

Diagnostic and possibly therapeutic nerve blocks have been given strong consideration in diagnosis and treatment protocols.[5]

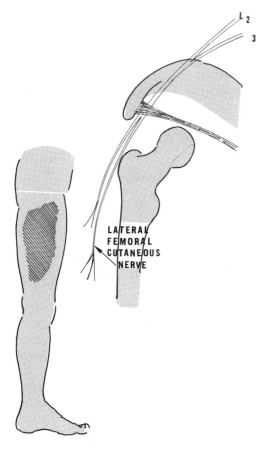

L 2
3

LATERAL
FEMORAL
CUTANEOUS
NERVE

Figure 11–18. Lateral femoral cutaneous nerve: meralgia paresthetica. The lateral femoral cutaneous nerve derives from L2-3 roots and subserves the dermatomal area of the lateral thigh (*left drawing*). When this area is painful and hyperesthetic, it is termed **meralgia paresthetica.**

Degenerative Arthritis

The most common painful disabling condition of the hip joint is degenerative arthritis. The cause and mechanism of degenerative joint disease of the hip remain elusive, however. The excellent dissertation by Trueta in 1963[7] has never been bettered. His statement that the "main cause of joint cartilage degeneration is the unsatisfactory adaptation of the femoral head to a socket which cannot cover all its surface, even in the most ideal anatomic condition."[7] The fossa, because it lacks cartilage, leaves the medial aspect of the femoral head without any chance of intermittent compression except when the femur is in extreme abduction, flexion, and external rotation.

The causes, therefore, of degenerative changes in the hip cartilage are excessive valgus (Fig. 11–19), some congenital, developmental problem such as an earlier subluxation, Perthes's disease or slipped epiphysis, and certain iatrogenic diseases following surgical intervention for fractures of the femoral neck.

Degenerative osteoarthrosis may occur with weakening of the trabecular structure of the femoral epiphysis such as exists in senile osteoporosis or after prolonged administration of corticosteroids.

Mechanical stress resulting from the current obsession with excessive jogging and running has been claimed as a major cause of later development of degenerative hip disease, but the assertion has yet to be confirmed. Mechanical stress from *repetitive impulsive loading* creates tensile fatigue of subchondral bone which remains a possible cause.[8,9]

Early hip pain probably develops as the stages of degeneration progress. Because cartilage has neither blood nor nerve supply, pain must emanate from other articular tissues which are the capsule, ligaments, and muscles.

Initially, synovitis is present with secretion of nociceptive elements that irritate the sensory nerve endings (Fig. 11–20). A secretion of lysosomes

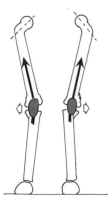
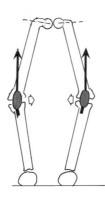

GENU VALGUS   GENU VARUS

Figure 11–19. Genu valgum and varum. The knee variations of valgum and varum have a significant effect on the femoral head orientation.

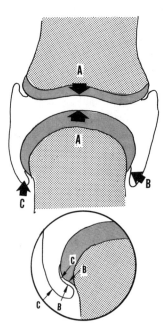

Figure 11-20. Synovial sites of inflammation in degenerative joint disease. (A) is the site of compression and the least prevalent in degenerative articular disease. (B) is a fold of synovium, which is the most frequent site of cartilage pathology. (C) The site of incipient osteophyte formation is under the fold of synovium.

causes degenerative changes, a mechanical deviation of the joint, and progression of the degeneration.[10]

Diagnosis. The history elicited is that of pain on weight bearing, impaired ambulation with limp, and even pain after prolonged standing. The pain is located in the region of the hip joint but that description is imprecise because pain can be in the groin, the front of the upper thigh, buttocks, or anywhere in the general area. It is also frequently referred to the region around the knee. Referred pain from the low back must be ascertained by an appropriate examination of that area.

Clinically, evidence exists of limited range of motion in joints as shown by Figures 11-10 through 11-13, and in an impaired gait. Initial radiographs may be negative. Bone scanning may reveal inflammation; ultrasound examination may be required for diagnosis.[11]

Treatment.

Nonsurgical. Rest, immobilization, traction, oral anti-inflammatory medication, both steroidal and nonsteroidal. Intra-articular injection of an analgesic with or without steroids (Figs. 11-21 and 11-22) is temporarily effective, as are nerve blocks of the articular branch of the obturator nerve (Fig. 11-23).

Use of a cane, or preferably crutches with severe, acute pain, is indicated. Positioning during bed rest is also desirable because flexion contracture is a frequent sequela and must be avoided. Frequently, lying prone stretches the

Figure 11–21. Technique and site of intraarticular injection. The needle is inserted 2 to 3 cm below the anterosuperior iliac spine and 2 to 3 cm lateral to the femoral artery pulsation. The needle penetrates in a posteromedial direction until bone is struck. After aspiration to eliminate arterial or venous injection, the steroid-anesthetic agent is injected.

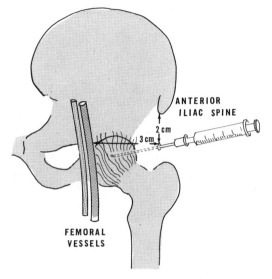

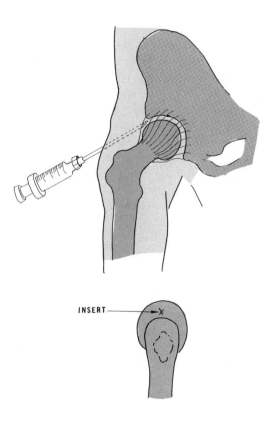

Figure 11–22. Technique and site of intraarticular injection into the hip joint. With the patient lying on the contralateral hip, the trochanter is located by palpation and the needle is inserted midline of the superior aspect of the femoral neck. The needle follows along the neck until the capsule is reached, then, after aspiration, the fluid is injected.

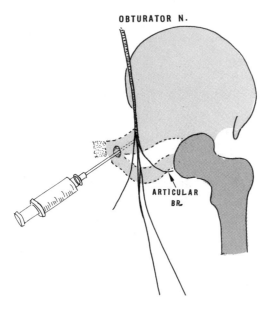

OBTURATOR N.

ARTICULAR BR.

Figure 11–23. Technique of obturator nerve block. With the patient supine and thighs separated, a wheel is raised 1 cm lateral to the pubic tubercle. A 22 gauge 8-cm needle is directed perpendicularly until the inferior ramus of the pubis is reached. The direction of the needle is then changed several centimeters into a lateral and superior direction parallel to the pubic ramus. After aspiration, 5 to 10 mL of an anesthetic agent is injected. An effective injection is ascertained by paresis of adduction and external rotation of the hip and *not* by an area of anesthesia.

hip flexors and positioning must be implemented by placing a pillow under the upper thigh while in the prone position, thus providing that the pillow itself does not cause symptomatic lumbar lordosis with concurrent low back pain. Traction immobilizes the joint and elongates the inflamed capsule (Fig. 11–24).

Exercises to regain or maintain hip range of motion are important and done preferably while the joint is non-weight bearing. Because hip flexion contracture is a prominent complication of hip pathology, this contracture must be minimized or avoided by proper exercise (Figs. 11–25 to 11–28).

Surgical. Numerous surgical interventions currently in vogue include:

1. Revascularization of bone procedures
2. Osteotomy to alter the alignment of the head to the acetabulum
3. Denervation procedures
4. Arthrodesis
5. Arthroplasty by cup
6. Total hip replacement

Arthrodesis causes a *stiff* hip, meaning a total change in gait with significant stress on the lumbar spine. Total hip replacement should be restricted to those patients with substantial pain and marked functional disability.[12] The choice of prosthesis and technique is beyond the scope of this book, but a gen-

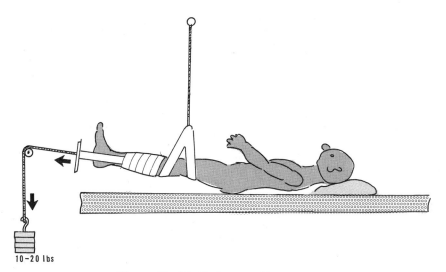

Figure 11–24. Technique of hip traction.

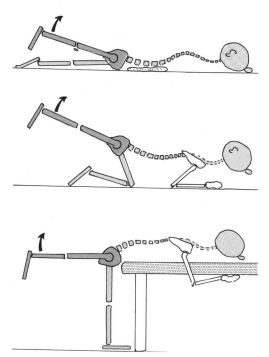

Figure 11–25. Hip extensor exercises. (*Top*) With patient prone, the leg is extended with and without resistance applied manually or with a weighted ankle apparatus. A pillow under the abdomen minimizes excessive lumbar lordosis. (*Center*) With the contralateral knee flexed and weight bearing, the involved leg is extended. (*Bottom*) With patient prone and over a table, the dependent leg stabilizes the pelvis and the involved leg extends actively and passively.

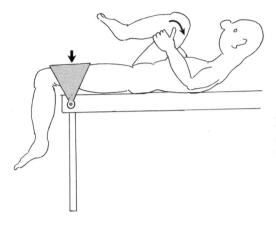

Figure 11–26. Hip flexor stretch exercise. With the afflicted leg held by a canvas strap, the opposite leg is gently and progressively flexed toward the chest. This action stretches the hip flexors.

eral decision is whether to use cement or not. The metallic part of the femoral shaft component does not form an intrinsic union with the femur, so that movement of the shaft within the femur becomes a source of pain after surgery in many patients. Wear or deterioration of the prosthesis requiring removal or replacement is also a dilemma familiar to most surgeons. A comprehensive rehabilitation program must be instituted after total hip replacement to maximize functional stability and mobility of the replacement hip to avoid the danger of dislocation.[13,14]

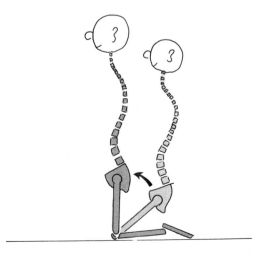

Figure 11–27. Hip extensor exercise kneeling. From the full kneeling position the patient arises to full erect posture. This stretches both hip flexors and strengthens the extensors.

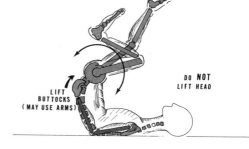

Figure 11–28. Bedroom bicycling. Assuming the supine position depicted, the legs are flexed as in riding a bicycle. This is a nonresistance non–weight-bearing flexibility exercise.

PELVIC TRAUMA

Trauma to the pelvis is common in today's society with severe vehicular injuries. Although most such trauma affect bony structures, an associated soft tissue component also merits attention. The proximity of sexual and urinary organs, as well as those nerves involved in lower extremity function, make early recognition and appropriate care mandatory.

The bony pelvis is an intact ring formed anteriorly and laterally by the innominate bones and posteriorly by the sacrum and coccyx. These bones are united by strong resistant ligaments which account for the pelvis's strength, support, and assistance in locomotion (Figs. 11–28 and 11–29).

When standing, body weight on the sacrum is transferred across the sacro iliac joints through the ilia and hip joints. When sitting, weight is borne by the ischial tuberosities.

Figure 11–29. Forces acting on the pelvis. The body weight is imposed on the fifth lumbar vertebra, which lies on the sacrum. This weight is transmitted through the sacrum, across the sacroiliac joints, through the ilia, into the acetabula, and then into the femora. The compressive forces of the femoral heads on standing are resisted by the superimposed pubic strut. In the sitting position, the forces (*white arrows*) tend to separate the ilia, which is resisted by the symphysis pubis and the sacroiliac ligaments (SI).

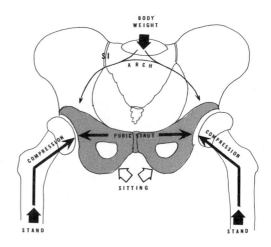

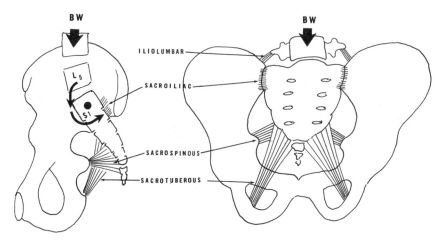

Figure 11–30. Ligamentous support of the pelvis. The side view of the pelvis indicates the stress of the superincumbent body (BW) on the fifth lumbar vertebra, which lies on the sacrum (S-1), causing it to rotate (*circular arrows*) to the extent permitted by the sacrospinous and sacrotuberous ligaments. Rotation of the pelvis is resisted by the sacroiliac ligaments. These ligaments are shown in the anterior view (*right*).

The normal pelvis forms a ring of resistance (Fig. 11–30), of which the strongest segments are the innominate bones; the weakest are the pubic rami, the symphysis pubis, and the sacroiliac joints. Fracture or dislocation located at any single site may disrupt the continuity of the whole ring. Any displacement of the segments may also disrupt the ring.

Isolated fractures of individual bones of the pelvis can occur without disrupting the ring (Fig. 11–31). Fractures are usually the result of direct trauma; with disruption of the ring, ligamentous structures are also violated (Figs. 11–32 and 11–33).

Separation of the sacroiliac joint as an isolated incident is rare without a concomitant fracture in the weaker bony portions of the ring (Fig. 11–34).

In the event of significant trauma, pain, and tenderness of the pelvic region, the pelvic ring should be tested manually. This is done by applying pressure to the pelvis. With both hands upon the anterior superior spines, downward and outward pressure indicates excessive motion and resulting pain. Placing the examiner's hands on both sides of the pelvis and compressing them may indicate disruption of the ring. Direct pressure upon the pubic rami and the symphysis pubis is also indicative. Confirmatory radiographs are diagnostic.

Forces on the normal pelvis (see Fig. 11–28) adversely affect these fractures and must be kept in mind during examination, treatment, and dealing with subsequent problems. The direction of the acetabuli may be altered by

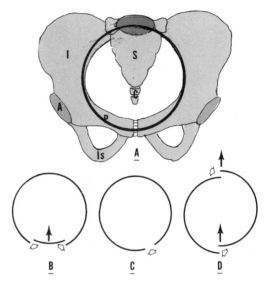

Figure 11–31. Pelvic ring. (A) The pelvic ring is bounded laterally by the ilia (I), anteriorly by the pubic rami, (P), and posteriorly by the sacrum (S) and coccyx (C). The ischia (Is) and acetabula (A) are depicted. Lower drawing B, C, and D depict various types of fracture-dislocations resulting from trauma (*white arrows*).

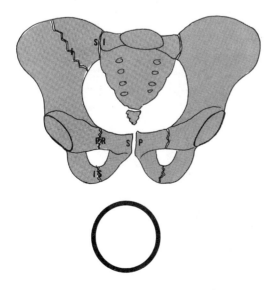

Figure 11–32. Sites of fracture with intact pelvic ring. An isolated fracture in the pelvic ring does not always disrupt the integrity of the ring. The sites noted are the pubic rami (PR), ilium (I), ischia (IS), and the sacroiliac (SI) and symphysis pubic (SP) joints.

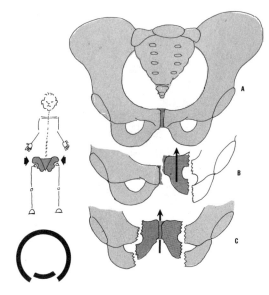

Figure 11–33. (A) Combined fractures within the pubic rami. These may be double fractures or single combined with separation of the symphysis pubis (B). The dislocation of the fragment is slight and only the anterior portion of the ring is disrupted (C).

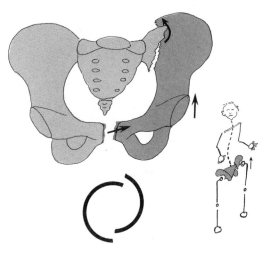

Figure 11–34. Combined sacroiliac and symphysis pubis separation. Injury resulting is combined separation of the symphysis pubis and the sacroiliac joints disrupts the pelvic ring. The fracture segment rotates posteriorly behind the sacrum and moves superiorly. The involved leg is clinically shortened.

having an effect upon the hip joint. The sacrum may suffer malalignment with subsequent lumbosacral pathology. Most in need of urgent attention are injuries to the urinary tract through a tear of the bladder or urethra. These are emergency conditions demanding immediate attention. Treatment of pelvic fractures may vary from conservative to operative intervention, depending on the site, extent, and complications.

REFERENCES

1. Basmajian, JV: Grant's Method of Anatomy, ed 8. Williams & Wilkins, Baltimore, 1971, p 393.
2. Inman, VT, Ralston, HJ, and Todd, F: Human Walking. Williams & Wilkins, Baltimore, 1981.
3. Sussman, A and Goode, R: The Magic of Walking. Simon & Schuster, New York, 1967.
4. Blount, WP: Don't throw away the cane. J Bone Joint Surg (A) 38:695, 1956.
5. Bonica, JJ and Spengler, DM: Painful disorders of the hip region. In Bonica, JJ (ed): The Management of Pain, ed. 2. Lea & Febiger, Philadelphia, 1990, p 1530.
6. Health Interview Survey: Prevalence of Selected Impairments United States 1977, Series 10, No. 134. National Center for Health Statistics, Hyattsville, Md., 1981.
7. Trueta, J: Studies on the etiopathology of osteoarthritis of the hip. Clin Orthop 31:7–18, 1963.
8. Rabin, EL: Mechanical aspects of osteoarthritis. Bull Rheum Dis 26:862–865, 1975.
9. Hettinga, DL: III. Normal joint structures and their reaction to injury. J Orthop Sports Phys Ther 1:178–185, 1980.
10. Chrisman, OD: Biochemical aspects of degenerative joint disease. Clin Orthop 64:77–86, 1969.
11. Bickerstaff DR, Neal LM, Booth AJ, et al: Ultrasound examination of the irritable hip. J Bone Joint Surg 72B:549–553, 1990.
12. Harris, WH and Sledge, CB: Total hip and total knee replacement. New Engl J Med 323:725–731, 1990.
13. Duncan, BF: The postoperative total hip—A patient-oriented rehabilitation program. Contemp Orthop 5:412–447, 1982.
14. Effekhar, NS: Dislocation and instability complicating low friction arthroplasty of the hip joint. Clin Orthop 121:120, 1976.

CHAPTER 12

Knee Pain

The knee, because of its composition and its frequent exposure to trauma, is probably the most vulnerable of all structures of the body to soft tissue injury with attendant pain and impairment. The knee joint is essentially unstable because its support is primarily ligamentous and muscular.

Two joints form the knee: the femorotibial and the patellofemoral (Fig. 12–1). The distal end of the femur has two convex condyles that articulate with the concave surfaces of the tibial plateau. The incongruous curvatures are thus unstable (Fig. 12–2). Although the interposed menisci add to the congruity, ligamentous support is still needed for stability (Fig. 12–3).

LIGAMENTS

The medial collateral ligament is three-layered (Fig. 12–4). The superficial layer is the major medial ligament. Inner layers of this ligament connect to the medial meniscus and the capsule. The deep layer of the major collateral ligament is divided into three sections with the inner extending anteriorly to stabilize the extensor mechanism (quadriceps), the middle laterally stabilizing the joint, and the posterior extending to the posterior popliteal capsule.

The lateral collateral ligament passes from the lateral epicondyle of the femur to the fibular head. The peroneal nerve passes the neck of the fibula behind the attachment of the biceps tendon.

The knee has maximum stability when in full extension because the collateral ligaments are taut (Fig. 12–5). Immediately on flexion, the collateral ligament relaxes, permitting slight lateromedial motion and rotation of the tibia on the femoral condyles. Upon full flexion, the collateral and cruciate ligaments regain their tautness (Fig. 12–6).

388

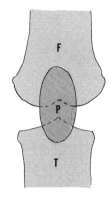

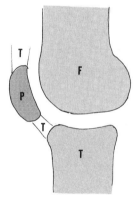

Figure 12–1. The joints of the knee. The upper view is an anterior view that depicts the femoral (F) tibial (T) joint with the superimposed patella showing the patellofemoral joint. The lower, lateral view shows the patellofemoral joint, wherein the patella (P) is connected by tendons (T).

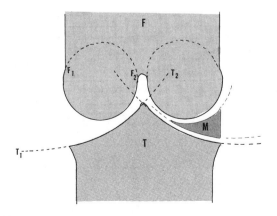

Figure 12–2. The incongruity of the femorotibial joint. The convex curves of the femoral (F) condyles (F1-F2) have a different curvature than the tibial (T) plateau (T1-T2), thus forming incongruous joints. The menisci (M) alter the adjacent curving surfaces, which approximates congruity.

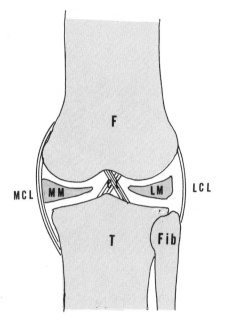

Figure 12–3. Ligamentous support of the femoraltibial joint. The medial collateral ligaments (MCL) connect the medial aspect of the femur (F) and the tibia (T) and are attached to the medial meniscus (MM). The lateral collateral ligament (LCL) attaches from the lateral aspect of the femur to the head of the fibula (Fib). It is not attached to the lateral meniscus (LM). The cruciate ligaments (CL) are shown.

These factors are important to the clinician in analyzing the position of the knee at the moment of impact or stress to determine which ligaments are injured.

The cruciate ligaments are paired and termed according to their attachment to the tibia (Fig. 12–7). The **anterior cruciate ligament** originates from the anterior tibial plateau and ascends to attach to the medial aspect of the lateral femoral condyle. By their origin and attachment the cruciate ligaments restrict shear (translation) motion of the tibia on the femur, but are also involved in flexion and extension of the knee.

The **posterior cruciate ligament** becomes taut when the tibia shears posteriorly during early flexion and becomes the fulcrum about which further knee flexion occurs. When the knee fully extends, the anterior cruciate ligament prevents knee hyperextension (Fig. 12–8).

The tibia rotates on the femoral condyles in flexion-extension: externally on extension and internally on flexion (Fig. 12–9). This is due to the relative difference in surface areas of the femoral condyles. As extension proceeds, the tibia *uses up* the surface area of the medial condyle—what remains causes external rotation. The same mechanism occurs in full flexion and causes internal rotation (Fig. 12–10).

The cruciate ligaments restrict excessive rotation as well as shear motion of the tibia on the femoral condyles (Figs. 12–11 and 12–12).

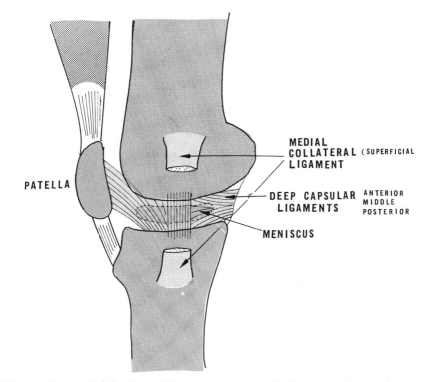

Figure 12–4. Medial collateral ligaments. The superficial medial collateral ligament attaches superiorly to the medial femoral condyle and attaches onto the tibia below the articular cartilage. The deep capsular ligament divides into anterior, middle, and posterior portions.

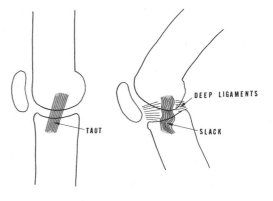

Figure 12–5. Collateral ligamentous tautness. The collateral ligaments are most taut on full knee extension (*left view*) and relax immediately on the knee flexion (*right view*). Deep ligaments do not undergo the same tautness and relaxation.

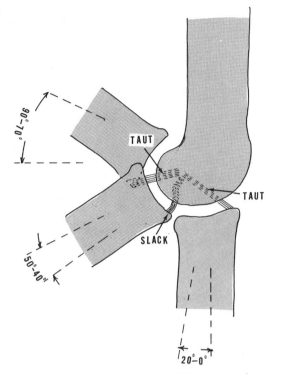

Figure 12-6. Ligamentous laxity and tautness of the cruciate ligaments during flexion-extension. The anterior cruciate ligament (ACL) is taut when the knee is fully extended and does not relax during the first 20° of flexion when it becomes slack until 70° to 90° of flexion. Rotation is permitted when the ACL is slack.

Beside giving mechanical support and restricting movement, the ligaments also supply proprioception to the joint. Proprioception of any joint, especially the knee, comes from the action of ligaments, capsule, muscle spindles, and the skin with the ligaments providing the predominant function. Proprioception depends on the age of the person[1] and the amount of amplitude and velocity of motion applied to the joint.[2] Impaired proprioception is a finding in degenerative joint disease and is considered causative.

The medial collateral ligaments are densely innervated with free-ending nerves and low-threshold mechanoreceptors, which have been considered to be activated as a protective ligamentomuscular reflex following injury. This thesis is now refuted, however, because these reflexes contribute to reflex coordination in *normal* movements. Such reflex actions are mediated through the gamma muscle spindles.[3] Increased tension in the collateral ligaments causes increased sensitivity in the muscle spindle afferents of the gastrocnemius soleus and semitendinosus muscles.

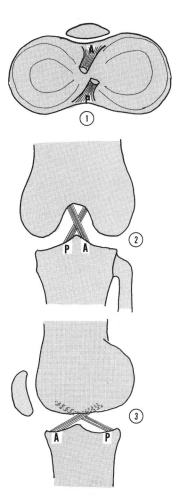

Figure 12–7. Cruciate ligaments. (1) Superior view of the tibial plateau showing the origins of the cruciate ligaments. A = anterior and P = posterior. (2) Anterior view of the cruciate ligaments. (3) Lateral view.

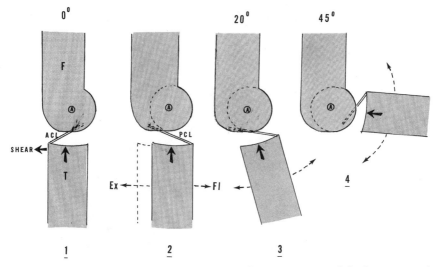

Figure 12–8. Effects of cruciate ligaments on flexion-extension of the knee. Normal flexion (Fl) of the knee is initially a posterior glide of the tibia (T) on the flat surface of the femoral (F) condyles *1* to *2*. The posterior cruciate ligament (PCL) stops further glide and becomes the fulcrum about which the tibia rotates about the axis (A) in *3* and *4*. In extension the final degrees of extension *2* to *1* is limited and shear is prevented by the anterior cruciate ligament (ACL).

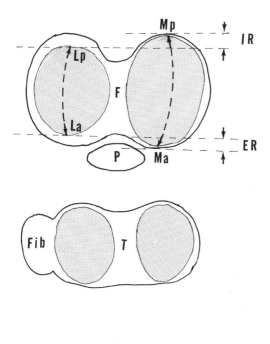

MaMp ⪢ LaLp

Figure 12–9. Basis of rotation of the tibia on the femoral condyles. The surface length of the femoral condyles are responsible for the rotation of the tibia on the femoral condyles in flexion and extension. The surface length of the medial condyle Ma to Mp is longer (ER and IR) than the surface length of the lateral condyles La to Lp in the upper drawing. In flexion and extension, the tibial articular condyles (*lower drawing*) glide on the femoral condyles and externally rotate during extension and internally rotate during flexion. The patella (P) depicts the anterior aspect of the drawings.

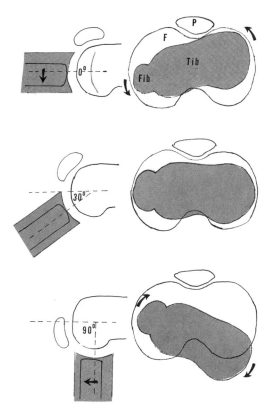

Figure 12–10. Rotational aspects of knee flexion-extension. Normally in full extension (*0°*) the tibia has rotated externally (*curved arrow*). In mid flexion (*30°*) the tibia is neutral. In flexion to 90° the tibia (*shaded area*) internally rotates (*curved arrow*).

The collateral ligaments are supplied by free-nerve, Ruffini, and Golgi endings. Ruffini endings have lower thresholds than the Golgi endings. Forces generated in other knee structures (capsule and cruciate ligament) are altered after rupture of the collateral ligament.[4] The proximal and distal ends of ligaments are most densely supplied with sensory endings with few receptors in the mid-portion of the ligaments.[5-8]

The medial collateral ligament (MCL) is the most commonly damaged ligament of the knee in sports-related injury (Figs. 12–13, 12–14, and 12–15). The proprioceptive action of the ligaments plays a major role in determining which type of treatment a torn ligament should receive for optimum ultimate functional recovery. Conservative (nonsurgical) treatment delivers good results in partial first and second degree tears.[9-11]

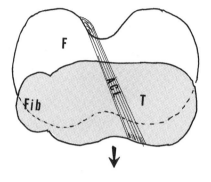

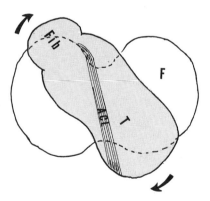

Figure 12–11. Cruciate ligament restriction of tibial rotation and anterior shear. The anterior cruciate ligament (ACL) originates from the anteriomedial aspect of the rim of the tibia (T) and inserts on the posteromedial aspect of the lateral femoral condyles of the femur (F). The upper drawing shows the anterior shear of the tibia being restricted by the ACL (*straight arrow*). The lower drawing shows how the ACL restricts external rotation (*curved arrows*) of the tibia on the femur. The fibula (Fib) reveals the lateral aspect of the knee.

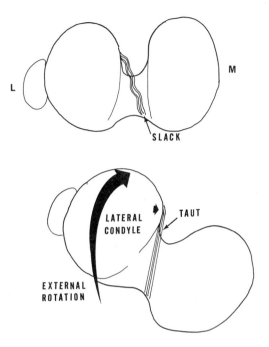

Figure 12–12. Cruciate ligamentous restriction of tibial rotation. Only the femoral condyles are shown with the cruciate ligament being reasonably slack with the knee in the neutral position. L = lateral and M = medial. With external rotation of the tibia on the femur, the cruciate ligament becomes taut and restricts further rotation.

MENISCI

The menisci are curved, wedged, fibrocartilagenous structures that lie between the femoral condyles and the tibial plateau. The medial meniscus is approximately 10 mm wide with its posterior horn portion wider than the anterior and middle portions. It forms a broader curve than the lateral meniscus which is rounder and O shaped. The outer margins of the menisci are thicker than the inner margins and taper toward the center.

The medial meniscus is attached around its entire periphery to the joint capsule and the medial collateral ligament (Fig. 12–13). Its anterior horn connects to the anterior intercondylar eminence, to the anterior cruciate ligament, and to the lateral meniscus through the ligamentum transversum.

The lateral meniscus is 12 to 13 mm wide with its anterior and posterior horns attaching directly to the intercondylar eminence, the posterior cruciate ligament, and the medial meniscus through the ligamentum transversum.

By its attachments, the medial meniscus moves directly with the tibia and femur during motion. It is therefore predisposed to mechanical injury. As the lateral meniscus rotates about its central attachment, it avoids mechanical entrapment.

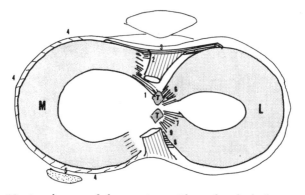

Figure 12–13. Attachment of the meniscus. The right tibial plateau viewed from above. (*1*) Fibrous attachment of medial meniscus (M) to tibial tubercle (T). (*2*) Connection to anterior cruciate ligament. (*3*) Transverse ligament, which connects to the anterior horn of the lateral meniscus (L). (*4*) Medial meniscus (M) is attached around the entire periphery to the capsule. (*5*) Attachment to semimembranous muscle tendon. (*6*) Lateral meniscus anterior horn. (*7*) Posterior horn attached to the eminentia intercondylaris (T) and attached to the posterior cruciate ligament (*8*). (*9*) A fibrous band attaches superiorly into the fossa intercondylaris at the femur.

The menisci have a unique blood supply (Fig. 12–14). Small blood vessels enter the periphery of the mensicus through a tortuous route and supply its outer third. They emanate from the middle genicular artery, a branch of the popliteal artery, which peripherally circumscribes the outer meniscus. The outer third of the meniscus has ample circulation, whereas the middle and inner thirds are avascular.

NERVE SUPPLY TO THE KNEE

The skin, synovial membrane, capsule, ligaments, muscles, and bursae are all supplied primarily by the femoral and obturator nerves with a smaller contribution from the sciatic nerve. The somatic nerve endings are myelinated and nonmyelinated and thus capable of carrying pain, as well as primary sensation and proprioception. Autonomic nerve supply innervates the blood vessels, hair follicles, and sweat glands, which are also capable of carrying nociceptive impulses as seen in reflex sympathetic dystrophy.

MUSCLES

The knee is stabilized and motored by extensors, flexors, adductors, and abductors with the extensors (i.e., quadriceps femoris muscles) being most prominent.

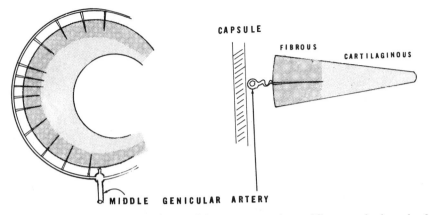

Figure 12–14. Intrinsic circulation of the meniscus. The middle genicular branch of the popliteal artery sends branches around the periphery of the meniscus under the capsule. Small tortuous nonanastomosing vessels enter the outer fibrous zone on the meniscus. Their tortuous state permits movement of the meniscus. The inner two thirds area of the meniscus is cartilaginous and avascular.

The quadriceps femoris is composed of four heads: rectus femoris, vastus medialis, vastus lateralis, and vastus intermedius. The rectus femoris muscle originates from the anterior iliac spine; the others come from the shaft of the femur. They all converge into a common tendon that attaches to the tibial tubercle. Within the patellar tendon is the patella itself, which provides mechanical leverage to the extensor mechanism. The quadriceps group is innervated by the femoral nerve, formed by the anterior divisions of L2, L3, and L4 roots. The extensor mechanism also has ligamentous attachments to the menisci, which permits them to move with the tibia during knee motions (Fig. 12–15).

The flexors of the knee are the posterior thigh muscles (Fig. 12–16). They originate from the ischial tuberosity. The semitendinosus muscle descends the medial aspect of the thigh and joins the sartorius and gracilis muscles to form a common tendon, the pes anserinus. This common tendon is joined by the semimembranosus, which divides into three tendinous inserts (Fig. 12–17), which move the medial meniscus and put tension on the joint capsule.

FUNCTIONAL ANATOMY

Knee function is multidimensional because flexion-extension occurs during rotation and glide initiated by muscular action and is thereby directed by the articular surfaces and the ligaments. The menisci participate in all such

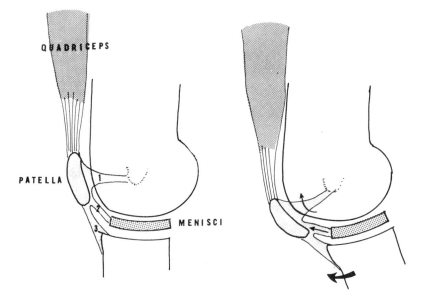

Figure 12–15. Quadriceps mechanism. The quadriceps muscle extends over the anterior knee joint through its tendon with three ligamentous extensions: (*1*) the epicondylopatellar portion, which attaches to the epicondyle eminence of the femur and guides rotation of the patella; (*2*) the meniscopatellar portion, which attaches to and pulls the meniscus forward during knee extension; and (*3*) the infrapatellar tendon, which attaches to the tibial tubercle and extends the knee on the femur.

movement. Injury can damage any of these structures and cause pain and dysfunction.

The knee flexes initially by having the tibia glide posteriorly on the femoral condyles. As the posterior cruciate becomes taut during this glide, the tibia begins gradual internal rotation about the axis described by the ligament. The menisci move with the tibia, always remaining within a controlled space between the plateaus of the femur and the tibia. The tibia is able to rotate because of relaxation of the collateral ligaments. The quadriceps, that is, the extensor mechanism, initially functions by supplying a decelerating force. Full flexion ends when the tibia's posterior edge has impinged on the femoral condyles and the cruciate and the collateral ligaments have again become taut.

Knee extension is possible when the quadriceps activates and the tibia glides forward on the femoral condyles in an external rotatory motion. During this extension, the posterior hamstring muscles act as decelerators.

This simplified analysis of knee function implies that all motions are part of a well-coordinated neuromuscular act when all tissues are physiologically intact.

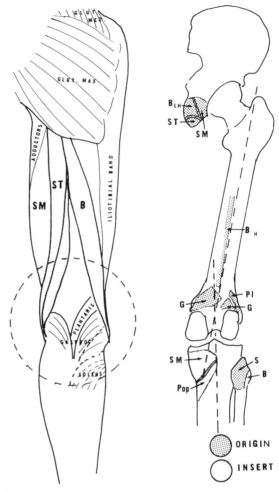

Figure 12–16. Posterior thigh muscles. The medial posterior thigh muscles are the semimembranous (SM), semitendinous (ST), and laterally, the biceps (B). All other posterior muscles are labeled. The right drawing indicates their origin (*dotted circle*) and their insertions (*clear circle*): Blh = biceps long head; Bsh = biceps short head; B = biceps; S = sartorius; Pl = plantaris; Pop = popliteal; G = gastrocnemius.

PATELLOFEMORAL ARTICULATION

The patella has a significant role in normal functional anatomy and is also a major source of pain and impairment. The patella is an ovoidal sesmoid bone located within the quadriceps tendon that enhances the extensor force of the quadriceps mechanism (Fig. 12–18).

The patella has a curved external surface and biplanar concave surfaces on its underside, which articulate with the femoral condyles. The facets of the patella are asymmetric with its lateral facet broader than its medial facet. A

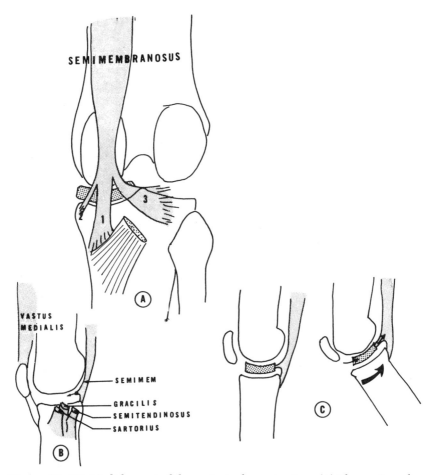

Figure 12–17. Medial aspect of the posterior knee structure. (A) The semimembranous muscle has three tendinous inserts. (1) The major insert that attaches to the posterior aspect of the tibia and sends fibers to the popliteus muscle. In its path, it has a branch that attaches to the posterior aspect of the medial meniscus. Branches 2 and 3 also attach to the tibia and attach to the capsule. (B) Indicates the insertional sites of the muscles. (C) The semimembranous muscle flexes the knee and simultaneously pulls the meniscus backward and causes it to rotate with the tibia.

third facet is termed the **odd facet** (Fig. 12–19). All facets are coated with cartilage.

The quadriceps muscle that inserts on the patella is also asymmetric in its action. The muscle has five bellies: rectus femoris, vastus lateralis, vastus medialis, vastus intermedius, and vastus medialis obliquus (Fig. 12–20).

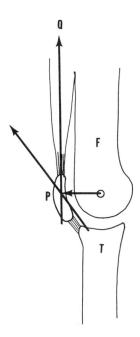

Figure 12–18. Parallelogram analysis of quadriceps mechanism. The pull of the quadriceps (Q) when it contracts (*vertical arrow*) elevates the patella (P), which attaches to the tibia (T) through an angled infrapatellar tendon (*oblique arrow*). Rotation about the axis (o) occurs at a distance (*horizontal arrow*) enhancing the force of the quadriceps. (From Cailliet, R: Knee Pain and Disability, ed 3. FA Davis, Philadelphia, 1992, p 144, with permission.)

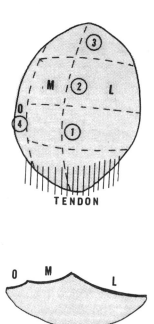

Figure 12–19. Facets of the patella. The cartilaginous surface of the patella has a broader lateral (L) surface than does the medial aspect (M). Each half (M and L) is further divided into three facets with the inferior facet attached to the inferior patellar tendon. The bottom drawing depicts the curving surfaces of the medial (M), lateral (L), and odd (O) facets viewed from above. (From Cailliet, R: Knee Pain and Disability, ed 3. FA Davis, Philadelphia, 1992, p 145, with permission.)

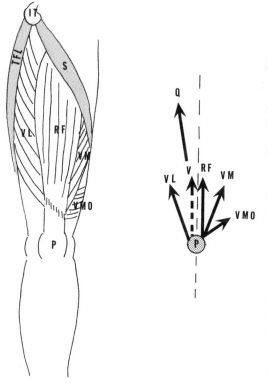

Figure 12–20. Quadriceps mechanism. The quadriceps mechanism comprises the rectus femorus (RF), vastus lateralis (VL), vastus intermedius (VI), vastus medialis (VM), and the vastus medialis obliquus (VMO). The vastus medialis obliquus does not essentially extend the lower leg but keeps the quadriceps in proper alignment (Q). All quadriceps muscles pull equally on the patella (P) to extend the knee or decelerate it. The vastus intermedius is shown in broken lines as it lies behind the rectus femoris. The ischial tuberosity is also shown (IS). The sartorius (S) and tensor fascia lata are not part of the quadriceps mechanism but are located in the anterior femur.

The origin-insertion of the quadriceps suggests an oblique action on the patella. This angulation is termed the **quadriceps angle** (Figs. 12–21 and 12–22). From this angulation, the patella tends to be moved laterally as well as superiorly, to cause greater stress on the lateral facets of the patella (Fig. 12–23). It is kept in reasonable alignment by the action of the vastus medialis obliquus muscle and the medial capsulomeniscal tissues (retinaculum) (Fig. 12–24).

CLINICAL EVALUATION OF KNEE PAIN AND DISABILITY

In eliciting a history of knee pain, the cause and mechanism of the injury and the results of the examination confirm the tissue involved. The history also elicits the nature of the external force or internal stress imposed by faulty neuromusculoskeletal mechanics (Fig. 12–25 and 12–26).

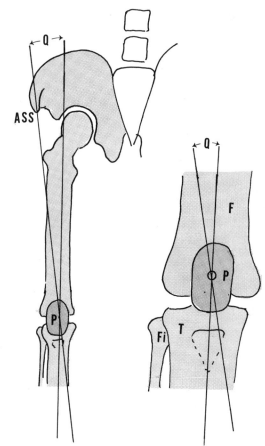

Figure 12–21. Quadriceps (Q) angle. A line drawn from the anterior superior spine (ASS) of the ilium to the tibial (T) tubercle (or from a midpoint of the patella [P]) forms an angle with a strictly vertical line. This angle is termed the "Q angle." Fi = fibula.

Most injured knee tissues involve the medial collateral ligament,[12] but the lateral collateral ligaments, cruciates, menisci, joint cartilage, and joint capsule may all be individually or collectively injured as well.

The initial injury may be only a simple sprain in which the ligamentous structure sustains a grade I or II injury with most collagen fibers remaining either intact or at worst stretched. The joint remains stable with little or no attendant effusion.

In a moderate sprain, some effusion is present (Fig. 12–27). Pain is elicited on actively stressing the joint in a valgus-varus motion. All signs of meniscus and collateral ligament injury must be proven to be negative.

Severe ligamentous injury implies tearing of ligamentous structures with

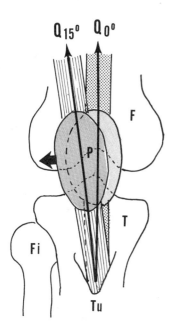

Figure 12–22. Q angle measured from the tubercle. The line from the anterior superior spine of the ilium (Q = 15°) to the tibial (T) and tubercle (Tu) is measured with the verticle line (Q = 0°). Fi = fibula, F = femur, and P = patella.

Figure 12–23. Effect of Q angle on the patella. (*1*) The Q angle (Q) is depicted. (*2*) The muscles that direct the quadriceps, vastus lateralis (VL), and vastus medialis (VM). (*3*) Due to lateral pull, the lateral patellar facet receives maximum compression and friction (*arrows*) on the lateral femoral condyle (L) as compared with the medial condyle (M).

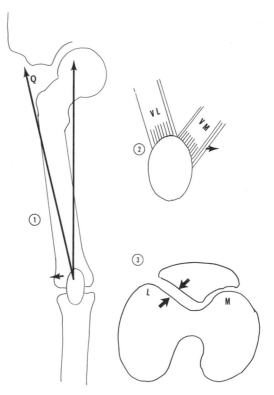

Figure 12–24. Anterior knee tissues guiding patellar motion. The patella has three facets on its inferior surface: lateral (L), medial (M), and odd (O). The vastus medialis (VLM) pulls the patella superiorly and laterally creating the Q angle (Qa) as measured with the quadriceps vertical pull (Q) through the suprapatellar tendon (SPT). The patella is attached to the tibial tubercle (Tu) through the inferior patellar tendon (IPT). The lateral retinaculum attaches to the lateral margin of the patella, which helps to stabilize its path. It contains proprioceptive and nocicpetive nerves. T = tibia and Fib = fibula.

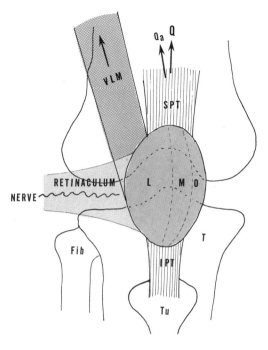

resulting instability and massive effusion. Aspiration of the effusion is indicated to rule out hemarthrosis which condition implies significant ligamentous injury and even possible bone involvement.

Collateral Ligament Injury

Examination for ligamentous injury is specific to determine the exact ligament injured and the extent of injury.

Medial Collateral Ligament

Although little pain is initially present, there is a feeling of *weakness*. Tenderness is present over the medial aspect of the knee (Fig. 12–28). The examination must be performed properly and accurately to be diagnostic. The knee must be slightly flexed and the quadriceps muscle totally

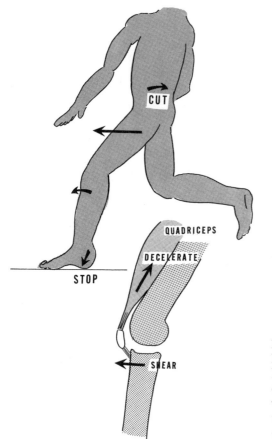

Figure 12–25. "Stop and cut" knee injury. A mechanism of knee injury is when the athlete comes to an abrupt stop with or without simultaneous rotation, thus placing severe shear stress on the ligaments.

relaxed. Active varus position of the knee must be arranged by the examiner to compare the injured knee with the opposite knee. Any pain elicited must be documented.

The treatment protocol of Indelicato[13] has been considered efficacious:

Phase 1: Knee is placed in a prefabricated orthosis that holds knee at 30° flexion. Isometric quadriceps exercises are done several times daily. Partial weight-bearing ambulation is permitted.

The mechanical healing behavior of tendons and ligaments is influenced by the component collagen fibers. Stress is a physical stimulus in the formation, alignment, and organization of collagen. Recovery is the return of a tendon to its original unruptured length.[13]

Between days 2 and 4, a clot forms in the wound with infiltration of connective tissue cells, including fibroblasts. Repair at this stage is very fragile.

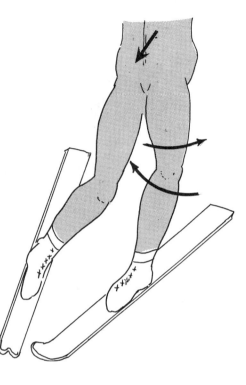

Figure 12–26. A mechanism of rotational knee injury. With the left leg fixed on the ground, sudden rotation of the body causes severe rotational stress on the knee ligaments: femur on the tibia.

Between days 5 and 21, fibroplasia increases with an associated increase in collagen fibers, which are highly active in the processes of synthesis and degradation. Motion permitted during this period has an impact on the remodeling of the collagen fibers.

Immobilization of several weeks duration is known to cause rapid atrophy and weakness of quadriceps function.[14]

Phase 2: After the second week, a hinge is inserted into the orthosis that permits motion only between 30° and 90°. Active isokinetic quadriceps exercises are instituted and full weight-bearing ambulation is allowed.

Phase 3: At the sixth week, the orthosis is completely removed and isokinetic exercises against resistance are begun.

Lateral Collateral Ligament Injuries

These injuries are less common but are potentially more ominous because they often indicate dislocation and have the potential to injure the peroneal nerve.

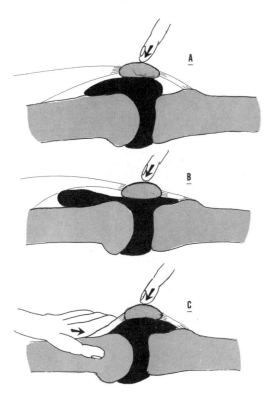

Figure 12–27. Ballottement test for effusion. (*A*) Fluid may not be visible and direct pressure on the patella causes no ballottement. (*B*) Direct pressure disperses the fluid superiorly and inferiorly. With a small amount of fluid a "negative" ballottement test may result. (*C*) Downward pressure on the suprapatellar tendon and direct pressure on the patella causes dispersal of the fluid laterally and medially: a positive ballottement test confirming the presence of fluid or blood and assisting aspiration.

In examination, excessive varus with a separation of 5 mm or more is considered diagnostic.

Cruciate Ligament Injuries

Injuries to the knee with involved cruciate ligament injury result in an unstable knee that often jeopardizes further athletic activities.

The purpose of the examination is to elicit instability of anterior-posterior shear action. With severe effusion present, the test is limited but once it has become possible, a positive *drawer sign* (Fig. 12–29) is diagnostic. With the knee flexed to approximately 30° to 45° and the foot fixed, anterior posterior translation of the tibia on the femur is performed and compared with the opposite side.

False negative tests have resulted from when hamstring spasm (Fig. 12–30) or a torn meniscus (Fig. 12–31) has occurred during the injury.

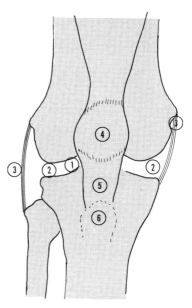

Figure 12–28. Tender sites of knee pathology. (1) The site of painful fat pads; (2) meniscal site of tenderness; (3) collateral ligament pain medial and lateral; (4) patellar pain and tenderness usually from pressure and quadriceps contraction; (5) infrapatellar bursal pain; (6) tibial tubercle pain.

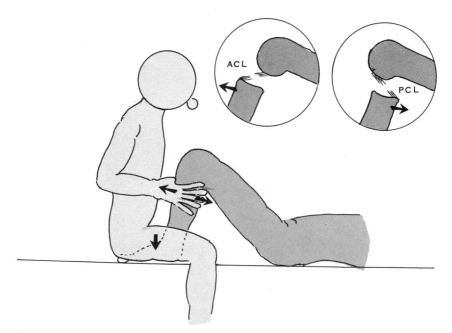

Figure 12–29. The drawer sign test. With the patient supine and the knee flexed to right angles, the examiner holds the foot down (*small vertical arrow*) and passively moves the lower leg forward and backwards on the femur (*small horizontal arrows*). Bringing the lower leg toward the examiner tests the anterior cruciate ligament (ACL). Pushing the leg away from the examiner tests the posterior cruciate ligament (PCL).

411

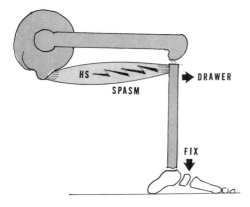

Figure 12–30. False negative drawer sign from hamstring spasm. Hamstring muscle spasm (HS) prevents translation of the tibia on the femur, which prevents motion thus creating a *negative* drawer sign, implying an intact cruciate ligament that may be damaged.

A more specific test for a torn anterior cruciate ligament (ACL) is the Lachman test.[15] This is performed (Fig. 12–32) with the patient supine on the table and the patient's leg next to the examiner. The knee is placed at 15° of flexion. The examiner stabilizes the thigh and applies firm upward force on the tibia (Fig. 12–33). Excessive motion is diagnostic and the possibility of a false negative test result is eliminated. Other tests for cruciate integrity include the

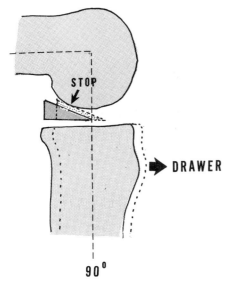

Figure 12–31. False negative drawer sign from a torn meniscus. A torn meniscus wedged between the femoral condyles and the tibial plateau may act as a wedge and prevent anterior translation of the tibia giving the idea that the anterior cruciate is intact when it may be torn.

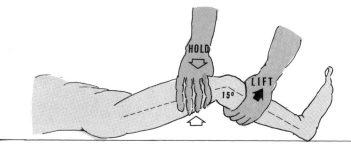

Figure 12–32. The Lachman tests. The knee is flexed approximately 15°. The thigh is held firmly and the lower leg is manually lifting the tibia. The distance is measured and compared with the other normal side, thus testing the anterior cruciate ligament.

reversed Lachman test (Fig. 12–34) and the rotatory instability test (Fig. 12–35).

Treatment of Anterior Cruciate Ligament and Collateral Ligament Injuries

Conservative nonsurgical treatment of ACL injuries remains favorable depending on the degree of tear. A complete tear determined during arthroscopic examination is best repaired surgically early on and before significant retraction of the ligament has transpired.

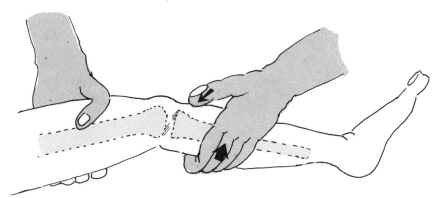

Figure 12–33. Position of the thumb in performing the Lachman test. The hand on the tibia is placed so that the thumb is on the tibial tubercle to measure the degree of translation more accurately.

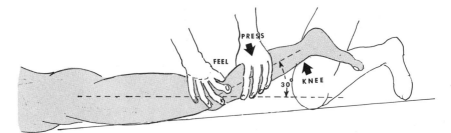

Figure 12–34. Reversed Lachman test. Performing a similar Lachman test has the patient prone and the lower leg flexed approximately 30°. The examiner's leg elevates and holds the lower leg in that position and the examiner's hand presses the lower leg downward stressing the anterior cruciate ligament. The examiner's other hand, placed in the popliteal space, determines the movement of the tibia.

The medial collateral ligament (MCL) is the ligament most commonly injured during sports-related activities.[12] A partial tear of the MCL, that is, a first or second degree sprain with little or no residual ligament laxity, derives excellent results from conservative treatment.[16,17] Whether a complete disruption of the MCL, for example, a third degree sprain, should be operated upon remains controversial, however.

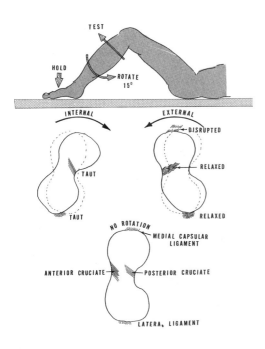

Figure 12–35. Rotatory instability test of the cruciate ligaments. With the examiner holding the patient's leg as in the drawer sign test (text) the examiner rotates the tibia internally and externally 15° testing the cruciate ligament while performing the drawer sign. With the tibia *internally* rotated, the posterior cruciate is taut. If *externally* rotated, the anterior cruciate is taut. Excessive motion indicates laxity or tear of a cruciate. The capsule and collateral ligaments also restrict motion.

The MCL of the knee are densely innervated with both mechanoreceptors and free-nerve endings. These receptors were previously assumed to initiate reflex periarticular muscle contraction intended to protect the knee from performing abnormal movement.[18-21] It has now been shown that these reflexes are too slow to prevent injury from inadvertent movements.[22-24] These ligament afferents are considered to contribute to reflex coordination in normal movements through the gamma muscle system rather than to initiate protective reflexes.[25,26]

A meaningful treatment program of injured collateral ligaments cannot be envisioned without recognizing the sensory (proprioceptive) role these ligaments play in regaining normal knee function.[27] Because ligamentous mechanoreceptors are known to signal within a limited traction force,[28-31] it is therefore crucial to re-establish the normal tension profile of the ligament.

The force generated in other knee structures (capsule and cruciate ligaments) are altered after rupture of a collateral ligament,[4] therefore failure to regain normality in one structure similarly plays detrimental havoc in all others.

An unsutured collateral ligament is likely to produce massive scar formation during healing, which many clinicians feel deters its functional properties. The proximal and distal ends of the cruciate ligaments are most densely innervated, with only a few receptors located in the midportions. These factors must all be taken into consideration when deciding which type of repair is most suitable—nonoperative, suture only, or full graft.

Decreased proprioception within a joint has been shown to predispose to ultimate osteoarthritic changes in a mobile joint. Objective measurement of proprioception remains primitive, instrumentations must still be developed to ascertain loss and the degree of hindrance of proprioception within a joint.[32]

Meniscus Injuries

Although the functions of the menisci remain conjectural, they apparently ensure congruity of the joint and thus increase stability. They also assist in lubrication of the joint between the femoral condyles and the tibial plateaus (Fig. 12–36).

The cartilage coating the medial tibial plateau is three times thicker than that of the lateral cartilage, making it more capable of absorbing impact. The diameter of the medial meniscus is larger than that of the lateral meniscus; its anterior horn is thinner and narrower than its posterior horn. The meniscus is divided into three distinct zones of collagen fibers (Fig. 12–37). The outer third is composed of circumferential fibers and is the only portion that has a

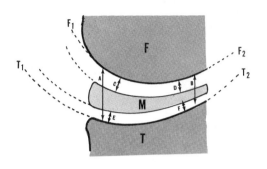

Figure 12–36. Hydrodynamic lubrication. The incongruous joint space between the femoral condyles F1-F2 in (F) and the tibial plateau T1-T2 in (T) is made more congruous by the insertion of the meniscus (M). The incongruous joint space are unequal at A and B. The space between the meniscus and femur is more equal at C and D and at E and F, which is the now congruous joint space.

blood supply. The inner two thirds contain fibers that run transverse and are divided by thickening layers termed the **middle perforating bundle** (MPB). The direction of these layer bundles are important in understanding how the meniscus is injured when torn.

The menisci move with the tibia on the femur in a well-coordinated manner. During aberrant movement, the menisci may be trapped between the opposing articular surfaces with injury resulting from torque, compression, or traction. Various knee activities have been suggested, but faulty femoral-tibial action is predominant (Figs. 12–38 and 12–39).

Clinical History and Findings. After injury is incurred, there is immediate, acute, severe pain, thereby stopping all activities, in which sense the mechanism differs from that of an acute ligamentous injury. Effusion is usual; hemarthrosis indicates more severe injury.[33]

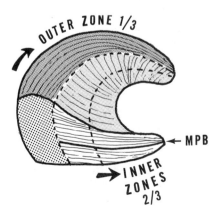

Figure 12–37. Microscopic structure of the meniscus. The meniscus is divided into three zones with the two inner zones having two layers. The collagen fibers forming the layers are circumferential in the outer zone and run radially in the inner two zones. The two inner layers are divided by a thin layer of fibers termed the middle perforating bundle (MPB).

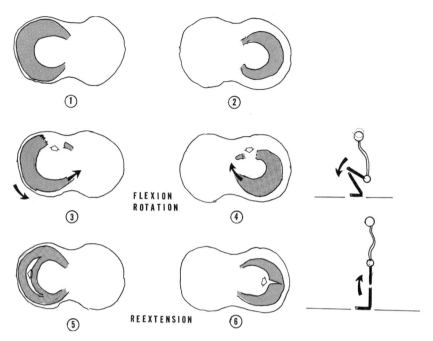

Figure 12–38. Mechanism of meniscus tears. (*1*) is the normal medial meniscus, (*2*) is the normal lateral meniscus, (*3*) is a tear (*white arrow*) of the anterior portion of the meniscus from internal rotation and flexion, (*4*) is an anterior lateral meniscus tear from flexion and external rotation, (*5*) is a "bucket handle" tear usually from reextension and derotation, and (*6*) is a radial tear. Rotation with flexion and extension must be in the unphysiologic rotation.

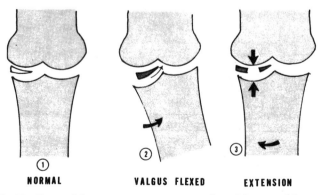

Figure 12–39. External force injuring meniscus. A forceful external force causing severe valgus may injure the meniscus on knee extension. (From Cailliet, R: Knee Pain and Disability, ed 3. FA Davis, Philadelphia, 1992, p 80, with permission.)

Tenderness is elicited along the entire medial meniscal line, whereas a tear of the lateral meniscus causes tenderness only above or below the joint line. Joint locking is rare until effusion increases, causing either gradual locking or significant limitation. Audible *clicking* may be noted. Shortly thereafter, atrophy may be seen in the quadriceps muscle. The concept that the vastus medialis obliquus atrophies first has been refuted.[17]

Numerous "meniscal signs" are propounded in which clicking, crepitation, limitation, and production of symptoms are elicited. All are based on mechanical changes in the contour of the meniscus from the tearing of its fibers as they move between the femoral condyles and tibial plateaus.

The type of tear can only be ascertained during surgery; whether open or arthroscopic, these procedures are illustrated in Figures 12–40, 12–41, and 12–42.

McMurray's Diagnostic Test. This is a time-honored test in which the patient is placed in a supine position with the hip and knee flexed at right angles. The examiner internally rotates the lower leg on the femur

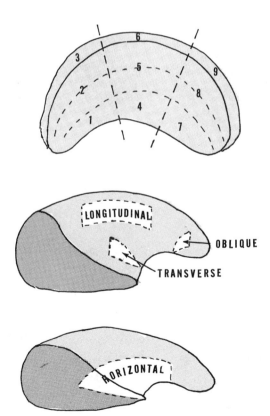

Figure 12–40. Primary meniscus tear patterns. The upper drawing depicts a method to specify the zone of the site of a lesion. The two lower drawings depict the type of tear that occurs in any of the specific zones and their designation.

Figure 12–41. Flap tears of the meniscus. Longitudinal or horizontal tears above the middle perforating bundle (MPB) may result in a superior flap or an inferior one. These tears may be identified using arthroscopy or magnetic resonance imaging.

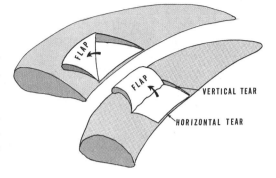

while slowly extending the leg (Fig. 12–43). Crepitation, pain, and limitation of action are considered *positive* for possible meniscus tear. If the lateral meniscus is suspected, the lower leg is externally rotated during the test.

Apley's Diagnostic Test. This test is similar to the McMurray's, but the patient is placed prone and the knee is flexed at a right angle (Fig. 12–44). The lower leg is rotated upon the femur with downward pressure and then traction. The knee is not extended during the test.

Many other tests, some involving standing as well as lying supine and prone exist, but they are all based on the same mechanism.

Confirmatory Tests. Arthroscopy and, more recently, magnetic resonance imaging (MRI) studies, have proven to be diagnostic. Although MRI studies are not invasive, during arthroscopic examination, any pathology found can be surgically addressed immediately.

Treatment Protocols. The healing process of a meniscus tear depends upon the site, type, and extent of the tear. Tears within the inner layers resulting from avascularity do not heal. Only when removal or modification of the torn fragment decreases friction on the articular cartilage will *recovery* be acceptable.

A locked knee resulting from a torn fragment must be reduced within 24 hours, because prolonged locking causes the meniscus to lose its elasticity and prevent its return to normal. Manipulation to unlock the knee has its advocates.[20,34]

The technique of manipulation is to apply longitudinal traction with simultaneous rotation in both directions and application of some valgus-varus force with the knee extended. If the medial meniscus is involved, extension of the knee with external rotational force is applied; internal rotational force is applied if the lateral meniscus is implicated.

Strengthening the quadriceps muscle group is initiated immediately using both isometric and progressively isokinetic exercises.[33]

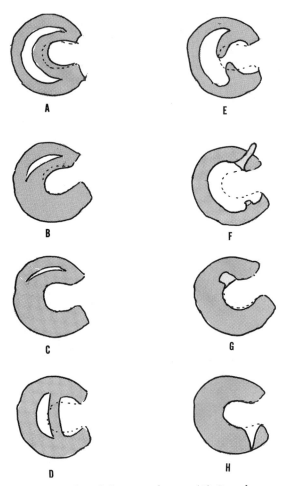

Figure 12–42. Varieties of medial meniscal tears. (*A*) Complete tear still attached. (*B*) Partial circumferential tear. (*C*) Partial tear remaining in situ and probably asymptomatic. (*D*) Partial tear encroaching into the joint (*bucket handle tear*). (*E*) Complete tear with detached fragments. (*F*) Complete tear with fragment forming a flap. (*G*) Torn flap with remainder of meniscus intact. (*H*) Vertical tear with retraction of the remaining meniscus.

Anterior Knee Pain

Pain and disability in the patellofemoral articulation is commonly known to be the most prevalent type of knee pain. It is considered that all people have sustained degeneration of the patellar cartilage by age 30. The term **chondromalacia patella** has been used indiscriminately for centuries as providing a meaningful diagnosis.

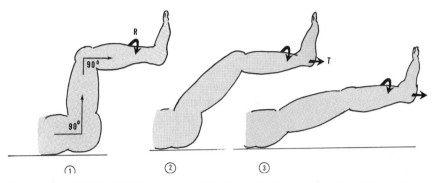

Figure 12–43. The McMurray test. With the patient supine and the hip and knee flexed at a right angle, the lower leg is internally rotated (to test the medial meniscus) and extended. To test the lateral meniscus the lower leg is externally rotated and extended. A *positive* test, indicating possible meniscus injury, elicits pain, crepitation, and limitation.

There are four stages of chondromalacia determined by the level of cartilage damage:

Stage I: Softening of the cartilage

Stage II: Blister formation

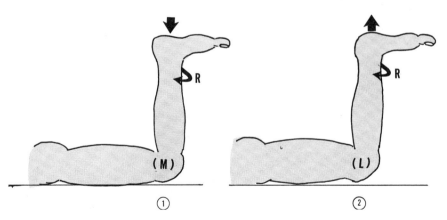

Figure 12–44. The Apley test. The Apley test is similar in method for testing meniscus tear but also is considered as a differential diagnosis of collateral ligamentous tear. (1) With prone patient's knee flexed at a right angle, pressure is placed on the foot (*small arrow*) and the lower leg is rotated (*curved arrow*) both internally (medial meniscus [M]) or externally (lateral meniscus [L]). (2) With patient in the same position, the leg is extended (*small arrow*) and the tibia rotated. This also tests the collateral ligaments.

Stage III: Ulceration

Stage IV: Crater formation and eburnation[35]

Usually trauma is the major cause of patellofemoral arthralgia. Such trauma takes the form of a sudden direct impact on the patella of a flexed knee. Repetitive minor trauma also commonly results from alterations from mechanical malalignment such as genu varum and valgum, patella alba, excessive Q angle, or tibial torsion.

Pain noted in the kneecap area is aggravated by activities requiring quadriceps action that increase patellar pressure during knee flexion-extension. Such actions include stair climbing and even more stair descending, deep knee bends, arising from a chair, and similar activities. Often the patient claims *stiffness* after prolonged sitting and feels the knee *giving way*. Crepitation is asserted by the patient; it usually can be elicited by the examiner.

Examination of a patient demands reproduction of the patient's patellofemoral pain. Significant normal movements of the patella on the femoral condyles such as lateral glide, tilt (Fig. 12–45), and sagittal motion exist. The latter (saggital) movement is performed by active contraction of the patient's knee while the pressure is applied directly to the patella; this test is diagnostic when the similar pain is elicited (Fig. 12–46) by the physician.

Radiologic examinations are usually not precise until marked degenerative articular change has occurred. Arthroscopic examination and MRIs are valuable, but the diagnosis is usually made by clinical means.

Treatment. Long periods of conservative treatment should precede a

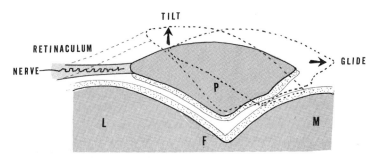

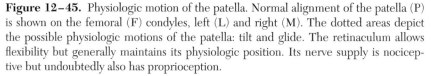

Figure 12–45. Physiologic motion of the patella. Normal alignment of the patella (P) is shown on the femoral (F) condyles, left (L) and right (M). The dotted areas depict the possible physiologic motions of the patella: tilt and glide. The retinaculum allows flexibility but generally maintains its physiologic position. Its nerve supply is nociceptive but undoubtedly also has proprioception.

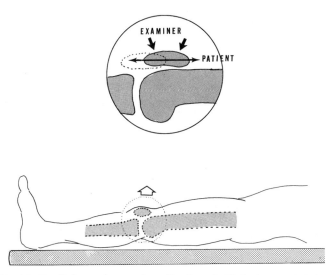

Figure 12–46. Patellofemoral pain clinically elicited. With the patient's leg extended and the quadriceps relaxed, the examiner presses down on the patella first in a downward, then an upward, direction. The patient's leg then slowly contracts and relaxes the quadriceps. Pain or crepitation is considered a *positive* test from articular pathology.

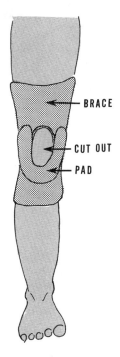

Figure 12–47. Arthrosis for patellofemoral pathology. A knee brace that prevents patellofemoral malalignment and abnormal *tracking* during contraction consists of an elastic-fitted webbing brace with a cutout over the patella and a pad around the inferior, medial, and lateral borders of the patella. This brace prevents the patella from migrating in non-physiologic directions during flexion and extension of the knee.

decision to resort to surgical intervention. Avoidance of pain-producing activities should be instituted, that is, stairs, deep knee bends, and squats, for example. Sports that aggravate or even initiate the pain should be curtailed. Arm-assisted arising from seated positions should begin.

With significant malalignment of the patella, an orthotic device to align the patella should be prescribed and implemented (Fig. 12–47). Isometric exercises for the quadriceps should be started. When acute pain occurs, the usual modalities of ice applications and oral nonsteroidal anti-inflammatory drugs provide symptomatic relief. Intra-articular injections of an analgesic and of an anti-inflammatory agent are effective in severe pain but are of more limited long-term value (Fig. 12–48).

Chronic pain occurs from degenerative arthritic changes or a neuroma within the retinaculum (Fig. 12–49), with the latter a possible consequence of

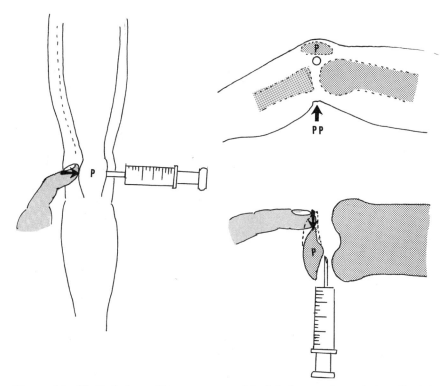

Figure 12–48. Technique of knee aspiration. The left drawing shows the patellas (P) being moved manually laterally to increase the injectible space between the patella and the femoral condyle. The right upper drawing shows the site of injection (o). Pressure on the popliteal space (PP) brings the intraarticular fluid toward the tip of the needle. The right lower drawing shows how manual movement of the patella increases the joint space.

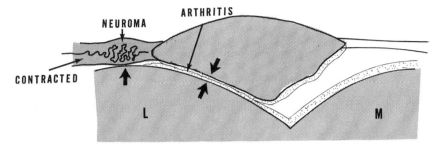

Figure 12–49. Degenerative arthritis and neuroma in patellofemoral disease. The predominant wearing of the patellofemoral cartilage occurs more frequently in the lateral (L) aspect (*small dark arrows*). A neuroma can occur in the contracted reticulum especially if surgical intervention has occurred to realign the patella.

surgical intervention. Details of the procedures are beyond the scope of this book, but include resurfacing the patella, resection of patellar plica, replacement with an orthosis, and even patellectomy. These surgical procedures are limited in their benefit but should be considered when severe disability persists and all more conservative measures have failed. An extensive lists of references is available.[36]

REFERENCES

1. Ferrell, WR, Crighton, A, and Sturroch, RD: Age-dependent changes in position sense in human proximal interphalangeal joints. NeuroReport 3:259–261, 1992.
2. Clark, FJ, Burgess, RC, and Chapin, JW: Proprioception with the proximal interphalangeal joint of the index finger. Brain 109:1195–1208, 1986.
3. Ekholm, J, Eklund, G, and Skoglund, S: On reflex effects from the knee joint of the cat. Acta Physiol Scand 50:167–174, 1960.
4. Shapiro, MS, Markoff, KL, Finerman, GAM, and Mitchell, PW: The effect of section of the medial collateral ligament on force generated in the anterior cruciate ligament. J Bone Joint Surg 73A:249–256, 1991.
5. Freeman, MAR and Wyke, B: The innervation of the knee joint. An anatomical and histological study in the cat. J Anat 101:505–532, 1967.
6. Andrew, BL: The sensory innervation of the medial ligament of the knee joint. J Physiol (Lond) 123:241–250, 1954.
7. Boyd, IA: The histological structure of the receptors in the knee joint of the cat correlated with their physiological response. J Physiol (Lond) 124:476–488, 1954.
8. Johansson, H: Role of knee ligaments in proprioception and regulation of muscle stiffness. J Electromyography Kinesiol 1:158–179, 1991.
9. Ballmer, PM and Jakob, RP: The non operative treatment of isolated complete tears of the medial collateral ligament of the knee. Arch Orthop Trauma Surg 107:273–276, 1988.

10. Bergfeld, J: First-, second- and third-degree sprains. Am J Sports Med 7:207–209, 1979.

11. Kannus, P: Knee flexor and extensor strength ratio with deficiency of the lateral collateral ligament. Arch Phys Med Rehabil 69:928–931, 1988.

12. Fetto, JF and Marshall, JL: Medial collateral ligament injuries of the knee: A rationale for treatment. Clin Orthop 132:206–218, 1978.

13. Indelicato, PA: Nonoperative management of complete tears of the medial collateral ligament. Pain Management 18:263, 1990.

14. Tillman, LJ and Cummings, GS: Biological mechanisms of connective tissue mutability. In Currier, DP and Nelson, RM (eds): Dynamics of Human Biological Tissues. FA Davis, Philadelphia, 1992, pp 1–44.

15. Arnoczky, SP, et al: Microvasculature of the cruciate ligaments and its response to injury: An experimental study in dogs. J Bone Joint Surg 61A:1221, 1979.

16. Gurtier, RA, Stine, R, and Torg, JS: Lachman test revisited. Contemporary Orthop 20:145, 1990.

17. DeHaven, KE: Diagnosis of acute knee injuries with hemarthrosis. Am J Sports Med 8:9, 1980.

18. Lieb, FJ and Perry, J: Quadriceps function: An anatomical and mechanical study using amputated limbs. J Bone Joint Surg 50A:1535, 1968.

19. Cyriax, J: Textbook of Orthopedic Medicine, vol 2: Treatment by Manipulation, Massage and Injection. Williams & Wilkins, Baltimore, 1971, p 366.

20. Petersen, I, Stener, B: Experimental evaluation of the hypothesis of ligamento-muscular protective reflexes. III. A study in man using the medial collateral ligament of the knee joint. Acta Physiol Scand 49(Suppl 166):51–61, 1959.

21. Johansson, H, Sjolander, P, and Sojka, P: Receptors in the knee joint ligaments and their role in the biomechanics of the joint. Crit Rev Biomed Eng 18:341–368, 1991.

22. Johansson, H, Sjolander, P, and Sojka, P: A sensory role for the cruciate ligaments. Clin Orthop 268:161–178, 1991.

23. Pope, MH, Johnson, RJ, Brown, DW, and Tighe, C: The role of the musculature in injuries to the medial collateral ligament. J Bone Joint Surg. 61(A):398–402, 1979.

24. Rack, PMH: Limitation of somatosensory feedback in posture and movement. In Brooks VB (ed): Handbook of Physiology. The Nervous System II. American Physiology Society, Bethesda, 1981, pp 229–256.

25. Stener, B and Petersen, I: Electromyographic investigation of reflex effects upon stretching the partially ruptured medial collateral ligament of the knee joint. Acta Chir Scand 124:396–415, 1962.

26. Johansson, H, Lorentzon, R, Sjolander, P, and Sojka, P: The anterior cruciate ligament. A sensory acting at the gamma-muscle-spindle system of muscle around the knee joint. Neuro Orthop 9:1–23, 1990.

27. Johnsson, H, Sjolander, P, Spjka, P, and Wadell, I: Reflex actions on the gamma-muscle-spindle systems of muscles acting at the knee joint elicited by stretch of the posterior cruciate ligament. Neuro Orthop 8:9–21, 1989.

28. Sjolander, P, Djupsjobacka, M, Johnsson, H, et al: Can receptors in the collateral ligaments contribute to knee joint stability and proprioception via effects on the fusiform-muscle-spindle system? Neuro Orthop 15:65–80, 1994.

29. Solomow, M, Baratta, R, Zhou, BH, et al: The synergistic action of the anterior cruciate ligament and thigh muscles in maintaining joint stability. Am J Sports Med 15:207–213, 1987.

30. Andrew, BL and Dodt, E: The deployment of sensory nerve endings at the knee joint of the cat. Acta Physiol Scand 28:287–296, 1953.

31. Skloglund, S: Anatomical and physiological studies of the knee joint innervation in the cat. Acta Physiol Scand 36(suppl 124):1–101, 1956.

32. Stener, B: Experimental evaluation of the hypothesis of ligamento-muscular protective reflexes. I. A method for adequate stimulation of tension receptors in the medial collateral liga-

ment of the knee joint of the cat and studies on the innervation of the ligament. Acta Physiol Scand 49(suppl 166):5–26, 1959.

33. Hall, MG, Ferrell, WR, Baxendale, RH, and Hamblen, DL: Knee joint proprioception: Threshold detection levels in healthy young subjects. Neuro Orthop 15:81–90, 1994.

34. DeHaven, KE: Diagnosis of acute knee injuries with hemarthrosis. Am J Sports Med 8:9, 1980.

35. Paterson, JK and Bunn, L: An Introduction to Medical Manipulation. MTP Press Limited, Boston, 1985, p 127.

36. Shahriaree, H: Chondromalacia. Cont Orthop 11:27–39, 1985.

37. Cailliet, R: Knee Pain and Disability, ed 3, FA Davis, Philadelphia, 1992, pp 176–178.

CHAPTER 13

Foot and Ankle Pain

THE FOOT

The injured foot represents a unique segment of human anatomy in that all its parts are directly accessible to visual examination, direct palpation, and mechanical evaluation. The patient states the history of onset, describes the pain and its relationship to motion, and directs the attention of the examiner to the precise site of injury.

The foot is composed of 26 articulating bones structured for weight bearing and ambulation. It is functionally divided into three units: anterior, middle, and posterior (Fig. 13–1).

The posterior segment lies directly under the tibia and literally supports the body. The talus articulates superiorly (Fig. 13–2) within the mortise formed by the tibia and the fibula (Fig. 13–3).

Viewed from above, the talus is wedge shaped with the anterior portion wider than the posterior. This is functionally significant because when the foot is dorsiflexed, the wider anterior portion wedges into the mortise allowing no lateral or rotational motion, hence creating stability. In plantarflexion, the narrower hind portion of the talus is in the mortise and allows significant lateral and rotational motion (Fig. 13–4).

THE ANKLE JOINT

The ankle joint depends on support from the medial and lateral collateral ligaments (Figs. 13–5, 13–6, and 13–7). The anterior talofibular ligament (ATFL) is the weakest and most often injured and has the greatest propensity for failure. The ATFL blends with the capsule, thus capsular tears occur fre-

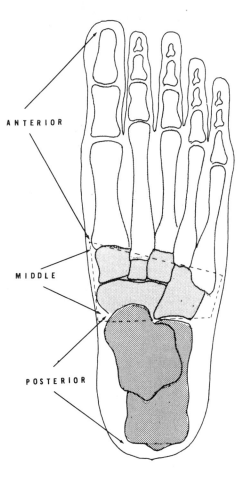

ANTERIOR

MIDDLE

POSTERIOR

Figure 13–1. The three functional units of the foot.

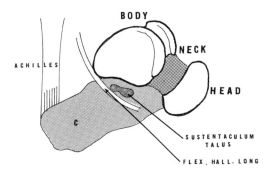

BODY

NECK

ACHILLES

HEAD

C

SUSTENTACULUM
TALUS

FLEX. HALL. LONG

Figure 13–2. The talus bone. Comprises a body, neck, and head. The body has two articulating surfaces that fit into the ankle mortise. The head articulates with bones of the middle segment. The entire talus sits on the calcaneus (C).

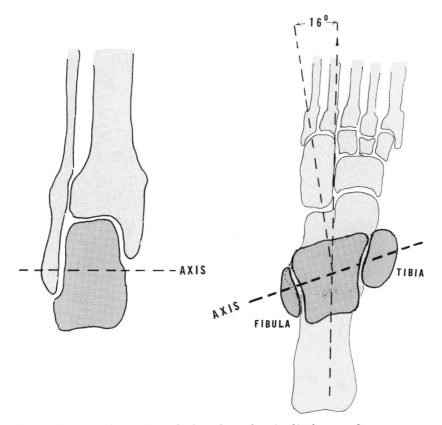

Figure 13–3. Ankle mortise and talus relationship. (*Left*) The axis of rotation passes through the fibula below the tip of the tibia. (*Right*) Viewed from above, the medial malleolus is anterior to the lateral fibula malleolus; and the axis of rotation forms a 16° toe-out stance. The talus is broader anteriorly than posteriorly.

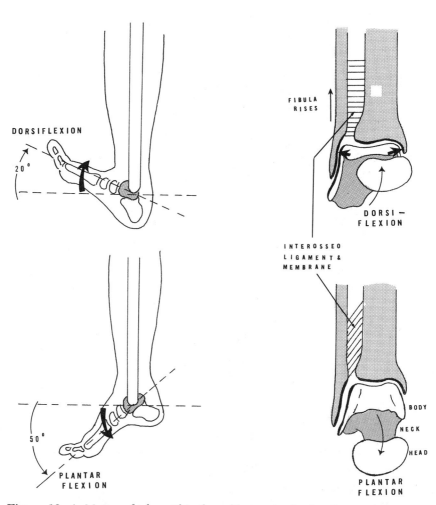

Figure 13–4. Motion of talus within the ankle mortise. In dorsiflexion, the anterior aspect of the talus, being wider, wedges into the mortise tightening the interosseous ligament. On plantar flexion, the narrower posterior portion of the talus allows the fibula to descend and relaxes the interosseous ligament. The mortise is also narrower and the talus less stable.

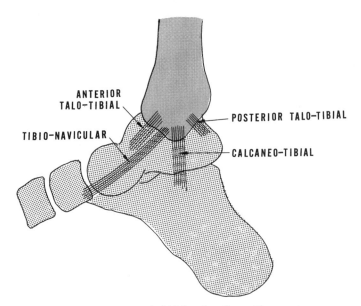

Figure 13–5. Medial (deltoid) collateral ligaments.

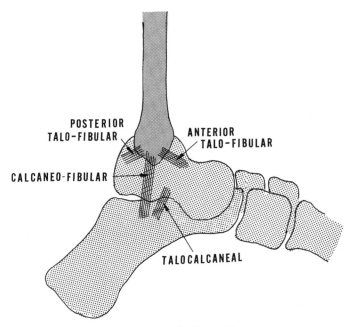

Figure 13–6. Lateral collateral ligaments.

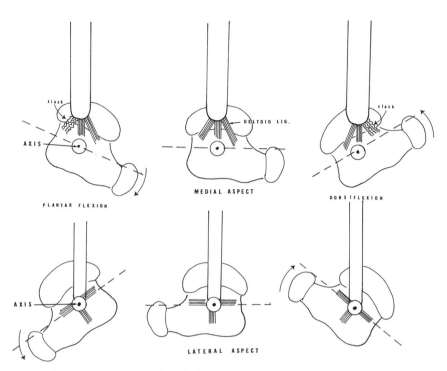

Figure 13–7. Relationship of medial and lateral collateral ligaments to axis of rotation of ankle. In medial aspect of the ankle, the axis of rotation is eccentric to the medial collateral ligaments and thus they vary in length during ankle motion as shown. Because the axis of rotation is central on the lateral side, the length of the ligaments does not vary.

quently with ligamentous injury. It normally tears in its midsubstance. The posterior talofibular ligament (PTFL) is $2\frac{1}{2}$ times stronger than the ATFL and thus is less often injured.

ANKLE INJURIES

Injury to the ankle is so prevalent that emphasis here is indicated. Mechanism of ligamentous injury is usually at the moment of impact of the foot to the ground when the foot is plantarflexed and supinated, which causes the greatest bony instability of the ankle. The ligaments absorb the major portion of the stress, because the peroneal muscles are unable to contract sufficiently rapidly to dampen the impact.[1]

Injury may vary from a simple strain, that is, mere elongation of the ligaments with microtrauma, to major injury with disruption of the ligamentous fibers with or without avulsion of the bone to which the ligaments are attached. The greatest traumatic injury is total dislocation of the ankle. Complete ligamentous tears occur in 75% of common ankle sprains associated with capsular tears.[2]

The severity of sprain frequently goes unrecognized that the statement of Watson-Jones[3] must be heeded "it is worse to sprain an ankle than to break it" implying that sprains are neglected or get inadequate treatment.

Ankle sprains have been classified:

Grade I: Partial interstitial tearing of ligaments

Grade II: More severe but incomplete tearing, with gross stability retained

Grade III: Gross instability of the ankle

Another classification has been proposed:

Grade I: Only lateral ligaments involved (Fig. 13–8)

Grade II: Both medial and lateral ligaments involved (Fig. 13–9)

Grade III: Both lateral and medial ligaments and the distal tibiofibular psuedoarticular (interosseous) ligament are involved

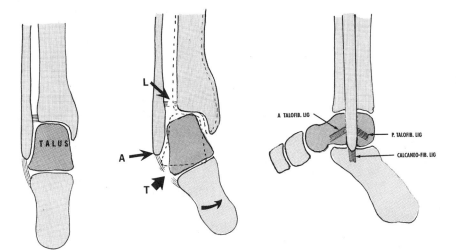

Figure 13–8. Lateral collateral ligament tear. The left drawing shows the normal ankle from anterior view and the right drawing shows the normal ankle from a lateral view. The middle drawing shows a severe inversion injury of the talus and calcaneus (*curved arrow*), which causes a talar tilt, a tearing the lateral collateral ligament (T), possible avulsion (A) of the fibular malleolus, and a possible tear of the interosseous ligament (L).

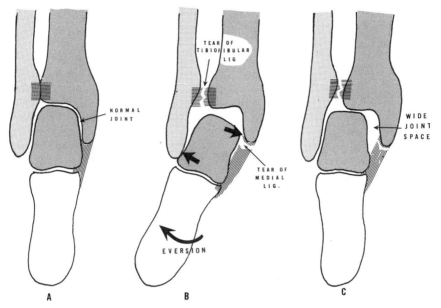

Figure 13–9. Medial collateral ligament tear. (A) The normal ankle and its ligaments. (B) A severe eversion injury (*curved arrow*) causing a talar tilt (*straight arrows*) and tears of the interosseous and medial ligaments. (C) The result of the injury is widening of the ankle mortise when the ligaments are torn.

Ligaments of the ankle are all amply supplied by sensory nerves, both nociceptive and proprioceptive. After injury, ankle instability is considered as being caused by neurologic damage to the ligaments and the capsule. This *deafferentation* can be treated successfully with tilting board exercises to restore proprioception.[4]

Damage to the lateral ankle ligaments is the most common sports injury.[5] It has also been considered the most common among cadets at West Point with a third sustaining ankle sprains within their 4 years.[6]

Injury Evaluation

Patients often describe the injury as a feeling of the ankle's *giving way* with the precise injury remaining unclear because it occurs so rapidly. Pain is usually present, along with swelling and ecchymosis. Such pain is increased with ankle inversion.

Diagnosis (of a lateral ligamentous injury) is made by (1) tenderness over the lateral ligaments; (2) pain asserted by inversion testing that is greater than inversion of the other ankle (Fig. 13–10); and (3) possibly a positive drawer sign (anterior stress test) (Fig. 13–11).

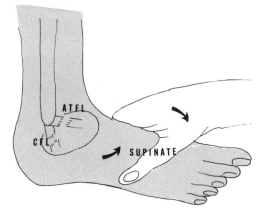

Figure 13–10. Inversion stress test of ankle. To test the integrity of the lateral collateral ligaments the inversion test supinates the foot (*curved arrows*), which causes excessive motion as compared with the normal foot. There is tenderness over the lateral malleolus where the ligaments—anterior talofibular ligament (ATFL) and the calcaneofibular ligament (CFL)—are located.

Finding of a 4 cm swelling about the lateral malleolus with tenderness indicates significant lateral ligamentous injury in 91% of patients.[7] Anterior drawer sign and inversion tests are often proven falsely negative if not done using general anesthesia.

Radiologic Evaluation

Clinical examination alone cannot rule out fractures about the ankle. Radiographs to measure stress and arthrography are confirmatory when clinical signs are present and disability exists.

Treatment—Acute Injury

Grades I and II ligamentous injuries usually do well with conservative treatment.

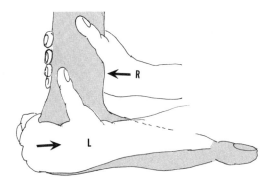

Figure 13–11. Saggital stress test of ankle: "drawer sign." Holding the lower leg with the right hand (R) the left hand (L) pulls the entire foot anteriorly. Excessive motion is a positive *drawer sign*, which indicates a tear of the anterior talofibular ligament when compared with the other normal side.

The first phase includes ice, elevation, and anklewrap, and crutches for first 24 hours. This is followed by compression stockings, cool whirlpool baths, and dorsiflexion–plantarflexion exercises. Gradual toe raises and inversion and eversion exercises against increasing resistance are next used.[6]

Acute treatment of grade III ankle sprain (complete ligamentous rupture) is more controversial. Young high performance athletes, workers who do heavy manual labor, and patients with avulsion fractures are considered good candidates for surgery.

Drez and colleagues[9] successfully treated patients with double ligamentous injuries with 5 to 6 weeks of short leg casting with the heel in slight eversion and a program, after removing the cast, of rehabilitation exercises of peroneal strengthening, heel cord stretching, and proprioceptive training (Figs. 13–12 and 13–13), but the majority of physicians favor surgical intervention in severe injuries in young active patients.

Rehabilitation[8] is considered to have three phases: (1) limitation of injury; (2) restoration of motion; and (3) regaining agility and endurance. Restoration of proprioception should be added to this program. The first is accomplished by intermittent pressure ankle splints and simultaneous ice packs. Peroneal muscle strengthening and heel cord stretching (Fig. 13–14) are beneficial.

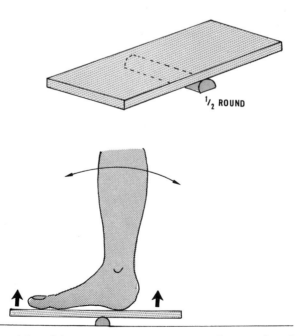

Figure 13–12. Tilt board for proprioceptive training. Standing on a board placed on a half-round, the person, by attempting balance, retrains proprioception.

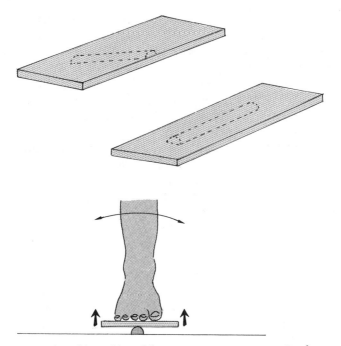

Figure 13–13. Tilt and lateral board for proprioceptive training. By changing the angle of the half-round under the board, added proprioceptive training is possible.

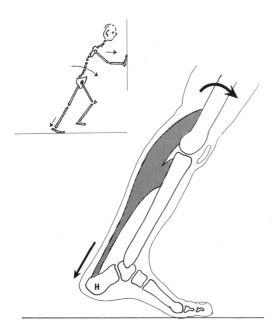

Figure 13–14. Heel cord stretching exercise. By leaning against a wall and maintaining the heel down, the gastrocnemius-soleus muscle gets stretched. Going up and down makes the exercise active as does bending the elbows. Starting farther from the wall increases the degree of stretch.

Initially partial weight bearing using crutches is permitted, gradually progressing to full weight bearing once heel-toe gait is possible. Step up exercises should be done first laterally, then with the patient facing the step as it moves up and down. For the athlete gentle jumping, hopping, then jogging are added.

Stress Fractures

With the current increase in avocational sports activities in reasonably under-conditioned people, there has been an increase in *overuse syndromes* and stress fractures. These appear in the fibula, tibia, calcaneus, and metatarsals.

Symptoms usually include *deep pain* and tenderness over the area of fracture, which recurs after resumption of the activity. Diagnosis is confirmed by early bone scan or radiographs done at a later date.

Treatment usually involves resting the part with local application of ice. A soft splint or an appropriate arthrosis in the shoe may be valuable.

SUBTALAR JOINT

The ankle joint has received substantial consideration in the literature because pathology in that area causes significant pain and disability. Scant concern has been shown for the talocalcaneal joint as related to the sprained ankle. It also causes impairment and so merits significant consideration.

The talocalcaneal joint has three facets with different planes of articulation; it is thus reasonably congruent and requiring little ligamentous support for the minimal motion permitted (Fig. 13–15).

A firm talocalcaneal ligament binds the two bones (Fig. 13–16), it runs the length of the tarsal tunnel, which is funnel shaped with the wider portion located slightly laterally and below the lateral malleolus (Fig. 13–17).

Chronic lateral instability of the ankle as a result of collateral ligament injury has received substantial attention, yet there has been little discussion of the relationship of subtalar instability.[10] In an ankle that remains unstable after repair and healing of the collateral ligaments, instability may recur because of talocalcaneal instability. This can be tested clinically and now may be verified radiologically. A method of holding the heel in a mechanical device and causing varus stress reveals a shift in the talocalcaneal joint by computed tomography.

The motion of this joint can be tested by dorsiflexing the foot, which stabilizes the talus within the ankle mortise. Manual passive motion of the calcaneous tests the mobility of the talocalcaneal joint.

Mechanism of subtalar ligamentous injury quickly becomes apparent.[11] In

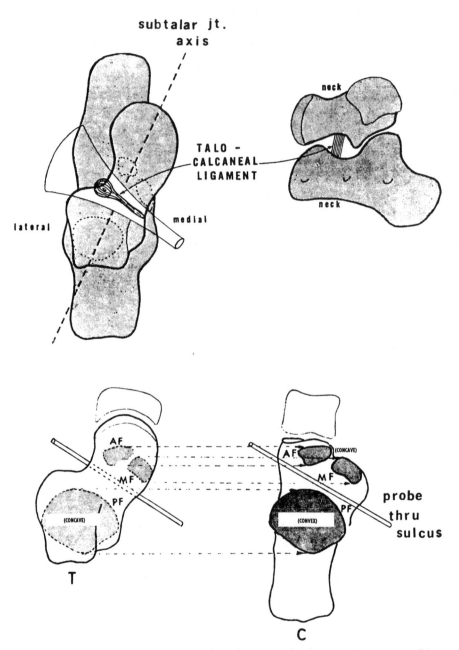

Figure 13–15. Talocalcaneal joint. The talus (T) and calcaneus (C) are joined by three facets: anterior (AF), middle (MF), and posterior (PF). The tarsal tunnel in its oblique course (sulcus) contains the talocalcaneal ligaments.

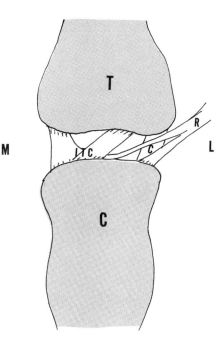

Figure 13–16. Ligamentous complex of the talocalcaneal joint. The talus (T) and calcaneus (C) form the talocalcaneal joint. It is connected by a capsule (not shown), the interosseous talocalcaneal ligament (ITC), cervical (c) ligament, and the retinaculum (R).

plantarflexion the anterior talofibular ligament is vulnerable to an inversion injury to the ankle, which, when severe, is followed by tearing of the talonavicular ligaments and the talonavicular capsule. The sustentaculum tali (see Fig. 13–2) becomes the fulcrum about which the foot moves (Fig. 13–18). The talus dislocates laterally whereas the calcaneus moves medially, thus tearing the lateral talocalcaneal ligament and capsule.

Rotation of the leg on the foot-ankle also predisposes injury to the talocalcaneal joint (Fig. 13–19). Severe injuries to the ankle joint may cause ligamentous disruption of the anterior talo-fibular ligament and the calcaneofibular, lateral talocalcaneal, cervical, and the interosseous talocalcaneal ligaments. Accurate diagnosis must be done with stress tomography, subtalar arthrograms, and fluoroscopy. After diagnosis, the treatment, whether surgical or conservative, must be determined.

THE PAINFUL FOOT

After discussing the ankle and subtalar pain and disability the remaining foot must be evaluated.

To be normal, the foot must conform with the following criteria:

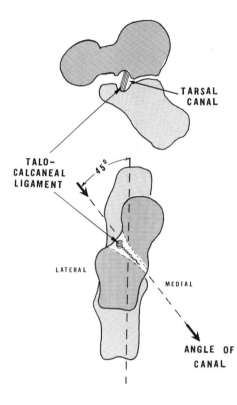

TARSAL CANAL

TALO-CALCANEAL LIGAMENT

45°

LATERAL

MEDIAL

ANGLE OF CANAL

Figure 13–17. The subtalar joint and tarsal canal. The talus and calcaneus form a canal, which forms a 45° angle with the anteroposterior axis of the foot. The lateral opening is under the lateral malleolus and is readily palpable. A firm ligament binds the two bones.

1. It must be pain free in its functions of weight bearing and ambulation.
2. It must have normal muscle function
3. The heel must be central and reasonably sagittal
4. The toes must have a straight alignment and be mobile
5. During gait and stance there must be three sites of weight bearing
6. There must be a normal nerve supply to the foot

Evaluation of the Painful Foot

Pain and difficulty in walking (kinetic) and standing (static) are the major complaints that patients present. The site of pain is usually directly indicated by the patient. The examiner must then anatomically and functionally evaluate the pain. The history indicates how the "injury" occurred, when the pain was initiated or aggravated, and how the pain will be relieved.

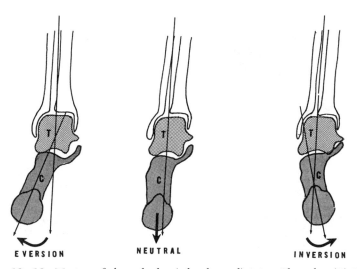

Figure 13–18. Motion of the subtalar (talocalcaneal) joint. The talus (T) is fixed within the ankle mortise and has no lateral motion. The calcaneus (C) has slight medial and lateral motion on the inferior surface of the talus. The degree of inversion and eversion is restricted by the talocalcaneal and collateral ligaments. Excessive inversion causes rotation about the sustentaculum shown in the left drawing.

Acute Foot Strain

Acute foot strain usually results from a specific activity, from excessive activity, or from persistence of activity to which the patient is unaccustomed. Pain and tenderness is usually either muscular, ligamentous, or periosteal, or all.

Rest of the part and avoidance of activities usually allows subsidence without recourse to medical attention. Local measures such as ice application, analgesic medications, and elevation usually afford relief.

Chronic Foot Pain

Chronic persistent pain and disability implies an anatomic deviation from normal, which denies normal function and thus restricts activity.

The static foot must be examined for structural deviations in bone, articular, muscular, and ligamentous structures. Stance and gait must be evaluated as well. Areas tender on palpation must lead to concept of an anatomic etiology (Fig. 13–20).

As an example the painful jogger's foot has several tissues that may be involved (Fig. 13–21).

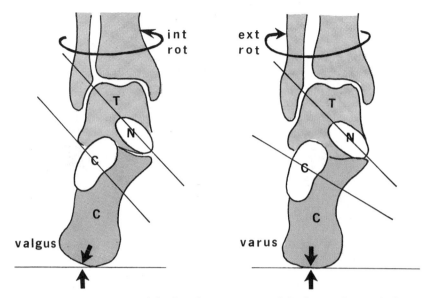

Figure 13–19. Supination of the foot during rotation of the leg. In the weight bearing stance, internal rotation causes valgus of the foot with *pronation* (*left drawing*). During weight bearing in the stance phase, external rotation (*right drawing*) causes the foot to rotate at the subtalar joint and thus *supinates* the foot for the ultimate swing-through phase. T = talus and C = calcaneus with their navicular (N) and cuboid (C) facets.

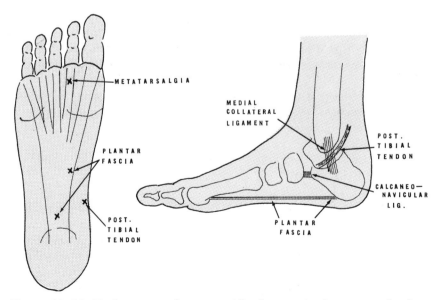

Figure 13–20. Tender areas in foot strain. All soft tissue that becomes tender from foot strain are pointed to by the patient and palpated by the examiner.

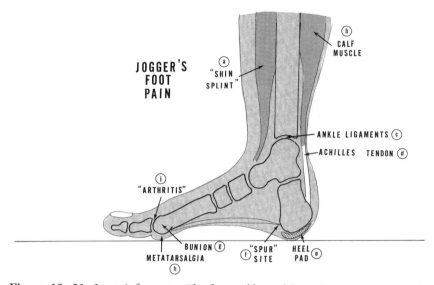

Figure 13–21. Jogger's foot pain. The foot, ankle, and lower leg pains sustained by joggers are listed. (*a*) "shin splints" (myositis of anterior tibialis muscle); (*b*) calf pain; (*c*) talotibial ligamentous strain; (*d*) Achilles tendon strain; (*e*) inflamed heel pad; (*f*) plantar fascia strain, which causes "spur-type" pain; (*g*) bunion pain if a hallux valgus exists; (*h*) metatarsalgia; and (*i*) arthralgia of the big toe's metatarsophalangeal joint.

The pronated foot is a frequent cause of foot strain because of its deviations from normal (Fig. 13–22). In these structural deviations, the foot is supported by muscular activity which becomes fatigued from excessive use or acute normal activity. In the pronated foot the heel everts causing the talus to slide medially. The forefoot abducts and broadens thus flattening and depressing the metatarsal arch. The three inner metatarsal heads become weight bearing (Fig. 13–23). The muscle most involved is the posterior tibialis, which is of the invertor type, in that, under stress it elongates, becomes tender, and is rendered functionally ineffective in weight bearing.

In prolonged pronation, lateral evertors shorten to take up the slack. Toe extensors change their alignment and become ankle-foot evertors. The talocalcaneal ligament, taut in supination, becomes inflamed and painful during stress. The longitudinal arch becomes flattened and stresses the plantar fascia with resulting heel and spur-type pain. The toes normally extended in weight bearing become flexed, thus resulting in *clawing*.

Each component of the effected painful foot must be evaluated in the course of a meaningful examination.

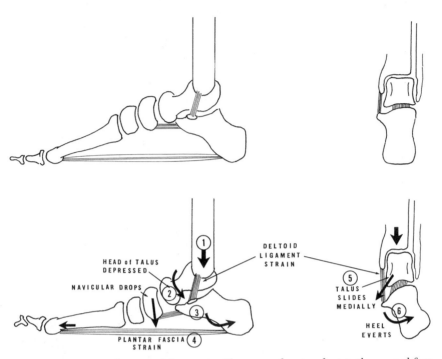

Figure 13–22. Mechanism of foot strain. The upper drawing depicts the normal foot with a central heel and a good longitudinal arch. In the lower drawing, weight bearing (*1*) on malaligned structures causes the talus (*2*) to slide forward and medially (*5*), and causes the calcaneus (*3*) to rotate posteriorly. The plantar fascia (*4*) elongates, which places strain at its calcaneal site of insertion. The resultant pronation causes the heel to evert (*6*), which strains on the medial (deltoid) ligament.

Heel Pain

Proceeding distally from the talocalcaneal joint is the heel, which is a frequent source of pain (Fig. 13–24), especially in athletes. The story is told[12] of a world class athlete training for the Olympics in the 1500m run who developed severe heel pain that prevented his running and defied every form of treatment: orthosis, shoe modifications, local therapies, medications, acupuncture, and hypnosis were tried without any success. Surgery followed, including fasciotomy and removal of the bony spur, which revealed that the spur was dorsal to the fascia and in the flexor brevis muscle. The nerve responsible for the pain proved to be the first branch of the lateral plantar nerve (Fig. 13–25). Only when the nerve was decompressed was the pain relieved.[13]

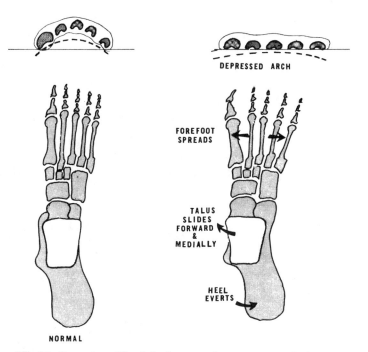

Figure 13–23. Pronation. The left drawing depicts a normal foot with a good metatarsal arch. The right drawing depicts a pronated foot, with the talus sliding forward and medially. This spreads the forefoot, which causes a depressed metatarsal arch.

There are other accepted causes of heel pain, many of which occur at the site where the plantar fascia and the intrinsic foot muscles attach to the medial calcaneal tuberosity. During gait there is repetitive traction stress of the plantar fascia on the periosteum of the os calcis (Fig. 13–26).

The plantar fascia is a multilayered fibrous aponeurosis originating from the medial calcaneal tuberosity and inserting into the plantar plates of the metatarsophalangeal joints, the flexor tendon sheaths, and the bases of the proximal phalanges of the digit. When the metatarsophalangeal joints are dorsiflexed (Fig. 13–27), a windlass-type tightening of the plantar fascia is present with traction on its insertions.

Over time microtears in the fascia and some tearing away of the plantar fascial attachment to the periosteum appear (Fig. 13–28). Fatigue fractures or periostitis may occur, which are viewed on bone scans and ultimately on radiographs.

Treatment is local before surgical intervention is undertaken. Because pronation of the foot causes excessive traction on the plantar fascia, it should

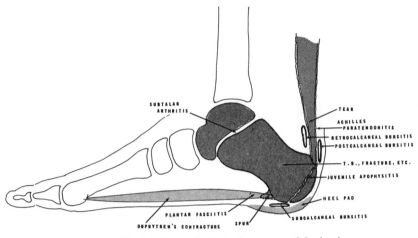

Figure 13–24. Sites of pain in the region of the heel.

be palliated by proper orthosis. Local injection of an analgesic agent, with or without steroids is effective (Fig. 13–29), whether fasciitis or entrapment of the nerve to the abductor digiti quinti. A hollow sponge pad inserted into the posterior portion of the shoe has provided some temporary benefit (Fig. 13–30).

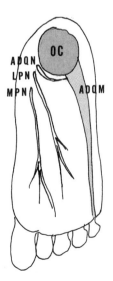

Figure 13–25. Nerve to the abductor digiti quinti muscle. The nerve (ADQN) to the abductor digiti quinti muscles (ADQM), which is the first branch of the lateral plantar nerve (LPN), also sensory innervates the os calcis (OC). The medial plantar nerve (MPN) innervates the medial aspect of the plantar surface of the foot.

Figure 13–26. Mechanism of plantar fascia on the longitudinal arch. (A) The large arrow depicts the body weight on the foot. The smaller arrow depict weight bearing on the heel (*left*) and the toes (*right*). (B) The arch is maintained by the articular structures with the plantar fascia merely reinforcing the strength of the arch.

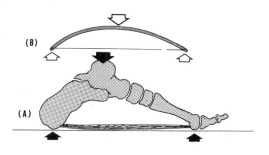

TRANSVERSE TARSAL JOINT

More distally and anteriorly to the talus are located the transverse tarsal joints: the talonavicular and the calcaneocuboid. These joints have the rounded head of the talus articulating with the concave joint of the navicular bone and the concave joint of the calcaneus articulating with the convex facet of the cuboid (Fig. 13–31). The former permits pronation and supination of the forefoot and the latter abduction and adduction of the forefoot. In supination, all joints are close packed and then loosened in pronation, which requires minimal ligamentous support.

Figure 13–27. Effects of toe motion on the plantar fascia. The lower drawing depicts the longitudinal arch, which flattens (*shaded area*) on weight bearing. The upper figure shows (A) toe extension (*curved arrow*), which places tension on the plantar fascia (B) and rotates the calcaneus (C). The longitudinal arch should enlarge (D) but superincumbent weight denies this elevation and instead strains the fascia.

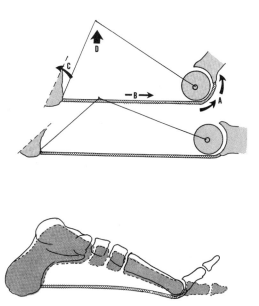

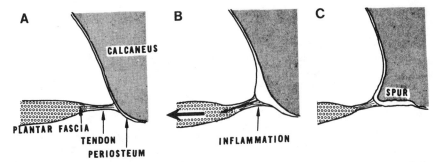

Figure 13–28. Mechanism of plantar fasciitis. (*A*) is the normal relationship of the plantar fascia with its tendon attaching to the calcaneal periosteum. (*B*) depicts traction (*arrow*) pulling the periosteum from the calcaneus. (*C*) Subperiosteal invasion of inflammatory tissue becomes ossified, thus forming a spur.

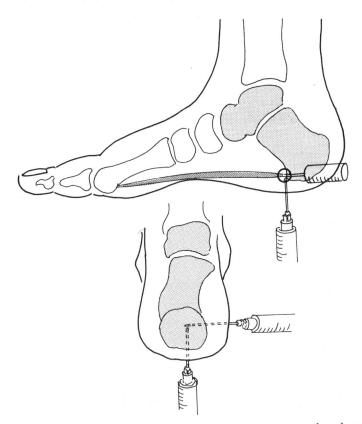

Figure 13–29. Technique of plantar fascial injection. Injection can be administered directly into the site of maximum tenderness through the heel pad. Injection can also be administered laterally but with less predictable results.

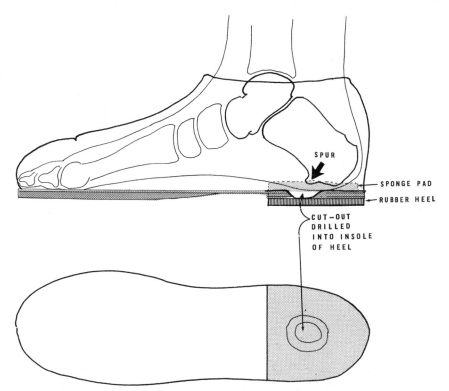

Figure 13–30. Shoe modification for the plantar fascial heel spur. A sponge pad inserted into the heel of the shoe decreases the pressure on the calcaneous. A cut out can be made into the insole of the heel of the shoe.

There are four arches of the foot: tarsal, metatarsal, metatarsal head (Fig. 13–32), and longitudinal (Fig. 13–33). The first two arches are fixed by their congruent joints; the metatarsal and longitudinal are more flexible.

Pain and impairment from the two posterior arches occur only with excessive ligamentous laxity of the arches, because they are ordinarily congruous and support themselves by their osseoarticular configuration. A connective tissue disease, for example, rheumatoid arthritis, can cause painful subluxation. Metatarsal arch deviation is a more frequent cause of metatarsalgia.[14]

In normal gait the foot supinates at the heel strike and remains so during the swing phase. It pronates during the stance phase (Fig. 13–34). Excessive pronation can require excessive weight bearing by the metatarsal heads and so cause metatarsalgia.

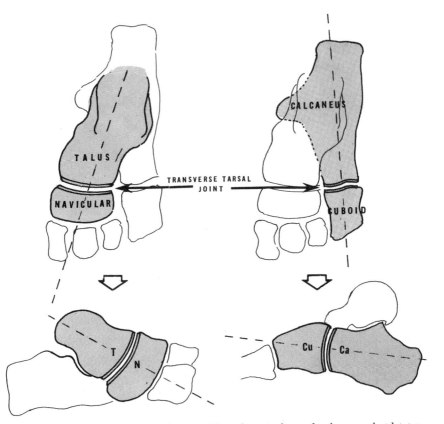

Figure 13–31. Transverse tarsal joints. The talonavicular and calcaneocuboid joints combine to form the transverse tarsal joint. The dashed lines depict the axis of rotation of each joint. These lines are parallel in a pronated foot and divergent in the supinated foot.

Metatarsalgia

Metatarsalgia is a well recognized but loosely defined entity in which pain is noted in the metatarsal heads.[15] When pain is noted in the four lateral metatarsals, it is termed **metatarsalgia**, whereas when noted in the metatarsoproximal phalanx of the big toe, it is termed **bunion, sesmoid disease**, or **localized arthritis**.

Metatarsalgia is associated with pain and tenderness of the plantar heads of the metatarsals. In normal gait, supination ensures an arching of the metatarsals, which causes weight to be borne by the base of the first (big) toe and the fifth metatarsal head. In a flattened transverse arch, excessive and abnormal weight is borne by the second, third, and fourth metatarsal heads,

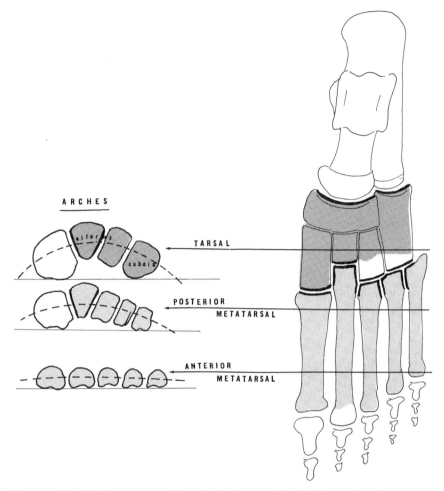

Figure 13–32. Transverse arches. *Left*, depicts the fixed tarsal and posterior metatarsal arches and the flexible anterior metatarsal arch. *Right*, depicts the receded second cuneiform, which creates a mortise for the seating of the base of the second metatarsal.

which are too poorly endowed with padding anatomically to minimize bone periosteal pressure (Fig. 13–35).

Pain and callus formation under the middle metatarsal heads result from altered biomechanics of weight bearing. Altered gait from a bunion, severely pronated feet that cause hammertoe, or clawed phalanges can cause metatarsalgia.

Examination uses manual pressure on the metatarsal heads to elicit tenderness similar to that noted by the patient. Care must be taken that the exam-

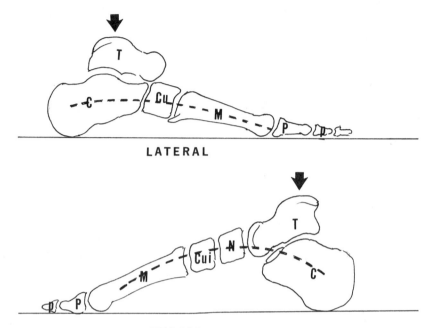

Figure 13–33. Longitudinal arch. The longitudinal arch is formed by contiguity of the talus (T) with the calcaneus (C) and anteriorly with the navicular bone (N). Medially viewed, the navicular bone articulates with the cuneiform bones (CU), thus with the metatarsals (M) and the phalanges (P). The plantar fascia is not shown.

ining pressure is not placed *between* the metatarsal heads where a condition of interdigital neuritis may exist, mimicking metatarsalgia.

Treatment is avoidance of weight bearing and correction of the flattened metatarsal arch. The calluses may be softened with warm water then abraded by scraping with a pumice stone. If severe, the callus may need to be surgically pared by a physician.

An orthotic shoe insert may be custom made to elevate the metatarsal arch and to supinate the foot with a cut out at the site of metatarsal callus.

Morton's Syndrome

This is not Morton's neuroma, but rather a metatarsalgia of the second metatarsal head (Fig. 13–36), which becomes weight bearing because the first metatarsal bone is too short. Examination reveals tenderness over the second metatarsal head and the diagnosis is verified by radiographic studies.

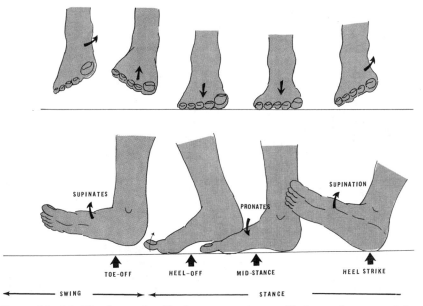

Figure 13–34. The foot and ankle during gait. At toe off, during the onset of the swing gait, the foot dorsiflexes and supinates. At heel strike, the foot is supinated and during stance phase, the foot becomes weight bearing and pronates with the forefoot slightly flattened.

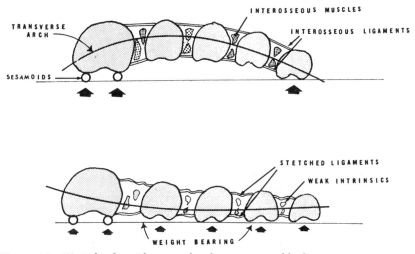

Figure 13–35. Splay foot. The normal arch is maintained by ligaments containing interosseous muscles within the compartments. As the arch depresses, weight bearing now is on the second, third, and fourth metatarsal heads, which causes metatarsalgia.

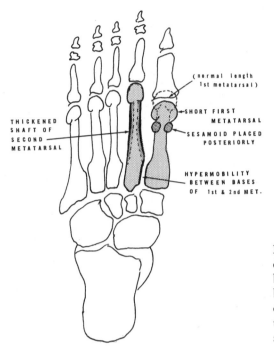

(normal length
1st metatarsal)

SHORT FIRST
METATARSAL

SESAMOID PLACED
POSTERIORLY

THICKENED
SHAFT OF
SECOND
METATARSAL

HYPERMOBILITY
BETWEEN BASES
OF 1st & 2nd MET.

Figure 13–36. Morton's syndrome. A short first metatarsal bone causes excessive weight bearing on the head of the second metatarsal, which thickens the shaft. Hypermobility of the second metatarsal may occur.

Treatment consists of placing an appropriate orthosis under the first metatarsal bone to relieve weight bearing pressure on the second metatarsal head. The pronated foot, if this condition is present, should also be addressed.

Interdigital Neuritis

An interdigital neuritis is frequently termed **Morton's neuroma** (Fig. 13–37). Because it is a fusiform swelling of a digital nerve, the term **neuroma** is used. It most commonly occurs between the third and fourth digits, but may also occur between the second and third. The neuroma appears between the metatarsal heads (Fig. 13–38), where the interdigital nerves are divided into two branches that supply sensation to the two digits.

The condition may arise from entrapment of the interdigital nerves as they pass under the transverse metatarsal ligament, perhaps due to pressure exterted by weight bearing and hyperextension of the toes (Fig. 13–39).

The condition occurs most frequently in middle aged women who may have worn constricting shoes with high heels for many years, but is also noted in other less characteristic situations.

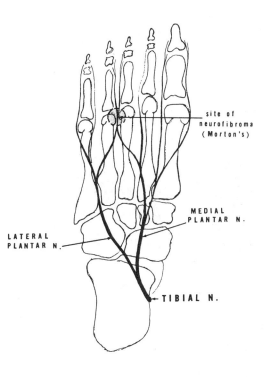

Figure 13–37. Morton's neuroma. A neurofibroma of the interdigital nerve. Its most frequent site is the third branch of the medial plantar nerve as it merges with a branch of the lateral plantar nerve to form a digital nerve between the third and fourth metatarsal heads. Pain occurs at the site, and there may be hypalgesia in the opposing areas of the foot.

site of
neurofibroma
(Morton's)

MEDIAL
PLANTAR N.

LATERAL
PLANTAR N.

TIBIAL N.

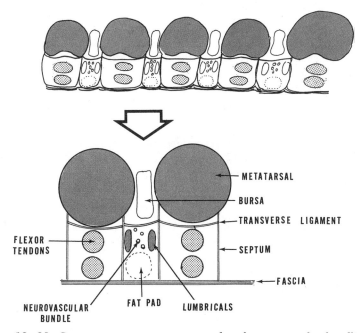

METATARSAL

BURSA

TRANSVERSE LIGAMENT

FLEXOR
TENDONS

SEPTUM

FASCIA

NEUROVASCULAR
BUNDLE

FAT PAD

LUMBRICALS

Figure 13–38. Compartments containing interdigital neurovascular bundles. The contents of the interdigital compartments are depicted.

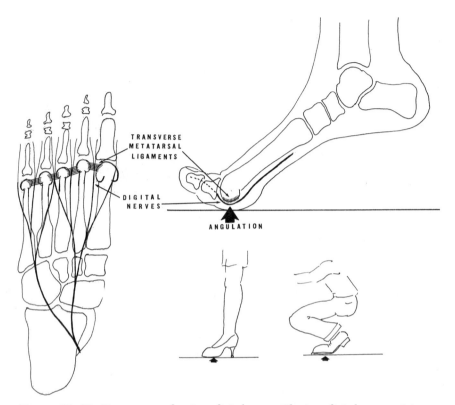

Figure 13–39. Entrapment of an interdigital nerve. The interdigital nerve originates from the plantar nerves in the sole of the foot and passes between the transverse metatarsal ligaments to supply sensation to the toes. If they become angulated at the ligaments by abnormal posture or activities, it can cause pain and numbness in the toes.

The approximating must reproduce pain from pressure *between* the metatarsal heads. Manually manipulating the metatarsal bones may evince the pain. Hypalgesia may be noted from a careful sensory examination of the skin between the involved toes.

Local injection of an analgesic agent is often both diagnostic and therapeutic. Treatment indicates the wearing of a shoe with a broad forefoot and full therapy to correct improper foot stance and gait.

March Fracture

March fracture (Fig. 13–40) is a stress fracture of a metatarsal shaft, initially so named because it was frequently noted after prolonged military marches. Pain and tenderness are evident over the suspected fracture site. Be-

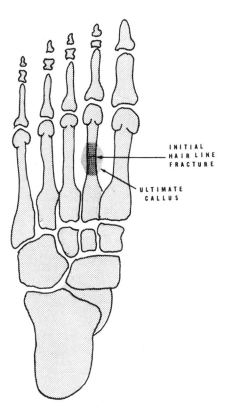

INITIAL
HAIR LINE
FRACTURE

ULTIMATE
CALLUS

Figure 13–40. March fracture. The initial fracture is often not observed in routine radiologic studies because they are hairline fractures. After 3 weeks of persistent pain, swelling, and local tenderness a callus forms that is evident radiologically.

cause it is a hairline fracture, initially it can only be confirmed by a bone scan because it does not become evident by radiography until a callus has formed around the fracture.

Treatment consists of avoiding weight bearing until symptoms subside. When pain is severe, a walking cast is indicated.

Hallux Valgus

Of the metatarsalgias, arthritic changes of the metatarsophalangeal joint of the big toe is a frequent, painful, and disabling condition, which includes bunion.

Hallux valgus is complex. There is lateral angulation of the proximal phalanx upon a medial (varus) condition of the first metatarsal bone (Fig. 13–41). Enlargement of the medial portion of the head of the first metatarsal bone ex-

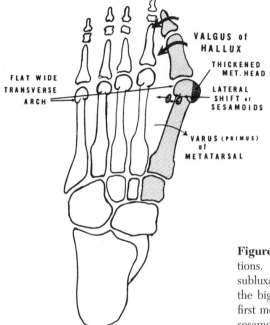

VALGUS of
HALLUX

THICKENED
MET. HEAD

FLAT WIDE
TRANSVERSE
ARCH

LATERAL
SHIFT of
SESAMOIDS

VARUS (PRIMUS)
of
METATARSAL

Figure 13–41. Hallux valgus conditions. Hallux valgus is essentially a subluxation of the two phalanges of the big toe in a valgus direction on a first metatarsal, which is in varus. The sesamoid bones migrate laterally.

ists, usually with concurrent inflammation of the overlying bursa at that joint. The second toe becomes encroached upon and overlies the third toe, deforming it with possible dorsal callus. The entire forefoot is widened.

Many concepts exist to explain the etiology of hallux valgus. Congenital factors predispose to later development of the syndrome. Varus or shortening of the first metatarsal bone is prevalent, as is obliquity of angle of the first cuneiform bone. Primary or secondary muscle imbalance may pull the first phalanx laterally and overcome an ineffectual abductor hallucis (Fig. 13–42).

Examination reveals the following findings:

enlarged forefoot (splayed)

thickened medial aspect of the first metatarsal phalangeal joint

palpable callus or thickened bursa

lateral deviation of the distal phalanx

crepitation on movement of the proximal metatarsophalangeal joint

Treatment depends on whether the complaint is typified by pain or merely cosmetic concerns. The need for a custom designed shoe with wide forefoot and narrow heel is expensive, yet effective. A cut-out of the shoe over

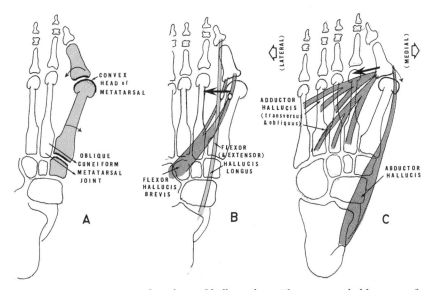

Figure 13–42. Concepts of etiology of hallux valgus. The most probable causes for hallux valgus are: (*A*) Excessive convexity of the head of the first metatarsal permits the phalanx to sublux laterally. There is also an oblique articular surface of the cuneiform, which causes the metatarsal to deviate in a varus direction. (*B*) As the phalanx deviates laterally, the flexor hallucis brevis and longus tendon on the plantar foot's surface and the extensor hallucis longus on the dorsal surface migrate laterally and act as a bow-string force. (*C*) Imbalance of the foot intrinsics have the adductors overpull and shorten. The imbalance overpowers the abductors, which elongate.

the bunion is effective, but cosmetically unacceptable to many people. Surgical remedies are numerous, but only and equivocally successful. These techniques are beyond the scope of this book.

Hallux Rigidus

The condition of hallux rigidus is manifested where the cartilage of the first metatarsoproximal phalanx is eroded or absent. The degenerative arthritic condition has many causes but it is the final clinical condition presented to the examiner.

In normal gait, as the toe extends at every step from midstance phase to heel off, a rigid big toe causes pain and impairment (Fig. 13–43). Examination reveals limited passive motion, if any, of the big toe at the proximal phalangeal metatarsal joint. Radiographs are diagnostic.

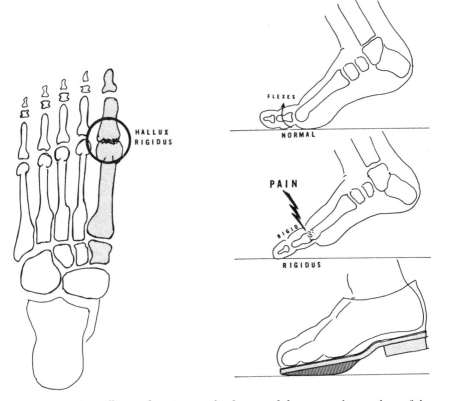

Figure 13–43. Hallux rigidus. As a result of repeated damage to the cartilage of the metatarsophalangeal joint of the big toe from numerous causes, the toe loses its ability to flex during gait and local pain results. A form of treatment is recommended in which a steel shank is placed in the sole, which prevents the shoe from flexing, and a rocker sole is applied.

Treatment requires wearing a rocker bottom shoe (see Fig. 13–43, bottom right). A steel shank in such a shoe prevents flexion of the sole during walking. Surgical intervention requires resection of the joint with application of an insert arthosis.

Hammertoe

The toes (phalanges) move in one plane: flexion extension (Fig. 13–44). The foot is mobilized by extrinsic muscles that originate from the lower leg and some intrinsic muscles originating from within the foot. The former include the gastrocnemius-soleus that causes plantarflexion, the peronei that

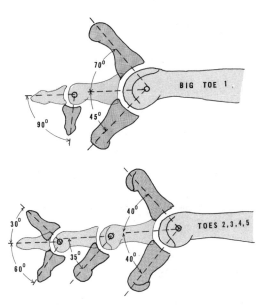

Figure 13–44. Range of motion of the phalanges. The passive range of motion of the phalanges are noted.

evert the foot, the posterior tibialis that plantarflex and invert, and the anterior tibialis that dorsiflex and invert the foot. In normal gait the gastrocnemius-soleus decelerates the foot in the stance phase. Toes are mobilized by both intrinsic and the extrinsic muscles (Fig. 13–45).

Hammertoe is a fixed flexion deformity of the interphalangeal joint occurring in any toe (Fig. 13–46).

Treatment includes avoiding pressure on the exposed joints and ankylosis

Figure 13–45. Muscular action on the phalanges. The flexor tendons of the big toe cross two joints and thus act to press the distal phalanx to the floor. The sesamoid bones are incorporated into the tendons of the short flexor, the flexor hallucis brevis (FHB), and act as a fulcrum. The flexor tendons of the other four toes cross three joints and act to grip the floor. This action is through the short flexor, the flexor digitorum brevis (FDB), and the long flexor muscles, the flexor digitorum longus (FDL).

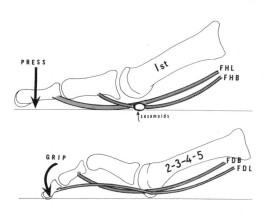

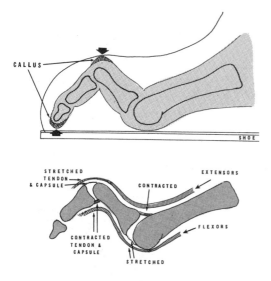

Figure 13–46. Hammer toe. Hammer toe is a flexion deformity of the interphalangeal joints with capsule and tendon contracture. The proximal phalanx is usually extended and the distal phalanx flexed and flexible. Pressure from shoe wear (*arrow*) with callus formation is frequent.

of the involved joints. Avoiding pressure requires the placement of properly cut and fitted pads over the involved joints or cutting away the offending portions of the shoe. Manual stretching of the joints will help to prevent contracture if it persists. When the condition is severe or disabling, surgical correction is indicated.

RUPTURE OF THE ACHILLES TENDON

In acute posterior calf pain as may be present after physical injury, the Achilles tendon may have been ruptured, requiring immediate diagnosis and medical attention. An audible "snap" is frequently noticed and pain is immediate. Depending on the site and extent of the tear, disability ensues.

The mechanism of tearing involves acute forceful extension of the gastrocnemius-soleus muscle tendon as a result of excessive or abrupt ankle dorsiflexion. Direct trauma to the Achilles tendon may be causative. Ecchymosis is often noted and a tear (Fig. 13–47), with retraction of the belly of the gastrocnemius-soleus muscle, may be palpable.

A test has been proposed to determine the completeness of the tear. With the patient prone and both feet hanging over the edge of the table, the calf muscles are squeezed. In the normal foot, the ankle plantarflexes, whereas with a completely torn Achilles tendon, no plantarflexion is present. In the erect position the patient cannot arise upon the toes of the affected leg.

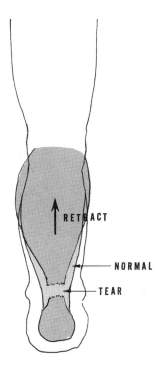

Figure 13–47. Tear of the gastrocsoleus Achilles complex. Most tears of the Achilles complex occur approximately 2 inches above the calcaneal insert. When complete, the calf muscle retracts toward the popliteal space and a "gap" can be palpated. The patient cannot arise on his toes.

Treatment of a complete tear remains controversial, but early repair is most promising. Therapy of placing the foot in extreme plantarflexion in a walking cast for 6 weeks, then using slow gradual rehabilitation has its advocates.

Clinical tests do not give positive results in measuring a partial tear; diagnosis is conjectural based on tenderness, localized pain, and aggravation from stretching the heel cord or arising on the toes. Treatment is primarily the avoidance of physical activities for at least 3 weeks. Use of a $\frac{3}{4}$-inch elevated heel relieves the stretch of the heel cord.

THE DIABETIC FOOT

In a patient with diabetes, foot problems must be carefully evaluated and eliminated with only appropriate care because complications of these conditions may be devastating. Hospitalizations for diabetic foot problems grew from 25% in 1965 to over 50% in 1985.[16,17]

The causes of foot damage resulting from diabetes are ischemia, neuropathic changes, and neuropathic arthropathy.[18] Ischemia may include large or small vessel disease and sensory, motor, or autonomic neuropathy.

Large vessel pathology with history of claudication and painful, nonhealing ulcers are the major presenting complaint. Diabetic ulcers have been classified;

Grade I: a superficial ulcer involving only skin and subcutaneous tissues

Grade II: ulcers extending to underlying tendon, bone, or joint capsule

Grade III: deep ulcers with associated osteomyelitis or abscess

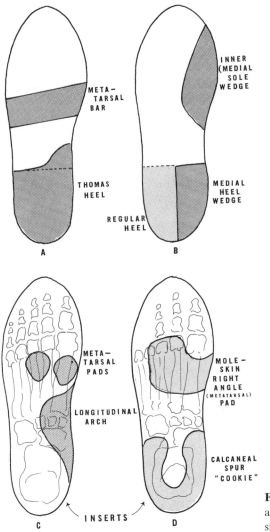

Figure 13–48. Shoe inserts and pads to minimize pressure sites.

Grade IV: gangrene of toe or distal forefoot

Grade V: midfoot and hindfoot gangrene

Treatment varies with these grade. Ulcers of Grades I and II usually respond to debridement, antibiotics, and wearing more appropriate shoes. Topical dressings used vary with the experience and opinion of the physician. Avoidance of pressure over the ulceration must be emphasized.

Ulcers of Grades III, IV, and V require correction of any or all underlying foot problems previously mentioned. Surgical debridement and possibly selective amputation may be required. Absolute control of diabetes is mandatory.

Prevention of complications of the diabetic foot is the desired goal because treatment of a lesion is limited in efficacy.

Patient education includes conveying that the foot must be inspected daily for signs of erythema, cuts, scratches, abrasions, blisters, or any build up of callus. Feet must be washed daily with a mild soap, dried carefully, and lubricated with a lanolin-based lotion. Thick socks without seams must be worn and any wrinkles in their fabric must be avoided. Astute avoidance of thermal, chemical, or physical irritating agents must be a major, and continuing concern.

ORTHOTIC DEVICES

In the discussion of various foot and ankle injuries and diseases, orthotic devices have been proposed as therapeutic or preventative. Not all types of devices can be discussed in a book of this scope, but several types can be illustrated (Figs. 13–48 through 13–51).

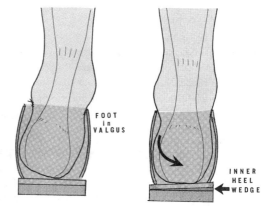

Figure 13–49. Shoe modification to correct heel valgus. (*Left*) A valgus deformity within the shoe. (*Right*) An inner heel wedge corrects this deformity.

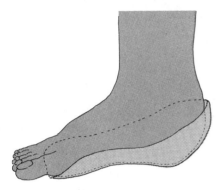

Figure 13–50. Molded orthotic device. The foot can be molded in the desired shape and supported by a molded plastic orthosis made from a plaster mold.

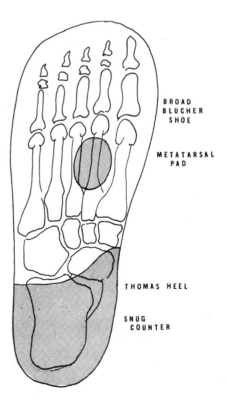

BROAD
BLUCHER
SHOE

METATARSAL
PAD

THOMAS HEEL

SNUG
COUNTER

Figure 13–51. Shoe modification in treatment of metatarsalgia. The placement of a metatarsal pad in the treatment of metatarsalgia is so important it needs specific instructions. The purpose of the pad is to elevate the heads of the second and third metatarsals to avoid weight bearing. The pad must be placed "behind" the heads to elevate the shafts and *not* the heads themselves.

REFERENCES

1. McConrey, JP: Ankle sprains, consequences and mimics. Med Sports Sci 23:39–55, 1987.
2. Brostrom, L: Sprained ankles. I. Anatomic lesions in recent sprains. Acta Chir Scand 128:483–495, 1964.
3. Watson-Jones, SR: Fractures and Joint Injuries. E & S Livingstone, Edinburgh, 1953.
4. Friedman, MAR, Dean, MRE and Hanham, IEF: The etiology and prevention of functional instability of the foot. J Bone Joint Surg 47B:678–685, 1965.
5. Machlum, S and Daljord, OA: Acute sports injuries in Oslo—a one year study. Br J Sports Med 18:181–185, 1984.
6. Jackson, DW, Ashley, RD, and Powell, JW: Ankle sprains in young athletes. Clin Orthop 101:201–214, 1974.
7. Funder, V, Jorgensen, JP, Anderson, A, et al: Ruptures of the lateral ligaments of the ankle: Clinical diagnosis. Acta Orthop Scand 53:997–1000, 1982.
8. Lassiter, TE, Jr, Malone, TR, and Garrett, WE, Jr: Injury to the lateral ligaments of the ankle. In Orthop Clin North Am 20:629–640, 1989.
9. Drez, D, Young, JC, Woldman, D, et al: Nonoperative treatment of double lateral ligament tear of the ankle. Am J Sports Med 10:197–200, 1982.
10. Rubin, G and Witen, M: The subtalar joint and the symptom of turning over on the ankle: A new method of evaluation utilizing tomography. Am J Orthop 4:16–19, 1962.
11. Cailliet, R: Painful Conditions of the Heel. In Cailliet, R: Foot and Ankle Pain, FA Davis, Philadelphia, 1968 pp 108–116.
12. Baxter, DE, Pfeffer, GB, and Thigpen, M: Chronic Heel Pain: Treatment Rationale. In Management of Foot Problems. Orthop Clin North Am 20:563–569, 1989.
13. Baxter, DE: Nerve entrapment as cause of heel pain. Presented to the Orthopedic Foot Clinic, New Orleans, May 1982.
14. Gould, JS: Metatarsalgia. Orthop Clin North Am 20:553–562, 1989.
15. Kitaoka, HB: Rheumatoid hindfoot. Orthop Clin North Am 20:593–604, 1989.
16. Pratt, TC: Gangrene and infection in the diabetic. Med Clin North Am 49:987–1007, 1965.
17. Selby, J, Showstack, J, and Browner, W: Indication to measure the prevention of amputation in persons with diabetes. Report for Division of Diabetes Control. Centers for Disease Control, Atlanta, 1985.
18. Harrelson, JM: Management of the diabetic foot. Orthop Clin North Am 20:605–619, 1989.

CHAPTER 14
Causalgia and Other Reflex Sympathetic Dystrophies

REFLEX SYMPATHETIC DYSTROPHY

The condition termed **Reflex Sympathetic Dystrophy (RSD)** encompasses various disabling neuromuscular and vasomotor conditions of both extremities: both lower and upper. This condition, more aptly termed a **syndrome**, is seen as possible to follow virtually any form of local injury; whether major or minor. The condition originally termed **causalgia** implied **burning pain** with associated neurovascular symptomatology. Further breakdown of this syndrome is more significantly seen in major and minor injuries wherein pain, whether burning or otherwise, need not be associated. By so delineating the condition, it is more apt to be recognized early and treated properly.

Bonica[1] divided RSD as major and minor using the following subdivisions:

Major	Minor
Causalgia	Shoulder-hand-finger syndrome
Thalamic syndrome	Postmyocardial infarct
Phantom limb syndrome	Postcerebrovascular attack
	Postinjection
	Postfracture, postcast, postsplint
	Postoveruse syndrome

It is apparent that in the above dystrophies considered minor, any trauma can be implicated, which in many patients could be an incident so insignificant that the causation is difficult to remember.

Major or minor RSD often occurs in the upper extremity. Because RSD is a major complication of any upper extremity impairment, both painful and painless, its recognition must be assessed in any complaint of the arm presented by the patient.

Reflex sympathetic dystrophy occurs so frequently in a post-traumatic patient, yet is so often overlooked by the uninformed, uneducated, or unaware physician that this entire chapter is being devoted to it because it is a frequent consequence of *soft tissue injury*.

RSD involves the lower extremities somewhat less frequently than the upper. This condition is seen more frequently during war, but with the increasing incidence of injuries similar to those seen on the battlefield in everyday life and as a result of auto-motorcycle accidents, RSD is increasingly being diagnosed.

RSD in the absence of causalgia is, however, often misdiagnosed and mistreated with severe disabling sequelae.

Perusal of the literature indicates that burning pain and associated symptomatology following peripheral nerve injury was noted by Pare[2] in the sixteenth century. It reached a great frequency during the Civil War in the United States when it was described in 1864 by Mitchell and colleagues.[3] They described the condition in wounded soldiers who developed *burning pain* following peripheral nerve injury, usually from gunshot wounds. Mitchell employed the term **causalgia** to describe the *burning* character of the pain. The condition he originally described is currently classified as *major reflex sympathetic dystrophy*.

Many clinicians followed with descriptions of this condition. Letievant in 1873[4] ascribed the condition as having a neurologic cause. Sudeck[5] published his classic 1900 description of the radiologic characteristics of bone osteoporosis following trauma, with subsequent RSD. Leriche[6] regarded the condition as a sequela of the breakdown of the sympathetic nervous system that leads to peripheral sympathectomy as a favored and successful treatment of RSD. Study of RSD was largely forgotten until World War II, when numerous cases were reported and the diagnosis of the clinical condition revived.

A number of terms to describe RSD have been used in the literature: **algodystrophy, sympathalgia, neurovascular reflex sympathetic dystrophy, traumatic angiospasm, traumatic vasospasm, Sudeck's atrophy, post-traumatic osteoporosis, post-traumatic painful osteoporosis, shoulder-hand-finger syndrome**, and many others. As pain persists, often after the initial trauma has subsided, in the peripheral nerve distribution through sympathetic nerve fibers, an enticing classification of this persisting pain has been termed using the acronym **SMP**, that is, **sympathetically maintained pain**. Where less evidence of sympathetic nervous system is involved yet persistent pain is manifest, the acronym meaning **sympathetic independent** pain (SIP) is used.[7]

All the above terms allude, in one way or another, to the clinical manifestations of RSD:

1. Persistent pain, variously described but, frequently as having a *burning* quality, although such a description is not necessarily diagnostic.
2. Vasomotor changes manifested as hyperthermia often followed by coldness.
3. Subcutaneous edema that becomes rapidly nonpitting.
4. Presence of sensory changes; first hyperesthesia, then hypoesthesia.
5. Ultimate trophic changes such as atrophy of the skin, muscle, and bone that causes functional impairment.
6. Significant osteoporosis.
7. Atrophic osteoarthrosis.[8,9]

Causalgia has been defined by the International Association for the Study of Pain (IASP)[10] as "a syndrome of sustained burning pain after traumatic nerve lesion combined with vasomotor and sudomotor dysfunction and later trophic changes." Amplification of the RSD syndrome now lists many conditions of RSD without the finding of burning pain, yet with all other vasomotor and sudomotor symptomatology and findings. This would conform to the diagnosis of SIP, as promulgated by Roberts. The basic mechanisms, pathophysiology, and symptomatology[11] are similar enough in any form of RSD to justify the diagnostic term and attendant therapies.

A definition of the terms of RSD plainly clarifies this disease entity. **Dystrophy** indicates wasting of the muscular and bony tissues of the region, as well as abnormal growth of the nails of the extremity and hyperkeratosis of the skin. **Sympathetic** includes vasomotor and sudomotor changes such as inappropriate sweating, coldness, and color changes of the extremity as a result of vasoconstriction or vasodilatation. **Reflex** because the signs emanate from sympathetic nervous system distribution to the extremity. Another confirmatory diagnostic test of RSD is its beneficial response to sympathetic interruption.

Onset of pain varies between major RSD (causalgia) and minor RSD in that the former has an immediate onset of pain or at least one within a short time, whereas minor RSD may have a delay of pain of several days to months. The character of pain must invariably have a burning quality to qualify the condition as RSD.

The site of this syndrome is distal in the extremity: either upper shoulder-hand-finger or lower knee-ankle-foot and toes.

Postulated mechanisms have varied from those first proposed by Mitchell:[3] "an inexplicable reflex in the spinal cord centers felt in remote regions outside the distribution of the wounded nerve . . . " This definition has been modified by me, but the sense of the idea has been retained. Many concepts have been posited but a more recent theory has been offered by Devor[12] in which he suggests that the injury damages or transects (i.e., cuts across) the involved nerve.

This appealing theory requires understanding the structure of nerve axons and the theory of axoplasmic transport. The hypothesis is illustrated in Figure 14–1.[13] Neuronal function is now considered to be axonal transport of protein and other materials needed by the tissues supplied by the nerve. Sensory impulses are also supplied by axonal transport.

The neuron cell body allows a high level of protein synthesis to be conveyed the length of the nerve fiber. This transport mechanism has been shown to be very dependent on adequate blood supply. Pressure on the nerve axon or its blood flow impairs axonal transport. The flow through the axonal microtubules and neurofilaments is similarly impaired. Variation of the components of the proteins of the peripheral nerve also determines the end result of axonal impairment.

After a nerve is constricted, the fibers may show collateral branching.[14,15] During recovery of the injured nerve, the exposed regenerating surface of the axon undergoes a greater than normal accumulation of receptors. These re-

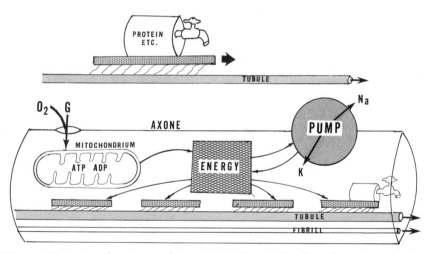

Figure 14–1. Axoplasmic neural transport: A theory. The flow of protein and other derivatives begins with entry of glucose (G) into the fiber. Glycolysis and phosphorylation occurs (O_2) in the mitochondria through metabolism of adenosinetriphosphate (ATP), which creates the energy to the sodium pump. This pump regulates balance of sodium (Na) and potassium (K) and determines nerve activity. The transport filaments move along the axon by oscillation and carry the nutritive protein elements along the nerve pathway. (Data from Ochs, S: Axoplasmic transport—A basis for neural pathology. In Dyke, PJ, Thomas, PK, and Lambert, EH (eds.): Peripheral Neuropathy. WB Saunders, Philadelphia, 1975, pp 213–230).

ceptors are alpha-adrenogenic, which results in abnormal electrical properties of that nerve.[16] These excessive, and possibly, abnormal, receptors become ectopic pacemakers that lead to spontaneous depolarization. These receptors bombard the central nervous system (CNS) and interfere with normal central processing of sensory information. The CNS is already in a state of hyperactivity and hyperreceptivity from previous bombardment by unmylelinated nerve fiber impulses and is now more accessible to persistent pain by this added excessive release of distal epinephrine impulses from these new branchings of the nerve fibers (Fig. 14–2).[17]

The peripheral stimuli are initiated because of the abnormal chemosensitivity and mechanosensitivity of the neurons; rather than as a result of otherwise physiologic stimuli.

Centrally the aberrant sensory processing from this barrage produces a sensation of pain (paresthesia) and altered sympathetic reflexes produce the somatic characteristics of RSD (Fig. 14–3).

Other theories postulate a peripheral nervous system mechanism rather than the CNS. At the site of the nerve injury, synapse occurs between efferent sympathetic and afferent pain fibers which causes a *short circuit* of sensory information.[18] This concept has been refuted because it does not explain why sympathetic nerve block placed distal to the lesion is effective. Another peripheral concept suggests liberation, at the involved area of algesic substances

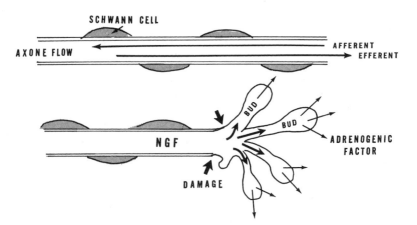

Figure 14–2. Axonal growth forming a neuroma. After a nerve injury with compression or partial to total severance, the nerve growth factor (NGF) stimulates the nerve to advance distally and to form "buds," which creates more endings than the normal nerve shown in the upper drawing. By virtue of the greater secretion of adrenogenic factors from these additional buds, the nerve becomes more sensitive to adrenogenic agonists and transmits greater numbers of potential pain fiber impulses to the spinal cord.

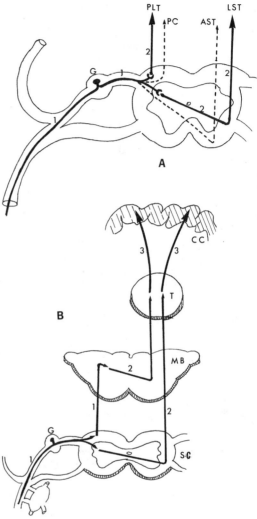

Figure 14–3. Neuronal pathways of pain. (A) The course of sensory fibers in a segmental nerve with its ganglion (G) in the dorsal root. On entrance into the spinal cord (SC), the fibers ascend (1) on the same side in the posterior lateral tract (PLT) and there they decussate to cross into the lateral spinothalamic tract: (2) indicates secondary neurons. The posterior column (PC) transmits position sense: the anterior spinal thalamic tract (AST) conveys tactile sensation. (B) 1 = first stage neurons to the cord; 2 = second-stage neurons through the midbrain (MB) into the thalamus (T); 3 = third-stage neurons and the thalamocortical pathways to the cerebral cortex (CC).

(nociceptive areas) that produces local hyperalgesia which, in turn, produces and sustains a vicious cycle.

Of the numerous *central* mechanisms postulated, the concept of bombardment of the dorsal horn cells in laminae IV to VI by the peripheral nociceptor substances is widely held (Fig. 14–4).

As stated by Rizzi and colleagues,[19] an unanswered question is posed as to why causalgia occurs most often with a *partial* instead of a complete lesion; and why there is such a low incidence of causalgia with many partial nerve lesions.

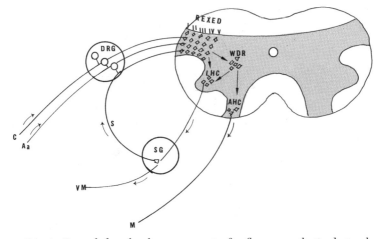

Figure 14–4. Central dorsal column concept of reflex sympathetic dystrophy. The sensory (C) fibers, mechano (A_a) and sympathetic sensory afferent fibers (S) enter the gray matter (dorsal horn) through the dorsal root ganglion (DRG) into the Rexed I, II, III, IV, and V layers. Layers I and II constitute the substantia gelatinosum. Within the cord the fibers connect to the dynamic wide range cells (WDR), which connect to the lateral horn cells (LHC) and the anterior horn cells (AHC). The sympathetic fibers originate from the lateral horn cells and become efferent as vasomotor impulses (VM) to the blood vessels. The anterior horn cells are efferent to the peripheral muscles (M).

The psychologic state of the individual at the time of injury has also been proposed as being significant. Much research is needed to ascertain the neuropsychologic–humoral susceptibility of individuals under extreme anxiety. Such predisposed patients with trauma are likely to develop causalgic RSD.

A hypothesis has been advanced[20] to answer why many patients with RSD develop it after a relatively minor trauma and why pain and other somatic symptoms are exacerbated by emotional stress. Ecker postulates that pre-existing anxiety or stress increases the release of norepinephrine, which increases arteriolar hyperactivity. The resultant vasospasm, ischemia, and nociceptor release on neural tissues already bathed by excessive norepinephrine from the anxiety and stress result in RSD.

Aggravation of the local pain and referred pain often from minor, unrelated, and reasonably innocuous stimuli are transmitted to the CNS through mechanoreceptors. These receptors and their afferent fibers normally do not transmit pain but with this condition, SMP, they enhance the pain. This concept is illustrated in Figure 14–5.

The original trauma transmits action potentials through C-nociceptive fibers to the dorsal root ganglion (DRG) where they are then transmitted to the cord in the region of the dorsal horn (Rexed layers). They bombard that region and form a hypersensitive set of neurons (termed **wide dynamic**

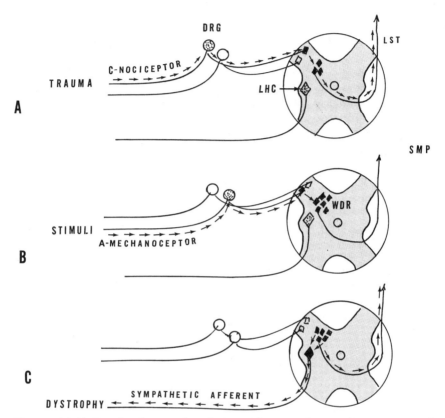

Figure 14–5. Postulated neurophysiologic mechanism of sympathetic maintained pain. The transmission through C-nociceptive fibers (A) of impulses derives from the peripheral tissues that have been traumatized with creation of peripheral nociceptive chemicals. These impulses pass through the dorsal root ganglion (DRG) to activate neurons within the Rexed layers in the gray matter of the spinal cord. When sensitized they activate the neurons within the wide dynamic range neurons (WDR). These neurons, in turn become receptive to impulses from the periphery transmitted through A-mechanoreceptor fibers (B), which normally transmit sensations of touch, pressure, vibration, and temperature but not pain. If the periphery is now stimulated the impulses maintain the irritability of the WDR. Further impulses continue cephalad through the lateral spinal thalamic tracts (LSTT) to the thalamic enters with resultant continued pain. The WDR impulses also irritate the lateral horn cells (LHS), which generate sympathetic impulses that innervate the vasomotor supplied peripheral tissues resulting in the symptoms and findings of dystrophy (C).

range [WDR] by Roberts). This WDR can then be bombarded by impulses through the mechanoreceptors from the skin, muscles, tendons, and ligaments that travel through A-mechanofibers of myelinated nerves. These latter impulses impinge on the already hypersensitive cord regions (WDR) which can spill over, or influence the proximal nerve cells (lateral horn) of the autonomic (sympathetic) nerves. This explains how innocuous unrelated touch, pressure, or movement intensify the pain, as mechanoreceptors and not nociceptors. These impulses then travel distally (efferent) to the periphery causing vasomotor reactions as well as stimulating sympathetic pain sensations.

The evolved vasomotor changes of the dystrophy are thus explained, as is the basis of sympathetic afferent impulses initiating the cycle which is then enhanced by mechanoreceptor irritants such as touch, stretch, and passive and active motion.

The diagnosis of RSD in the upper extremity has received significant attention in the literature, making the diagnosis more frequent in that area (Fig. 14–6), but avoided or dismissed when the lower extremity is affected. It will thus receive detailed attention here.

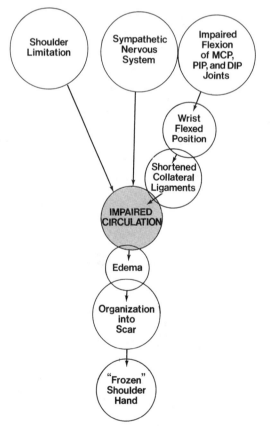

Figure 14–6. Development of reflex sympathetic dystrophy "frozen shoulder-hand-finger syndrome." Sequence of events causing the frozen shoulder-hand-finger syndrome.

REFLEX SYMPATHETIC DYSTROPHY IN LOWER EXTREMITY

In the symptomatic lower extremity, RSD lesions that eventually develop a minor or major RSD, the etiologic concept may remain unanswered but its occurrence demands attention, both diagnostic and therapeutic, to minimize the disabling sequelae.

Whereas major RSD causalgia occurs post-traumatically in lower extremity injuries, by definition, a partial nerve lesion must be present to have RSD and causalgia occur. In conditions such as fractures, dislocations, and hemiparetic lower extremity lesions after strokes, no nerve lesion is needed to develop RSD. The minor RSD lesion of knee-ankle-foot syndrome, regardless of its etiology, usually does not have a partial nerve lesion nor will it develop a painful causalgia. All the other sequelae of RSD do develop.

LEG-ANKLE-FOOT RSD SYNDROME

In this condition, dysfunction of the sympathetic nervous system is present, but from a different physiologic basis and from a different etiologic entity. As a rule, such RSD is mechanical, resulting from nerve pressure and neurovascular response. The somatic nerve supply to the lower extremity is accomplished by sympathetic nerves (Figs. 14–7 and 14–8).

Normal circulation of the lower extremity can be simplistically divided into arterial and venous segments, both of which have a mechanical component.

1. The arterial component is the cardiac *pumping* action, major arterial tone, and constriction-relaxation cycle, and the gravitational forces that propel the arterial blood flow to the distal portions of the upper extremity. The blood flows through the major arteries, then the arterioles to end in the capillaries where diffusion into the tissues takes place.
2. The return of the circulation to the heart and lungs is through the venous and lymphatic channels by virtue of pump action. The muscles of the calf and anterior compartment literally pump the blood proximally with the assistance of gravity. The affected leg must frequently be held above heart level for gravity to be effective. The lower leg muscles thus act as a pump in this activity. The thigh, knee, and ankle muscles move the leg, ankle, and foot in every direction as well as pump the venous lymphatic blood elements toward the heart. This exercise thus elevates the upper extremity above the level of the heart (Fig. 14–9).

Repeated contraction and relaxation of muscular action of the leg muscles pumps the blood and lymphatic fluid proximally. Failure of either of these

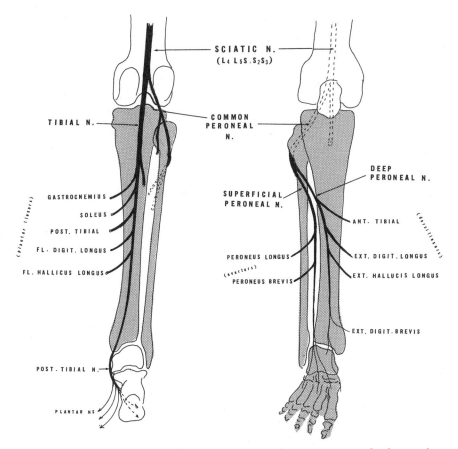

Figure 14–7. Innervation of the leg and foot. The sciatic nerve divides at the popliteal angle to form the tibial nerve and the common peroneal nerve.

pumps to function adequately may lead to a painful and disabling condition termed **leg-ankle-foot syndrome** (LAF syndrome). Loss of the ankle's alternating flexion-extension eliminates the distal pump. As is well known, a fracture dislocation of the knee, with or without application of a cast, may initiate this condition.

Pain from this syndrome varies from an ache, deep discomfort, tenderness, painful movement, to even a mild burning sensation. Pain usually does not occur initially nor even necessarily early in this entity, but instead may only be noticed several days to weeks after onset. Most often other functional impairments of function besides pain are present, which is why the condition is rarely diagnosed early in many patients.

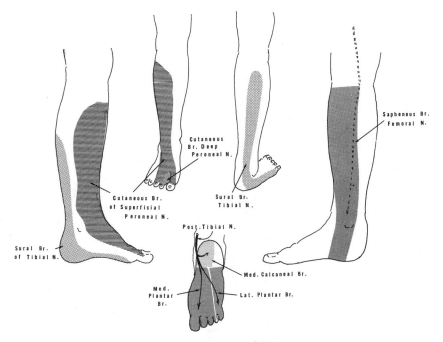

Figure 14–8. Sensory patterns of the lower extremity.

Mechanism of LAF Syndrome

The sequelae of the LAF syndrome from whatever initial condition occur because the muscular pump does not function. The knee, ankle, and foot fail to move appropriately and there is ultimately failure of elevation above the level of the heart. Inadequate hip and knee motion impairs the upper pump action, with attendant diminution of venous lymphatic flow.

There are many factors that may initiate limited motion:

1. Meniscal tears
2. Ligamentous tears, collateral and cruciate
3. Fracture dislocation of the bones of, and those adjacent to, the knee joint
4. Posthemiplegic knee, foot, and ankle impairment
5. Postoperative casting
6. Soft tissue surgical procedures

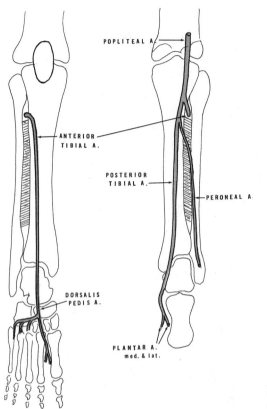

POPLITEAL A.

ANTERIOR
TIBIAL A.

POSTERIOR
TIBIAL A.

PERONEAL A.

DORSALIS
PEDIS A.

PLANTAR A.
med. & lat.

Figure 14–9. Arterial supply of the leg and foot.

Diagnosis

The knee or ankle may become *stiff*, that is, have limited passive and active range of motion. The cause of this limitation must be discerned and addressed. Most of these causes have been discussed elsewhere in this book and will not be repeated here but in addition to the many knee problems elicited the following must also be considered:

1. Systemic paresis, such as in Guillain-Barré syndrome, and poliomyelitis.
2. Spinal cord injury with paraplegia or quadriplegia
3. Inappropriate immobilization from casting or sustained position.

The onset of the RSD LAF syndrome is the first noted in the foot where there appears subtle edema on the dorsum and in the toes. The skin becomes *shiny*, smooth, and pale. At first, pitting may be elicited, although the degree of pitting is usually so minimal as to escape attention.

Full ankle plantarflexion and dorsiflexion are decreased, along with the active and passive ranges of motion of the toes. Careful evaluation here requires close attention because the degree of limitation is so minimal it must be compared with the opposite foot, ankle, and toes or else its presence may escape attention. This limited range of motion is the subtle beginning of the loss of the distal "pump." Limitation of the toes and the ankle results from edema under the corresponding tendons.

The skin, at first edematous, is also ischemic; it thickens then ultimately becomes atrophic. Clinically, early hyperhydrosis (excessive sudomotor activity) is present. The foot is moist. It may be either pale or with slight rubor. Color changes depend upon impaired vasomotor tone and whether vasodilatation or vasoconstriction is present. The foot is thus moist, pale, cold, or warm. When it is compared with the other, normal, foot, the vasomotor-sudomotor abnormality can be noted early in the condition.

Although affected skin in RSD is more often cold (vasoconstriction) than warm (vasodilatation), blood flow is increased in subcutaneous tissues,[21] muscles,[22] and bones.[23] This increased blood flow to the bone may account for the increased activity noted in results of radioactive bone scans in RSD. This increased deeper blood flow may also initiate a transient arteriovenous shunt with decreased superficial blood flow, hence creating the ultimate dystrophy.

The hair follicles thicken (hypertrichosis) from excessive sudomotor activity; the nails also thicken. All these sudomotor vasomotor changes are subtle, at first, but gradually progress. The stage at which they are discovered and when treatment is started determines the correctability or reversibility of the structural changes.

Stages of LAF Syndrome:

Stage I: Vasomotor signs of hyperhydrosis with edema:
1. Limited ankle toes range of motion (with or without pain)
2. Swelling of dorsum of foot and ankle; at first, with pitting
3. Skin becomes shiny, either dry or moist
4. Limited range of motion of foot ankle and toe flexion
5. Pain on ankle dorsiflexion and plantarflexion

Stage II: Most significant change: firmer edema; cannot be dimpled by pressure.
1. Foot and ankle pain may subside; slight increase of active and passive range of motion; edema of foot appears to subside, with less pitting
2. Skin less elastic
3. Toes stiffen
4. Nails and hair coarser
5. Skin less sensitive
6. Osteoporosis evident on radiographs

Stage III:
1. Progressive atrophy of bones, skin, and muscles
2. Limited passive range of motion at the ankle and toes
3. Nails brittle and grooved. The hair follicles larger, more brittle
4. Pain minimal or absent except when passive motion attempted

Radiographs that reveal bone atrophy (osteoporosis) may be noted early even at stage I but usually it is only noted at Stage II. Radiographs, made for diagnostic purposes, should always include the opposite foot for comparison because early changes are subtle and easily missed. Bone density studies have currently been developed that differentiate and grade the degree of osteoporosis but they are more academic because it must be stated the initial diagnosis must not be made on finding changes in bone density foot radiographs. By that point, stage III is in its early onset.

During the progression of LAF syndrome, ultimately atrophic articular changes occur. The cartilage of the tarsal, metatarsal, and phalangeal bones, by virtue of the ischemia resulting from vasomotor abnormality, impairs circulation of the joints—atrophic arthritis results and no active or passive motion is possible. Although without pain, the condition allows no function of the ankle, foot, and toes.

Stages I and II are considered reversible to a practical functional degree. Stage III has many irreversible structural changes that make functional recovery limited, if feasible at all.

This diagnosis should be considered where subtle skin changes of the foot occur in any condition of the lower extremity where there is also:

1. Pain and limitation involving an ankle "problem"
2. Pain or limitation of the foot
3. Pain and limitation of the digits of the foot
4. Trauma to the lower extremity such as surgery, injection, a sprain, or strain
5. A systemic condition with referred pain to the lower extremity

Treatment

Treatment of RSD varies only slightly whether causalgic pain is present or not. Causalgic pain must obviously be addressed forcefully and energetically until overcome or at least significantly minimized. Without relief of causalgic pain, the syndrome can be neither remediated nor moderated. Treatment of the sequelae of RSD must also be simultaneously and energetically addressed as well, concurrently with treatment of causalgic pain. To relieve the pain but still have a hand involved in residual stage III would ill serve the patient.

Interruption of sympathetic hyperactivity is universally indicated. For

RSD of the lower extremity, at one point, a chemical block of the sympathetic nervous system using caudal block was considered both diagnostic and therapeutic. Other forms of sympathetic intervention have subsequently been advised but use of the chemical caudal block initially still prevails.

White and Sweet[24] suggested that, because of emotional factors being so commonly associated with this condition, a placebo diagnostic test should be considered. After getting relief with a local anesthetic but getting no response from sterile saline solution, sympathetic interruption should be considered. Because the condition is so ominous and caudal block (Fig. 14–10) is relatively simple and safe, initial active treatment should be considered and undertaken. If severe emotional problems play a role, therapy in that direction becomes a part of the treatment regime.

Series of epidural blocks should be considered, usually a minimum of four, but a greater number have been undertaken beneficially before surgical extirpation of the sympathetic ganglia is considered. The decision is based on subjective and objective results of the chemical sympathectomy and the duration of the benefit. This is a clinical judgment based on the experience of the attending physician.

The following treatment procedures based on the current understanding of the pathomechanics of the syndrome have been advocated:[25]

1. Early recognition
2. Early active therapeutic involvement of the patient, a therapist, and a family member
3. Early patient involvement indicating a meaningful explanation in understandable terms regarding symptoms and findings, and their significance
4. Local application of ice or heat as tolerated by the patient, depending on presence of vasodilatation (rubor and warmth) or vasoconstriction (cold and blanched)
5. Passive and active range of motion of the extremity
6. Elevation of the involved extremity as often and as long as feasible
7. Passive and active removal of edema with compression dressings and available vasoconstrictive devices
8. Injection of local *trigger* areas with an anesthetic agent, with or without soluble steroid
9. Vasocoolant spray followed by stretch of any restricted myofascial tissue
10. Application of a transcutaneous electrical nerve stimulation (TENS) unit if pain is significant enough to curtail active patient participation in therapeutic modalities[26]
11. Specific somatic nerve blocks[27] of the involved area
12. Interruption of the sympathetic nervous system to the area. Can be

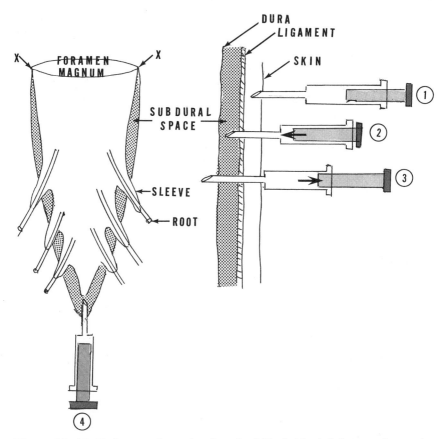

Figure 14–10. Technique of causal and epidural block. The left drawing depicts the dural sac with closure at the foramen magnum and the nerve root sleeves following the nerve roots through the intervertebral foramena. (*1*) Penetration the spinal needle through the skin. (*2*) Penetration through the ligament into the subdural space with resultant vacuum that pulls the plunger into the syringe. (*3*) Penetration of the dura into the canal from which the spinal fluid forces the plunger from the syringe. This is no longer an epidural injection. (*4*) Site of needle entrance as an epidural injection through a caudal block.

caudal or epidural. [28,29] A 6% to 7% phenol application to the sympathetic ganglion [30]

Various medications have also been suggested:

1. Nonsteroidal anti-inflammatory drug (NSAID) use is often advocated and although it may have short-term value, long-term it has been more disappointing.
2. Oral steroids (60 to 80 mg prednisone) in a short (2-wk) course, followed by gradual tapering, has proven beneficial.
3. Heterocyclic antidepressants[31] such as amitriptyline[31] 10 to 50 mg HS or trazadone 50 to 150 mg HS have some clinical benefit albeit not known of their pharmacologic rationale.
4. Carbamazepine[32] initially 200 mg then monitored—effective in trigeminal neuralgia, has been valuable in some RSD patients.
5. Beta blockers (propranolol) allegedly invoked in the vasomotor component of RSD have been proposed, as well as alpha adrenergic blockers (prazosin)[33] and phenoxybenzamine.
6. Topical application of capsaicin[34] often relieves hypersensitivity of the affected region in many patients.

REFERENCES

1. Bonica, JJ: Causalgia and other reflex sympathetic dystrophies. In Bonica, JJ, Liebeskind, JC, and Albe-Ferrand, D (eds.): Research and Therapy, vol 3. Raven Press, New York, 1979, p 141–166.
2. Paré, A: Oeuvres. 2:115, 1840.
3. Mitchell, SW, Morehouse, GR, and Keen, WW: Gunshot wounds and other injuries of nerves. JB Lippincott, Philadelphia, 1864.
4. Letievant, E: Traité de Section Nerveuses. JB Bailliere et fils, Paris, 1873.
5. Sudeck, P: Uber die akute entzundlike knockenatrophie. Arch Clin Chir 62:147, 1900.
6. Leriche, R: De la causalgie envisagée comme une nevrite du sympathique et son traitment par la denudation et l'excision des plexus nerveuses periarteriées. Presse Med 24:178, 1916.
7. Roberts, WJ: A hypothesis on the physiological basis for causalgia and related pains. Pain 23:297, 1986.
8. DeTakata, G and Miller, DS: Posttraumatic dystrophy of the extremities. Arch Surg 46:469, 1943.
9. Miller, DS and DeTakata, G: Post-traumatic dystrophy of the extremities (Sudeck's atrophy). Surg Gynecol Obst 75:538, 1943.
10. Merskey, H: Classification of chronic pain: Description of chronic pain syndromes and definitions of pain terms. Pain(suppl)3:285, 1986.
11. Tahmouth, AJ: Causalgia: Redefinition as a clinical pain syndrome. Pain 10:187, 1981.
12. Devor, M: Nerve pathophysiology and mechanism of pain in causalgia. J Autonom Nerv Syst 7:371, 1983.
13. Ochs, S: Axoplasmic transport. A basis for neural pathology. In Dyke, PJ, Thomas, PK, and Lambert, EH (eds): Peripheral Neuropathy. WB Saunders, Philadelphia, 1975, pp 213–230.
14. Perroncito, A: La rigenerazione delle fibre nervose. Boll Soc Med Chir Pavia 4:434, 1905.

15. Garfin, SR, et al: Compressive neuropathy of spinal nerve roots: A mechanical or biological problem? Spine 16:1991.
16. Shawe, GDH: On the number of branches formed by regenerating nerve fibers. Br J Surg 42:474–488, 1955.
17. Wirth, FP and Rutherford, RB: A civilian experience with causalgia. Arch Surg 100:633–638, 1970.
18. Doupe, J, et al: Post-traumatic pain and the causalgia syndrome. J Neurol Neurosurg Psychiatry 7:33–48, 1944.
19. Rizzi, R, Visentin, M, and Mazzetti, G: Reflex sympathetic dystrophy. In Bendedetti, C (ed): Advances in Pain Research and Therapy, vol 7. Raven Press, New York, 1984, p 451.
20. Ecker, A: Norepinephrine in reflex sympathetic dystrophy: An hypothesis. Clin J Pain 5:313, 1980.
21. Christensen, K and Henricksen, O: The reflex sympathetic syndrome and experimental study of sympathetic reflex control of subcutaneous blood flow in the hand. Scand J Rheum 12:263, 1983.
22. Sylvest, J, Jenson, EM, Siggard-Anderson, J, Pederson, L: Reflex dystrophy: Resting blood flow and muscle temperature as diagnostic criteria. Scand J Rehab Med 9:25, 1977.
23. Ficat, T, Arlet, J, Lartigoe, G, Aujol, M, Trans, M-A: Trans M-A. Algodystrophies réflexes post-traumatique. Rev Chir Orthop 59:401, 1973.
24. White, JC and Sweet, WH: Pain and the Neurosurgeon: A Forty Year Experience. Charles C Thomas, Springfield, Ill, 1969, p 87.
25. Pratt, RB and Balter, K: Posttraumatic reflex sympathetic dystrophy: Mechanisms and medical management. J Occup Rehab. 1:57–70, 1991.
26. Richlin, DM, Carron, H, Rowlingson, JC, et al: Reflex sympathetic dystrophy: Successful treatment by transcutaneous nerve stimulation. J Pediatr 93:84, 1978.
27. Fink, BR: History of local anesthesia. In Cousins, MJ and Bridenbaugh, PO (eds): Neural Blockade. JB Lippincott, Philadelphia, 1980, pp 3–18.
28. Ladd, AL, DeHaven, KE, Thanik, J, et al: Reflex sympathetic imbalance: Response to epidural blockade. Am J Sports Med 17:60–67, 1989.
29. Dirksen, R, Rutgers, MJ, and Coolen, JMW: Cervical epidural steroids in reflex sympathetic dystrophy. Anaesthesiology 66:71–73, 1987.
30. Payne, R: Neuropathic pain syndromes with special reference to causalgia and reflex sympathetic dystrophy. Clin J Pain 2:59–73, 1986.
31. Max, MB, Culnane, M, and Scafer, SC, et al: Amitriptyline relieves diabetic neuropathy in patients with normal or depressed mood. Neurology 37:589–596, 1987.
32. Taylor, JC, Brauer, S, and Espir, MLE: Long term treatment of trigeminal neuralgia with carbamezine. Postgrad Med J 57:8–16, 1981.
33. Abram, SE and Lightfoot, RW: Treatment of long standing causalgia with prazosin. Reg Anaesth 6:79–81, 1981.
34. Simone, DA and Ochoa, J: Early and late effects of prolonged topical capsaicin on cutaneous sensibility in neurogenic vasodilatation in humans. Pain 47:285–294, 1991.

CHAPTER 15

Psychologic Concepts of Soft Tissue Pain

Of the various types of soft tissue pains, the pain of the low back is the most prevalent. "Pain, the barking watchdog of our health, is normally temporary. It immobilizes the damaged muscle, tendon, or ligament so that healing can occur. This acute or subacute pain usually passes quickly and is completely forgotten after it has."[1]

Admittedly the *specificity theory* of pain still prevails in today's medical education. This theory suggests that pain is a *specific* sensation and that its intensity is proportional to the degree of peripheral tissue damage. This concept has been gradually modified in that the perception of pain, in addition to the degree of peripheral tissue damage, is influenced by attention, anxiety, suggestion, prior conditioning, learning, and other variables.[2] This change in thinking in no way demeans the newer neurophysiologic, neurohormonal, pharmacologic, and mechanical aspects but does significantly influence the approaches to pain management.

Pain is not considered merely sensory, because it has motivational affective consequences.[3] Behavioral and physiologic studies[4] have proposed the following sequence in appreciating pain:

1. A precise evolution of neurophysiologic aspect of the mechanism of pain (see Chap. 2).
2. Activation of the reticular and limbic systems through ascending neuropathways that involve emotional aspects of neurophysiology by studying these neurologic sites
3. Involvement of higher centers implicating powerful motivational drives such as suggestion, learned responses, anxiety, and fears that exert control over physiologic activities.

489

Acute pain is usually responsive to a *specific* approach, but chronic pain is a totally different matter. The presence of pain with no discernible *organic* etiology presents a concern. The **benign aspect of pain** is a term that denotes the enigma of disabling pain proceeding from a relatively innocuous etiology. Treatments often fail to diminish such pain and may even enhance it. Disruption of the nerve tracts that are recognized as mediators of pain often do not relieve pain. Patients who fail to respond to *specific* treatment become depressed, resentful, and suffer further from being dismissed as *malingerers*, or *neurotics*, rather than diagnosed.

Responses to *placebo* therapy have also further categorized patients in this manner.[5] Placebo responses were initially discredited but now that design flaws have been eliminated, it has proven to be an effective tool in controlling pain. Suggestion is one example of this enhancement,[6] and it is now recognized that multiple approaches are more effective.[7]

An approach envisioned by Melzack was called an *alpha-training procedure*, because it used electroencephalo graphic (EEG) alpha technology. The patient was placed in a trance, that is, a meditational state, using EEG alpha documentation.[7] It employed distraction of attention from the painful body site; strong suggestion; relaxation; and development of voluntary control over the pain by the patient. Many other stimuli have been found to suppress pain such as *audio analgesia* wherein pain (such as during dental drilling) could be modified by intense auditory stimulation (loud music or noise). This modality combined with suggestion has proven effective.

Chronic pain has frequently grown progressively worse when the inferred pathologic cause has been removed. It persists day after day and night after night leading to an endless circle of sleeplessness, depression, agony, and social isolation. Pain, formerly, merely a symptom has now become a disease. Scientific attempts to explain chronic pain are incomplete. Although many claims have been advanced regarding liability of specific personality traits and genetic hereditary factors, none have withstood time and subsequent studies.

A recent hypothesis[8] is that muscular responses of a injured part (in this case, the low back) persist due to a psychobiologic mechanism. This learned cortical process (memory) responds to stressful events that trigger the latent increased state of muscular tension.[9,10] Muscles that undergo prolonged muscular tension are those in the region of the initial tissue site, that is, the low back.

Moderate levels of muscle tension may induce pain in both healthy subjects and patients with chronic pain.[11] In people prone to reactive stress, these muscles fail to relax to baseline levels in a normal time, which causes them to become the site of pain (Fig. 15–1).[12,13] This implies a central mechanism, because electrophysiologic and imaging studies have demonstrated (experimentally) that pain activates cortical and other central nervous system (CNS) structures.[14,15]

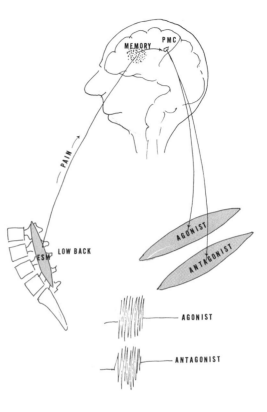

Figure 15–1. Concept of sustained muscle contraction from pain memory. Pain ascending from the low back with extensor muscle spasm (ESM) creates a memory of the pain, which, when stimulated by any event, causes activation of the premotor cortex (PMC), which causes muscle contraction. The agonist and antagonist muscles cocontract (*lower drawing*) rather than undergo reciprocal relaxation, and pain from the sustained muscle contractions may result.

A supporting paper[16] has shown electromyographically that patients with carpal tunnel syndrome and low back pain initate cocontraction of the agonist and antagonist muscles simultaneously and that the antagonists fail to reciprocally relax. This may well explain the onset and persistence of low back pain in individuals prone to it. This *proneness*, however, remains unclear in terms of neurophysiologic causes.

Each individual appears to have (have had) a breaking point under stress, after which their coping mechanism has failed. Learned maladaptive coping mechanisms have emerged.

Brena[17] postulated the five consequences of chronic pain in what he termed the **Five "D" Syndrome**:

1. Drug misuse and abuse
2. Dysfunction
3. Dependency
4. Depression
5. Disability

The importance of psychosocial factors as determinants of back pain and resultant disability has become increasingly prominent in the literature.[18] Frymoyer[19] developed a model based on the experience of numerous experts in determining the resulting disability from low back pain. He concluded that the following factors had equal weight: physical requirements and job satisfaction were equal to stress, Minnesota Multiphasic Personality Inventory (MMPI) scores, and psychologic symptoms.

In those patients with chronic low back problems who do not respond to rehabilitation efforts, there was evidence of depression, anxiety, distress, and pain behaviors.[20-24] To rehabilitate work-injured patients studies discerning pertinent factors needing correction have been studied.[25] Physical work load reduction has been accepted, but recent studies emphasize avoidance of sick leaves of long duration and early initiation of rehabilitation measures in poorly educated injured people.

A qualitative study[26] emphasized the fact that people sustaining a low back injury perceive their back problem as being a lifelong one to which they remain susceptible. This indication highlights the need to indoctrinate and educate initially the injured person about the cause, significance, and prognosis of the given musculoskeletal problem using meaningful and easily understood terminology.

PANIC AND ANXIETY DISORDERS

Undoubtedly chronic pain is prevalent in patients who develop acute pain and panic about the threatening symptoms. Anxiety disorders are among the most prevalent forms of psychiatric illness in the United States. They are more prevalent in women and in both genders in lower socioeconomic groups.

Differentiation must be made between significant anxiety and everyday normal episodic anxiety associated with upsetting life experiences. A clinically significant anxiety reaction literally interferes with a person's ability to function and thus can be considered an illness.

The diagnostic distinctions are codified in the American Psychiatric Association's *Diagnostic and Statistical Manual of Mental Disorders, Third Edition, Revised (DSM-III-R)*.

The following is a listing of anxiety disorders, phobic neuroses, and panic disorders with and without agoraphobia:

1. At some time during the disturbance, one or more panic attacks (discrete periods of intense fear or discomfort) have occurred that were unexpected, that is, did not occur immediately before or on exposure to a situation that almost always previously caused anxiety, and not triggered by situations in which the person was the focus of another's attention.
2. Either four attacks, as defined in criterion (1), have occurred within a 4-

week period, or one or more attacks have been followed by a period of at least a month of persistent fear of having another attack.

3. At least four of the following symptoms developed during at least one of the attacks:
   a. Shortness of breath
   b. Dizziness, unsteady feelings, or faintness
   c. Palpitations or accelerated heart rate (tachycardia)
   d. Trembling or shaking
   e. Sweating
   f. Choking
   g. Nausea or abdominal distress
   h. Depersonalization or derealization
   i. Numbness or tingling sensations (paresthesias)
   j. Flushes (hot flashes) or chills
   k. Chest pain or discomfort
   l. Fear of dying
   m. Fear of going crazy or doing something in an uncontrolled manner (attacks involving four or more symptoms are **panic attacks**: attacks involving fewer than four symptoms are **limited symptom attacks**)

4. During at least some of the attacks, at least four of the (3) level symptoms developed suddenly and increased in intensity within 10 minutes of the beginning of the first (3) level symptom noticed in the attack.

5. It cannot be established that any organic factor initiated and maintained the disturbance, for example, amphetamine or caffeine intoxication or hyperthyroidism.

There are subtypes designated: as being present with and without agoraphobia.

Agoraphobia: is a term denoting fear of being in public or open places or situations from which escape might be difficult (or embarrassing) or in which help might not be available in the event of a panic attack. This includes patients in whom persistent avoidance behavior originated during an active phase of panic disorder, even if the person does not attribute cause of the avoidance behavior to fear of having a panic attack.

As a result of this fear, the person either restricts travel or needs a companion when away from home, or else endures agoraphobic situations despite intense anxiety. Common agoraphobic situations include being outside the home alone, being in a crowd, standing in line, being on a bridge, and traveling in a bus, train, or car.

Associated anxiety disorders also include*:

---

*Source: DSM-III-R, American Psychiatric Association 1987.

300.22 Agoraphobia without history of panic disorder

300.23 Social phobia

300.29 Simple phobia

300.30 Obsessive-compulsive disorder

309.89 Posttraumatic disorder

300.02 Generalized anxiety disorder

300.00 Anxiety disorder not otherwise specified

The biologic basis of anxiety is an abnormality in chemical neurotransmission. Presynaptic neurons normally transmit impulses both electrically and chemically. These neurotransmitters are both fast signal and slow signal. Fast signals are mediated by glutamate ("on") and gamma-aminobutyric acid (GABA) ("off"). The slow signals are mediated by monoamines and peptides.

Effective chemical treatment of anxiety disorders, in recent decades, has clarified much of this chemical interplay. The discovery of benzodiazepine receptors and delineation of reciprocal relationships between benzodiazepines and GABA have evolved. Their effect on the locus coeruleus has been postulated. Besides GABA and norepinephrine, current evidence shows that serotonin is also implicated in mood disorders and anxiety disorders, as well as in obsessive-compulsive disorders. Anxiety has been considered as a disorder caused by a serotonin excess. Higher levels of serotonin have also been found in most obsessive-compulsive disorders, whereas aggressive impulsive patients may suffer from lower serotonin levels. This dichotomy is conceptualized as characterizing *harm avoidance* in the patient where serotonin levels are high in situations with a concern about danger and lower when the patient worries too little about the impending harm.

A protocol for treating a panic disorder has been offered:[27]

1. Rule out medical conditions causing anxiety, such as hyperthyroid disease.
2. Initiate antipanic psychotherapy by a therapist competent in disorders of behavior and cognition.
3. Begin therapy with an antipanic drug, such as imipramine or desipramine.
4. Start behavioral psychotherapy in conjunction with medication, if panic states persist.

Three essential features of panic attacks must be addressed: (1) the actual panic attack; (2) the anticipatory anxiety; and (3) anxiety about avoidance of the phobic events. The last usually fails to respond to medication, but often disappears if the other two aspects are under control. Panic attacks can usually be controlled and is thus a self-limited factor, although one prone to recurrence.

PAIN BEHAVIOR

Evaluation of pain behavior to indicate the presence and severity of pain has been the starting point for behavioral psychologists in their management of pain.[28] Such patient behaviors have been verbal, nonverbal, related to medications, emotional attitudes and postures, and evidence in facial expressions.[29] In an attempt to document behavior objectively, electromechanical devices are being developed to record activity and gait patterns.[30]

Pain behaviors are most frequently observed directly and are so recorded. Observations can be modified depending on whether the action is being performed in a natural situation or a regulated one, which may simulate the natural production of pain and may be videotaped for further clinical evaluation.[31]

Objectivity is a challenge to the trained observer. Most criteria are considered too simplistic and focus on behavior that denies the presence of pain and questions whether such behavior is an expression of pain or merely a mechanism for coping.[32]

Albeit a valid method of documenting pain it may be grossly misapplied and its value questioned.[33]

Facial Expression of Pain

After onset of pain, physical effort is made to withdraw from the source of trauma, a nociceptive type of reflex, accompanied by guarded movements, postures, and characteristic grimaces. Vocalization, including crying and moaning may be elicited but facial expression is often ignored.[34]

Nonverbal signs of physical distress have been noted for centuries. Shakespeare commented in *Macbeth* (I/4): "There's no art to find the mind's construct in the face." Physicians have actually claimed to be able to determine the location of pain more accurately through analyzing nonverbal expression of pain than through verbal information.[35,36]

The quantification of pain has eluded the clinician. Most quantifications of severity have been based on verbal statements by the patient,[37] which implies that much information may be missed.[38]

Nonverbal expression of pain may provide collateral and confirming information; it may also contradict the credibility of the verbal complaint, however. Empassioned display of agony may accompany calm verbal information.

The manner of verbal expression of pain is also influenced by experience, interpretation, significance, and degree of psychosocial loss for which appropriate descriptions are found.

A Facial Action Coding System (FACS) is emerging in pain research[39] in which patients videotaped or filed; results are then compared with objective standards. The conclusions gained from this testing is that facial expression is a major nonverbal factor, especially when accompanied by verbal expression. The latter is more subjective and so nonverbal factors are considered more accurate. These hardly exemplify truly objective quantification.[40]

The need for accurate measurement of pain was well documented when Wilse[41] performed a double-blind study and confirmed that patients who had minimal psychologic findings did better postoperatively, even with objective finding of lumbar discogenic disease, than did those who had severe hypochondriacal and conversional findings.

The "Undesirable Patient"

Many patients whose pain complaints present with significant or suggested psychopathology become examples of "undesirable patients."[42] A patient so stigmatized by his physician can create a catastrophic situation. This patient is apt to have less than adequate study and care.

Such undesirable patients include:

1. Socially unacceptable including patients with alcoholism, old people, dirty people, the uneducated, and the very poor. Often the perceived undesirability may be based on religion, race, social class, or country of national origin.
2. Attitudinal undesirables are examplified by the ungrateful patient, the too inquisitive patient (i.e., who knows too much), or one who is arrogant in the physician's office.
3. Physically undesirable because the absence of positive findings and a failure to respond to treatment creates doubt in the physician's mind.
4. Circumstantial undesirability—the patient arrives late, the chart or laboratory studies are not available, the physician is tired or ill.
5. Distraction undesirability in which the patient presents a medical problem outside the expertise or interest of the physician.

Any of these other forms of undesirability may interfere with adequate patient study, care, or concern; both patient and physician suffer. Labeling that patient rather than providing a meaningful diagnosis may be the result.

PSYCHOLOGICAL TESTING IN PATIENTS WITH CHRONIC PAIN

Pain has traditionally been considered a stimulus-evoked response with the response being equivalent to the stimulus. Relief of pain should therefore follow removal of the noxious stimulus. Repeated stimuli over time, however, modifies, diminishes or eliminates the relationship of time to stimulus and the response becomes dependent upon other factors.[2]

Through generalized stimuli, sensations similar to the original noxious stimulus acquire the ability to elicit a pain response. These stimuli are then considered to be *conditioned* and *learned*. The pain response loses its correspondence with the original stimulus, which was *unconditioned* and becomes a response to a variety of stimuli[43] not necessarily similar to the original.

The phenomenon of pain can be conceptualized as a *behavior* controlled by the initial unconditioned (pathologic) stimulus and conditioned (ecologic) stimuli that follow.[44] Tissue pathology initiates the noxious stimulus that is transmitted throughout all neural mechanisms following which a given pain behavior evolves.

Pain must be measured to achieve objective documentation, verification, and quantification of the emotional and psychologic aspects influencing the complaint of pain, especially chronic complaints. The usual index of pain, that is, the patient's verbal report, is a poor correlation of pathology with subjective complaint.

In a patient with minimal objective findings, measurement remains a significant concern to practitioners treating the patient with pain. A confirmable and reproducible "Pain Indicator" has been and continues to be sought. A physiologic indicator that quantifies verbal reporting is the quest of algologists. Some sort of "dolorimeter" is needed.[45]

There are several potential uses for psychologic testing:[46]

1. Screening of patients considered to have a large psychologic component of their complaints of pain
2. Affirming and confirming precise psychiatric diagnosis
3. Acquiring a basis for appropriate treatment protocol
4. Initiating a research program
5. Giving a base for outcomes assessment of treatment modalities and protocols. Long-term follow-up has been lacking in most recommended procedures.

Numerous tests for substantiating and quantifying pain are being reported in the literature. Only a few of these tests will be discussed here because all have some validity, level of acceptance, and worth as outcomes assessments. Any test must be used carefully to diagnose a patient with pain. The initial assumption of the existence of a psychologic basis, which may then be therapeutically pursued, must be validated; treatment, as well as diagnosis, must not be based solely on the outcome of such a test.

Treatment that ensues from the interpretation of any test must also be based on the age, sex, cultural background, educational level, and potential secondary gains, including economic (e.g., litigation), as well as acceptance by the patient. The competence of the therapist must be measured, as well.

A test that has had acceptance for many years is the MMPI (Fig. 15–2).[47] This test has a self-administered true-and-false format. It consists of either a 550-question form or an abbreviated 399-question form. The test, in its original form, had statements requiring an answer of "true or false." The test is computer-scored and computer interpreted. It is a checklist of physical and emotional symptoms, both at the time of examination and in the past.

Scores vary in patients with acute pain and those with chronic pain. In the latter, patients score lower in hypochondriasis (HS), depression (D), and hysteria (Hy), whereas patients in acute pain score higher in hypochondriasis (Hs) and hysteria (Hy). Because patients with both acute and chronic pain are preoccupied with the significance of their pain they express agitation (i.e., elevated Ma score), which mitigates when the pain becomes chronic, and depression (D) rises.

Rejection of the MMRI test was based on the fact that the study group used to determine normal or average behaviors was not a good cross-section of the general public. The original group had 700 men and women, all white and all residents of Minnesota. The average members of the group interviewed were semi-skilled workers or farmers with an eighth grade education. The phrasing of the statements was considered awkward and unclear. Many topics such as drug abuse, alcoholism, and suicidal tendencies were not addressed. The revised MMRI-2 corrected these flaws and now consists of 567 items,

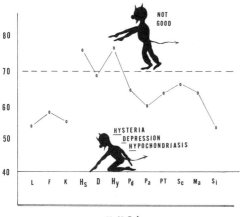

M. M. P. I.

Figure 15–2. Minnesota Multiphasic Personality Inventory.

which include a post-traumatic stress scale and a gender role scale; this revision is being evaluated to determine its efficacy.

In evaluating an MMPI scale, the physician cannot determine whether the scores were elevated before or after onset of chronic pain.[48] Another disadvantage is the length of time needed for the patient to take the test and the differing interpretation placed on its scores by psychologists.

The Eysenck personality test (EPI) measures mental stability versus neurosis and introversion versus extroversion.[49] This test primarily indicates the stability of the patient's reaction to stress and the tendency for the patient to break down. A direct relationship of susceptibility to the N score exists. A high N score does not indicate neurosis but merely susceptibility; it indicates an introverted person. Extroverts allegedly complain more freely than introverts but have a higher threshold to pain. The EPI test is not of as much help in therapy as it is in evaluating the patient's susceptibility to decompensate under stress.

The Beck Depression Inventory[50] test consists of 21 items, is self administered and can be taken in 5 minutes. Each item relates to a factor connected with depression but not to other psychologic factors that may aggravate pain.

Hendler[51,52] proposed an excellent test validating the complaint of chronic pain but it has been used only for low back pain. Its value to substantiate other types of chronic pain, such as that likely to result from surgical successful intervention in low back pain, remains untested.[53]

An approach to pain estimate has been advocated by Brena and Koch[44] in which pain (i.e., noxious stimulus) is held constant with the type of categorized pathology; the recorded pain response from which the relative pain behavior is calibrated.

In this model, objective pain is based on a physical examination, radiologic studies, and laboratory studies which, in themselves, cannot be fully accepted as purely "objective." Pain assessment is in turn based on (1) semantic inventory; (2) activities checklist; (3) drug use rating scale; and (4) MMPI results. On the basis of these findings, a rating is derived to relate objective damage to the degree of expressed pain. Just as the objective evaluation of significant pathology is questionable, so too are the factors of pain assessment—the semantics of pain inventory as verbalized by the patient and interpretation of the MMPI results by the physician are its variables. What is pertinent and valuable in this model is measuring the activities that remain possible "in spite of pain" and before resorting to drugs. The scale that documents this model is depicted in Fig. 15–3.[44]

All numeric components in the model have a derivation which can be acquired in the proposal. Each component, such as the semantic inventory, is numbered, as are the activity checklist, the drug rating scale, and the MMPI. All are obviously variable and most are also subjective.

The strong emotional component of any significant pain and the proportion of the emotional component frequently remains obscure, often to the

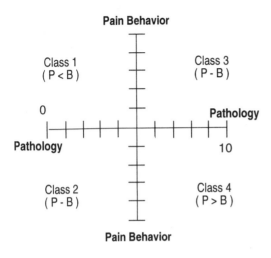

Figure 15–3. Emory University Pain Clinic "Pain Estimate Chart." (From Brena, SF and Koch, DL: A "pain estimate" model for quantification and classification of chronic pain states. Anesthesiology Review 2:8, 1975.)

detriment of the patient and to the frustration of the therapist. Cultural and educational factors in today's society imply potential ominous sequelae of any pain with possible mitigating psychologic involvement.

That psychologic factors are prevalent in patients complaining of orofacial pain is the conclusion of this relationship in the psychiatric-psychologic medical literature. The International Association for the Study of Pain (IASP) and the American Psychiatric Association (APA) both have classified orofacial pain as having psychogenic origin. The IASP literature asserts that orofacial pain is psychogenic only if no known physical cause or pathologic function can account for the pain and if other contributing factors are undeniably present.[53] The APA originally[54] classified orofacial pain as a "psychogenic pain disorder" and later[55] redefined it as a "somatoform pain disorder." This variation may also be applied to pain from soft tissue.

Considering these claims and implications, it is evident that many soft tissue pains, as subjective complaints, with little, if any, confirmatory, objective findings, tend to be labeled psychogenic. Failure of the patient to respond to what is considered appropriate treatment lends further support to a psychogenic basis for pain rather than an organic basis. Accusation, rather than diagnosis, ensues. Pain becomes chronic, resilient, and intractible. Inappropriate exotic treatments are pursued in search of another solution that fails and thus further frustrates the patient.

Patient-physician rapport and communication are the keystone of appropriate examination, diagnosis, and treatment. "Listening" to the complaint and interpreting it properly is the initial basis of diagnosis and the beginning of effective treatment. The examiner should have knowledge of the presence of the underlying psychologic aspect of any, if not all, pain complaints, especially when evaluating soft tissue pain.

The use of understandable "words" in explaining the cause and effects of a patient's pain is mandatory. It can never be denied that a patient's cooperation in receiving benefit from any treatment begins with the patient's clear understanding of the problem. The presence of a psychologic component to the acceptance of pain—either causative or as an aggravation—can and must be conveyed to the patient. Its acceptance is the beginning of relief and even cure.

The validity of psychologic testing has not been demeaned but its proportion of etiology needs clarification before a treatment protocol is initiated and evaluated. In too many chronic pain centers, the psychologic aspect is stressed even where it is not used to the exclusion of other modalities. *The* exact psychologic test remains to be accepted and management of *the* psychologic abnormality needs to be outcomes assessed. Use of a standard test and conventional treatment protocol, regardless of "specific" diagnosis for the individual, inevitably will lead to failure.

SECONDARY GAIN CONCEPT

Nowhere is the term **secondary gain** so rampantly used than in therapy for pain and disability resulting from soft tissue disorders. In a recent article, Fisbain[56] noted the term secondary gain was mentioned in 163 articles by authors of various specialties and disciplines.

The definition of secondary gain, however, remains unclear. Whether it is consciously or unconsciously motivated remains undetermined; its relationship with malingering needs clarification. Even the concept of malingering remains undefined; it is unaccepted by some physicians.

Gain was first noted as a psychoanalytic concept by Freud in 1917,[57] who described two types of gain from illness: primary and secondary. He defined primary gain "as a decrease in anxiety brought about through a defensive operation that had resulted in the production of the symptom of the (an) illness." He termed this **intrapsychic**. Freud considered secondary gain as "an interpersonal (social) advantage attained by the patient as a consequence of the illness."

Barsky[58] also defined primary gain as "a reduction in intrapyschic conflict and the partial gratification accomplished by the defense operation." He defined secondary gain as "acceptable or legitimate interpersonal advantages that result when one has the symptoms of a physical disease." DSM-III-R[55] defined primary gain as "the gain achieved from generating conversion symptoms that results in keeping an internal conflict or need out of awareness." Secondary gain was defined as "gain achieved from the 'conversion' symptom in avoiding a particular activity that was noxious to the patient or enabled the patient to get support from the environment that might otherwise be forthcoming, or both."

Freud and Barsky related gain to illness, whereas DSM-III–R relates specifically to a conversion disorder. Both primary and secondary gain are considered to result from unconscious mechanisms.[58–60]

Tertiary gains were described and defined by Dansak[61] as gains sought or attained by someone other than the patient from the patient's illness.

The operant conditioning concept claimed that "reinforcers" enhanced the concept of gain.[29,62] Operant behaviors were considered as "rewards" that maintained and promoted chronic pain behavior. Some of these behaviors were:

1. Rest, excessive and inappropriate
2. Relief from pain including medications taken as needed
3. Avoidance of responsibility
4. Compensation, including financial compensation
5. Avoidance of sexual activities
6. Approval and justification from physician
7. Pending litigation and its rewards
8. Little job satisfaction before injury and consequent avoidance of work
9. Poor relationship with employer

The relationship between secondary gain concept and operant reinforcers has never been clearly defined. Fordyce[62] believes that although reinforcers can maintain pain behavior, they do not necessarily produce that behavior and further believes that reinforcers do not necessitate real or imaginary pain. Fordyce's theory is that observed behavior is merely a response to reinforcers, whereas psychodynamic gains have an unconscious meaning and motivation. Cameron[63] claims that secondary gains are the result of a neurotic process and not its cause. It is apparent that the relationship between secondary gains and reinforcers remains unclear.

If a patient responds from secondary gains, the subsequent behavior generally results in secondary losses.[64]

Some of these losses are:

1. Loss of earnings
2. Loss of meaningful social relationships
3. Loss of recreational activities
4. Loss of community approval
5. Guilt over disability
6. Social stigma

The secondary gain concept unfortunately has been associated with malingering. According to recent definitions, the presence of unconscious secondary gain is a somatoform disorder and not an example of malingering. Also confusing the issue is the fact that financial rewards are often associated with disability.[65] The mere presence of litigation or disability benefits can be considered as secondary gain. The medical profession has done very little to resolve the problem,[66] stressing mostly secondary loss and not secondary gain, in fact defining secondary gain as "whatever advantages the patient gets out of being neurotic, once his neurosis has been established."[63]

Chronic pain patients are usually only *sick* for a short time, after which they develop their subsequent impairment and disability, which becomes a *disability role*. The *sick-role* concept now differs from the disablement concept. Studies have not been published to determine whether secondary gain necessarily has an etiologic or a reinforcing effect on the chronic pain.

The conscious-unconscious dichotomy regarding secondary gain is critical to establish a clear definition. This is particularly true of patients involved in litigation.[67]

Fishbain[56] states that "at issue is whether secondary gain concept should not be entirely abandoned until there is objective scientific study data that supports the concept." This concept must become a diagnosis and not be an accusation or inference of malingering.

Secondary gain may help or harm the patient[68] because there are unanswered terms of insinuation such as **unfulfilled dependency** or **unconscious motivation**, which may be difficult to define.

The concept of *advantage of illness* relates loosely to the secondary gain concept. **Advantage** was used by Freud,[69] when he used that term rather than "gain." He further stated that "yet another kind of advantage" of illness exists that supervenes later than that borne with the initial symptoms.

Observed reinforcers are suggested to represent "rewards for secondary gain behaviors or perceptions"[70] which rewrites the definitions of operant psychology.[29] Fishbain concluded that the secondary concept was abused and problematic and should thus be "buried." It has instead infiltrated every aspect of medicine, especially disciplines dealing with pain. The concepts of conscious and unconscious motivation remain unclear and largely unaccepted, because they have no treatment utility. The use of reinforcers probably has a clearer basis and may eventually replace the secondary gain concept.

In the consideration of the relationship between soft tissue pain and disability, because it often lacks definition and acceptance, much abuse and argument has come from physicians, insurers, attorney, and claims adjusters. Only the patient, however, is experiencing suffering.

REFERENCES

1. Brom, B: Corticalization of chronic pain. APS Journal 3:131–135, 1994.
2. Melzack, R: The Puzzle of Pain. Basic Books, New York, 1973.
3. Melzack, R: Psychological Concepts and Methods for the Control of Pain. Advances in Neurology, vol 4. Raven Press, New York, 1974, pp 275–280.

4. Melzack, R and Casey, KL: In (ed.): The Skin Senses. Charles C Thomas, Springfield, Ill., 1968, p 423.
5. Beecher, HK: Measurement of Subjective Response. Oxford University Press, New York, 1959.
6. Turk, DC, Wack, JT, and Kerns, RD: An empirical examination of the "pain behavior" construct. J Behav Med 8:119–130, 1985.
7. Sternbach, RA: Acute versus chronic pain. In Wall, PD and Melzack, R (eds): Textbook of Pain. Churchill Livingstone, London, 1984, p 606.
8. Flor, H and Birbaumer, N: Acquisition of chronic pain: Psychophysiological mechanisms. APS 3:119–127, 1994.
9. Flor, H, Birbaumer, N, and Turk, DC: A diathesis-stress model of chronic back pain: Empirical evaluation and therapeutic implications. In Gerber, WD, Miltner, W, and Mayer, K (eds): Behavioral Medicine: Results and Perspectives of Empirical Research. Edition Medizin, Weinheim, 1987.
10. Flor, H, Turk, DC, and Birbaumer, N: Assessment of stress-related psychophysiological reactions in chronic back pain patients. J Consult Clin Psychol 53:354–364, 1985.
11. Borgeat, F, Hade, B, Elie, R, and Larouche, LM: Effects of voluntary muscle tension increases in tension headaches. Headache 24:199–202, .
12. Christensen, LV: Physiology and pathophysiology of skeletal muscle contraction. Part I, Dynamic activity. J Oral Rehabil 13:451–461, 1986.
13. Christensen, LV: Physiology and pathophysiology of skeletal muscle contraction. Part II, Static activity. J Oral Rehabil 13:463–477, 1986.
14. Backonja, M and Miletic, G: Somatosensory cortical neurons on mononeuropathy model. Soc Neurosci Abst 19:1074, 1993.
15. Kenshalo, DR Jr and Willis, WD, Jr: The role of the cerebral cortex in pain sensations. In Jones, PA (ed): EG: Cerebral Cortex. Plenum Press, New York, 1991, pp 153–212.
16. Donaldson, S, Romney, D, Donaldson, M, and Skubick, D: A Single Blind Randomized Study of the Application of SMU Training Principles to Chronic Low Back Pain personal contact (1994). Publication pending.
17. Brena, SF: Chronic Pain: America's Hidden Epidemic. Atheneum, New York, 1978.
18. Linton, SJ, Althoff, B, Melin, L, et al: Psychological factors related to health, back pain, and dysfunction. J Occup Rehabil 4:1–10, 1994.
19. Frymoyer, JW: Predicting disability from low back pain. Clin Orthop Rel Res 279:101–109, 1992.
20. Jensen, MP and Karoly, P: Pain-specific beliefs, perceived symptoms severity, and adjustment to chronic pain. 8:123–130, 1992.
21. Keefe, FJ and Williams, DA: Assessment of pain behaviors. In Turk, DC and Melzack, R (eds): Handbook of Pain Assessment. Guilford Press, New York, 1992, pp 275–294.
22. Truner, JA, Robinson, J and McCreary, CP: Chronic low back pain: Predicting response to nonsurgical treatment. Arch Phys Med Rehabil 64:560–563, 1983.
23. Jensen, MP, Turner, JA, Romano, JM, and Karoly, P: Coping with chronic pain: A critical review of the literature. Pain 47:249–283, 1991.
24. Feuerstein, M and Thebarge, RW: Perceptions of disability and occupational stress as discriminators of work disability in patients with chronic pain. J Occup Rehabil 1:185–195, 1991.
25. Kemmlert, K and Lundholm, L: Factors influencing ergonomic conditions and employment rate after an occupational musculoskeletal injury. J Occup Rehabil 4:11–21, 1994.
26. Tarasuk, V and Eakin, JM: Back problems are for life: Perceived vulnerability and its implications for chronic disability. J Occup Rehabil 4:55–64, 1994.
27. Gorman, JM: The Essential Guide to Psychotropic Drugs, St. Martin's Press, New York, 1990.
28. Keefe, FJ and Dunsmore, J: Pain behavior: Concepts and controversies. APS Journal 1:92–100, 1992.
29. Fordyce, WE: Behavioral Methods for Chronic Pain and Illness. CV Mosby, St. Louis, 1976.

30. Keefe, FJ and Hill, RW: An objective approach to quantifying pain behavior and gait patterns in low back pain patients. Pain 21:153–161, 1985.
31. Follick, MJ, Ahern, DK, and Aberger, EW: Development of an audio-visual taxonomy of pain behavior: Reliability discriminate validity. Health Psych 4:555–568, 1985.
32. Turk, DC, Wack, JT, and Kerns RD: An empirical examination of the "pain behavior" construct. J Behav Med 8:119–130, 1985.
33. Keefe, FJ: Behavioral measurements in pain. In Chapman, CR, and Loeser, JD (eds): Advances in Pain Research and Therapy. Raven Press, New York, 1989.
34. Craig, KD: The facial expression of pain. Better than a thousand words? Focus. APS J 1:153–162, 1992.
35. Johnson, M: Assessment of clinical pain. In Jacox, AK (ed): Pain: A Source Book for Nurses and Other Health Professionals. Little, Brown, Boston, 1977, pp 130–166.
36. Rosenthal, R: Skill in nonverbal communication: individual differences. Oelgesschlager, Gunn & Hain, Cambridge, Mass., 1979.
37. Max, MB, Portenoy, RK, and Laska, EM (eds.): The Design of Clinical Trials: Advances in Pain Research and Therapy, vol 18. Raven Press, New York, 1991.
38. Gracely, RH: Pain psychophysics. In Chapman, CR and Loeser, JD (eds): Issues in Pain Measurement. Raven Press, New York, 1989, pp 211–230.
39. Ekman, P and Friesen, W: Facial Action Coding System: a technique for the measurement of facial movement. Consulting Psychologists Press, Palo Alto, Calif., 1978.
40. LeResche, L and Dworkin, SF: Facial expressions of pain and emotions in chronic TMD patients. Pain 35:71–78, 1988.
41. Wiltse, LL and Rocchio, PD: Predicting Success of Low Back Surgery by the Use of Preoperative Psychological Tests. Presented at annual meeting of American Orthopedic Association, Hot Springs, Virginia, June 1973: to be published in J. Bone Jt. Surg.
42. Papper, S: The undesirable patient. Editorial. J Chron Dis 22:777–779, 1970.
43. Fordyce, WE, Fowler, RS, Lehman, JF, and Delateur, BJ: Some implications of learning in problems of chronic pain. J Chron Dis 21:179, 1968.
44. Brena, SF and Koch, DL: A "pain estimate" model for quantification and classification of chronic pain states. Anesth Rev, February 1975, 8–13.
45. Hardy, JD, Wolff, HG, and Goodell, H: Studies on pain: A new method for measuring pain threshold: Observations on spatial summation of pain. J Clin Invest 19:649, 1940.
46. Rome, HP, Harness, DM, and Kaplan, HJ: Psychological and behavioral aspects of chronic facial pain. In Jacobson, AL, and Donlon, WC (eds.): Headache and Facial Pain. Raven Press, New York, 1990.
47. Dahlstrom, WG, Welsh, GS, and Dahlstrom, LE: An MMPI Handbook, vol 1. University of Minnesota Press, Minneapolis, 1960.
48. Naliboff, BD, Cohen, MJ, and Yellen, AN: Does the MMPI differentiate chronic illness from chronic pain? Pain 13:333–341, 1982.
49. Bond, MR: Personality and Pain. Churchill Livingstone, Edinburgh, 1984, pp 45–50.
50. Beck, AT, Ward, CH, Mendelson, M, et al.: Arch Gen Psychiatry 4:561–571, 1961.
51. Hendler, NH: The four stages of pain. In Hendler, NH, Long, DM, and Wise, TN (eds): Diagnosis and Treatment of Chronic Pain. John Wright, PSG Publishing, Boston, 1982, pp 1–8.
52. Hendler, N, Viernstein, M, Gucer, P and Long, D: The Hendler Ten Minute Screen Test For Chronic Back Pain Patients. The Chronic Pain Treatment Center, The Johns Hopkins Hospital, Baltimore, 1978.
53. Mersky, H: Classification of chronic pain descriptions of chronic pain syndromes and definitions of pain terms. Pain 3(suppl):S1–S225, 1986.
54. American Psychiatric Association Committee on Nomenclature and Statistical Manual of Mental Disorders, ed 3. American Psychiatric Association, Washington D.C., 1980.
55. American Psychiatric Association: Diagnostic and Statistical Manual of Mental Disorders, ed 3, rev. American Psychiatric Association, Washington D.C., 1987.

56. Fisbain, DA: Secondary gain concept: Definition problems and its abuse in medical practice. APS J pp 3:264–273, 1994.
57. Freud, S: Introductory Lectures on Psychoanalysis (1917). Hogarth Press, London, 1959, pp 378–391.
58. Barsky, AJ and Klerman, GL: Overview: Hypochondriasis bodily complaints and somatic styles. Am J Psychiatry 140:273–282, 1983.
59. Colbach, EM: Hysteria again and again and again. Int J Offender Ther Comp Criminology 31:441–448, 1987.
60. Sarwer-Fonger, GJ and Dancy, TE: The psychodynamic basis of compensation: A contribution to the study of ego defenses. Can J Psychiatry 4:125–132, 1959.
61. Dansak, D: On the tertiary gain of illness. Compr Psychiatry 14:523–534, 1973.
62. Fordyce, WE, Fowler, RS, Lehmann, JF and DeLateur, BJ: Some implications of learning in problems of chronic pain. J Chron Dis 21:179–190, 1968.
63. Cameron, N: Personality Development and Psychopathology. Houghton Mifflin, Boston, 1963, pp 273–274.
64. Bienoff, J: Traumatic neurosis of industry. Industr Med Surg 15:109–112, 1946.
65. Finneson, BE: Modulating effect of secondary gain on the low back pain syndrome. Adv Pain Res Ther 1:949–952, 1976.
66. Thompson, DL: Secondary gain, a second look: Issues in counseling the industrially injured worker. NARPPS J News 6:59–63, 1991.
67. Weissman, HN: Distortions and deceptions in self-presentation: Effects of protracted litigation in personal injury cases. Behav Sci Law 8:67–74, 1990.
68. Gallagher, RM: Secondary gain in pain medicine. APS J 3:274–278, 1994.
69. Freud S: Introductory lectures on psycho-analysis, ed 2. Hogarth Press, London, 1937.
70. Whitehead, W and Kuhn, WF: Chronic pain: an overview. In Miller, TW (ed): Chronic Pain Vol 1, International Universities Press, Madison, WI, 1990, pp 5–48.

CHAPTER 16

Workers' Compensation

In the field of workers' compensation a prevalence of work-related musculoskeletal disorders may lead to disability. These causes are also related to the rising cost of insurance premiums, employer indemnity, and the cost of the incurred medical services themselves.

The prevalence of occupational musculoskeletal disorders (OMD) continues to increase because of repetitive motion factors, receiving the greatest (18%) concern in 1981 in Bureau of Labor statistics.[1] Among OMDs, low back and upper extremity disorders together account for 60% of total claims.[2] These and other OMDs are *soft tissue injuries* which is why they are being considered in this book.

PROBLEMS WITH THE SYSTEM

Standardized comprehensive health care, timely and easily accessible, of the injured worker is unfortunately not the case in most states. This is owing, in large part, to the failure of the medical delivery system to be aware of soft tissues, their mechanisms, their symptoms and physical findings and thus the inadequacy of treatment and appropriate recording.

Injured workers traverse through a complex adversarial system of legal and health care.[3] Many do not receive appropriate medical evaluation, treatment, and rehabilitation, even after waiting many weeks and even months before receiving whatever treatment they ultimately get. This delay compounds the problem by causing the injured worker to become angry, depressed, discouraged, dependent on drugs, and deconditioned, resulting in a diminished desire to return to work producing further physical impairment and susceptibility to reinjury. Tissue healing is delayed, if it is not aggravated, and the psychologic component results in chronic pain with persistence of disability.

With failure to benefit, or even receive adequate care for the sustained injury there is recourse to a second medical opinion termed **independent medical evaluation** (IME), which often interposes a second provider no more competent than the original. Failure to recognize soft tissue injury and the resulting impairment and disability often prevails in these IME reports.

Many medical reports regarding the incurred injury use terminology that if not meaningless is at least noninformative to the employer, the insurer, and the injured worker. Employers have a poor understanding of the diagnostic terminology, objective impairment and subsequent disability, expected outcomes, and time factors involved in the entire process. Treatment protocols are often based on relief of symptoms rather than recognizing and addressing *impaired function*.

Prevention is given scant concern; thus the cause of possible further injury has not been addressed. Rehabilitation, if it is taken into consideration, also often merely identifies symptoms rather than functions and thus incurs meaningless therapeutic modalities.

Preventive programs are also inadequate even when implemented. Cost saving programs on a case basis have indicated a benefit when appropriate, accepted, and implemented.[4]

Health-care costs associated with work-related injuries have increased more rapidly than other medical costs. Between 1980 and 1987, workers' compensation–related health-care costs rose by 150%, compared with a rise of 101% in overall health-care costs.[5,6]

The reason for this cost increase is difficult to estimate unless, as is claimed, injured workers as a group require more intense treatment, which finding is hard to explain. The allegation that injured workers are more demanding, less educated, less motivated, and more involved in psychosocial allied problems also needs investigation and confirmation.

Guidelines for diagnostic procedures and treatment are being developed in many states to decrease these exorbitant costs.[6] Comprehensive programs that include all pertinent factors are needed.[7] Many employers have neither disability management plans nor standardized health-care management protocols, especially for musculoskeletal disorders. Finally, no *objective* markers exist for quality assurance for treatments given the injured worker.

PROPOSED REMEDIES

Standards of health care for injured workers are indicated in the preceding chapters including those related to injuries to spine and extremities but should be codified into *standards* for consideration and use by all diagnostic and therapeutic personnel.

These standards should be based on a broad understanding of the etiology (mechanisms) of musculoskeletal pain, impairments, and resulting disabilities. These factors involve medical (orthopedic/neurologic), psychologic, and social demands. It becomes apparent, that in fully evaluating and addressing a worker disability claim, that this decision is not solely concerned with medical processes. Environmental, attitudinal, and behavioral factors may also initiate injury, prolong or intensify disability, and aggravate subsequent pain.

Terms of recovery must be defined and acceptable to both worker and employer. Keystone of this recovery is usually considered to be *return to work* with ramifications concerning return to the same work, similar but more limited work, or different work altogether.

Standards should be based on scientific data such as those developed by the Quebec Task Force on Spinal Disorders,[8] or the State of Minnesota Treatment Parameters.[9] These standards should preferably be derived from efforts by multidisciplinary groups which include physicians representing every specialty, physical therapists, chiropractors, psychologists, nurses, vocational rehabilitation counselors, insurance specialists, ergonomists, and even workers. To get such a multidisciplinary group together is a formidable task but one which would be beneficial.

Standardized diagnostic tests should be formulated. It is apparent in daily clinical practice that many diagnostic procedures such as computed tomographic (CT) scanning, magnetic resonance imaging (MRI), and electrodiagnostic procedures are often done without any significant purpose; too often the results of such tests constitute *the* diagnosis when they may reveal only an insignificant or an irrelevant condition. Diagnostic procedures should only be done to confirm what is suspected in the clinical diagnosis or to reveal a condition suspected during examination that has not otherwise been confirmed by the diagnostic procedures. Procedures such as thermograms and isokinetic muscle testing may have research significance but are currently of questionable clinical value. Value of the routine radiography is also to be deplored.

Treatment protocols are also being questioned as being placebos, that is, comforting but not therapeutic. Many treatment modalities are aimed at relieving pain and discomfort but have no bearing in restoring function. Many are also sufficiently passive that their implementation incurs both physical disuse and psychological debility in the patient.

The duration of therapy as well as finding the precise modality are also abused. Continuation of a questionable modality and its failure to achieve significant response must always be taken in consideration. Competent chiropractors and osteopaths condemn repeated "adjustments" over long periods without sustained benefit.

Prompt attention to the injured worker by a skilled and interested provider is always the norm. Delay of attention causes prolongation of impairment; delayed healing; imposition of disuse; muscle wasting; loss of flexibility, strength, and endurance; and psychologic deterioration. These matters have been discussed in Chapter 1.

Discouragement and disgust encourage litigation by the patient to correct the neglect. Failure to provide a meaningful and prompt report to the employer and the insurance carrier also contribute to the breakdown of appropriate care and rehabilitation.

Workplace safety must be addressed in all injuries to prevent their recurrence. Employers should be mandated to develop and implement a comprehensive prevention program that addresses the many factors leading to injuries of workers. The factors must include ergonomics, existing medical problems of workers, psychologic factors, socioeconomic factors, work environment, worker-employer relationship, and competence and awareness in supervisor-worker relationships.[10,11]

Programs should be investigated at each employer site and be consistent with workplace procedural protocols. These programs should follow the Occupation Safety and Health Administration's (OSHA) *Guidelines for Prevention of Occupational Musculoskeletal Disorders*.[12] After being initiated, outcomes assessment should be instituted to ascertain compliance and benefit.[13]

A favored concept of injury prevention has been the establishment of a *Back School*, in which the worker is trained in proper back mechanics in standing, bending, lifting, and squatting, wherein the psychologic aspect of proper function is emphasized. Numerous concepts and inclusions inform the *Back Schools* of the United Stated without outcomes' assessment of their efficacy and determination of which aspects are most efficient.[14]

Back schools are operated under the precept that workers accept responsibility for their own management to prevent injury. Most programs include training in functional anatomy, physical fitness, and nutrition. These courses emphasize stress management, coping with pain, relaxation, avoiding drug dependency, and maintaining job satisfaction. Schools vary in methodology from audiovisual education[15,16] to hands-on information.[17] Education may be preventive (primary) or preventive of recurrence (secondary).

The variations in outcomes' assessment are those of methodology involving pretest and posttest measurement, types of education, patient involvement, and job task designs. Most evaluations claim benefit from the institutions of these programs but do not quantify value in terms of time and financial benefit.

Ongoing education must be afforded the employer, the injured worker, and the worker who has returned to work. It is presumption, but accurate to avert that there should also be ongoing education of the insurance provider to update medical knowledge, and ensure effective adherence to protocols of treatment and documentation of procedures.

The choice of provider ought to be that of the injured worker and the employer, but such choice must be limited to complete trained physicians or therapists skilled in evaluating and treating whatever musculoskeletal impairment creates disability. Many competent, scrupulous, conscientious physicians and therapists skilled in their primary care capacities are unskilled, even if they are interested, in evaluation and management of many musculoskeletal lesions. Such care providers must be constantly re-educated and their skills and compliance reassessed.

Outcomes' assessment must be instituted, implemented, and constantly updated to ensure that the procedures advocated are effective, that costs are contained, and that acceptance by all parties is total.

DISABILITY AND IMPAIRMENT

Much of the confusion in evaluating the injured worker and the programs of prevention and care exists in confusion between the terms **disability** and **impairment**.[18]

The American Medical Association (AMA)[19] defines *impairment* as a medical concept involving a person's change in health status resulting from disease or illness. Impairment, thus, is a loss of, loss of use of, or derangement of any part, system, or function. *Disability* is a nonmedical phenomenon affecting the person's ability to function, thus essentially, it is a concept related to vocation. As defined by the AMA, disability is limiting loss or the absence of the capacity of an individual to meet personal, social, or occupational demands, or to meet statutory or regulatory requirements. "Disability may be caused by medical impairment or by non medical factors."[21]

Physicians are frequently asked "Can Mr. Smith work?" and "Is Mr. Smith totally or partially disabled?" The physician cannot answer these questions objectively. Only the injured person or the employer are in a position to do so. Most physicians cannot answer this question because no objective criterion exists to inform such decision.

Disability implying inability to perform a *specific* function depends upon a work-specific situation. A total finger amputation can permanently and totally disable a pianist, whereas it will not significantly impair a bus driver. The *impairment* is identical, whereas the disability resulting from it is totally different.

Only a few physicians have addressed this problem. McBride in 1956[20] initiated a Committee on Rating of Physical and Mental Impairment and helped to produce the AMA guidelines.[21,22]

Because of this difference, only appropriate employer intervention and definition can sufficiently clarify the situation to benefit the injured worker and to make the worker's treatment and rehabilitation meaningful. A Disability Management Program (DMP) must evolve.[21]

Besides the ability to work, being able to pursue the **Activities of Daily Living** (ADL) are important to the injured worker. These include:

1. Self care and personal hygiene including urination, defecation, brushing teeth, combing hair, dressing self, and eating

2. Communication including writing, typing, seeing, hearing, and speaking
3. Normal postures when standing, sitting, and lying down
4. Ambulation including climbing stairs
5. Traveling
6. Nonspecific hand activities such as grasping, lifting, tactile sensation
7. Sexual activities
8. Sleep to provide restoration of normal function
9. Ability to participate in social and recreational activities

These factors must be assessed in disability evaluation because they are pertinent to psychologic as well a physical rehabilitation.[16]

MEDICAL REPORT

As stated, the entire process of appropriate injured worker's care and rehabilitation demands a pertinent report to the employer and the insurer so that care is neither disrupted nor delayed. Contents of the report must include:

1. Narrative history of the event(s) and symptoms subsequently sustained
2. Relevant physical findings including supportive tests such as radiologic studies and laboratory studies, and their interpretation in *meaningful manner*
3. Assessment of current impairment and the relationship to resultant disability
4. Meaningful diagnosis
5. Recommended treatment, its basis, and expectation of outcome
6. Estimated expected date of recovery, full or partial, date of expected return to work and at which level of re-employment
7. Summary of the impact of the medical condition on the worker's lifestyle and employment. Prognosis as to extent of recovery, persistence of impairment and disability, expected response to treatment, consideration of possible need for rehabilitation, and vocational modification.

These guidelines must evolve into a standardized report concerning impairment, disability, treatment advocated, prognosis, and complicating factors.[19-24] Brevity must not sacrifice the need for detailed information needed by the worker, the employer, and the insurer.

ERGONOMIC APPROACHES FOR THE CLINICAL ASSESSMENT OF OCCUPATIONAL MUSCULOSKELETAL DISORDERS

Pain related to the musculoskeletal system is the most frequent cause of visits to the primary care provider.[25-27] The workplace can and does play a significant role in initiating, exacerbating, or maintaining pain and disability. A high percentage of occupational illnesses are related to damage to the tendons, tendon sheaths, related bones, muscles and nerves of the hands, wrists, elbows, arms, shoulders, low back, and legs; all are related to *soft tissue*.[1] These disorders are commonly associated with forceful exertions, awkward postures, and repetitive motions.[8,10,28,29]

As the current economic trend insists on return to work, emphasis on *recovery of function* is therefore stressed more often than complete pain relief.[30-32] Feuerstein in 1991[10] proposed a model of these broad factors:

1. Medical status of the individual (musculoskeletal, neurologic, and cardiovascular)
2. Physical capabilities (strength, endurance, flexibility, and aerobic capacity)
3. Work demands (biomechanical and psychologic)
4. Psychologic and behavioral factors (i.e., readiness to return to work)

As stated, these factors contribute to work disability and so each must be assessed. Unfortunately these factors are usually inadequately addressed in the consideration of pain and resultant disability. Most medical and psychologic factors have been addressed in previous chapters but the concept of work demands (i.e., ergonomics) needs emphasis.

Ergonomics has been defined[33] as "that branch of science and technology that includes what is known and theorized about human behavioral and biologic characteristics that can be validly applied to the specification, design, evaluation, operation and maintenance of products and systems to enhance safe, effective, satisfying use of individuals, groups and organizations."[31]

References abound in the literature regarding workplace factors;[34] they highlight the following factors:

1. Forceful exertions
2. Awkward work postures
3. Localized contact stresses
4. Whole body or segmental vibrations
5. Temperature extremes

6. Repetitive motions or prolonged activities
7. Psychosocial stresses[35] of the job

Forceful exertions are whole-body exertions involving the low back, arms, and legs in acts of lifting, pushing, and pulling an outside object. The size, weight, shape of the load, and position at beginning and end[36] of the task are all factored, with distance, speed, and frequency of motion into the equation.

The expectation of the person who exerts these efforts plays a major role because the person's mind must initiate the exertion needed to accomplish the intended task.[37] Lifting an object thought to be heavy will be damaging if the object actually weighs little or nothing, because too much effort will be used. Sudden unexpected maximal efforts have been shown to be harmful to the low back.[36]

Normal neuromusculoskeletal action is subjected to internal and external forces. Of the *internal* forces involved, *perturbers* have been suggested as impairing normal neuromusculoskeletal action. These perturbers include fatigue, distraction, anger, impatience, boredom, anxiety, and depression.[38]

Awkward postures have also been blamed for many neuromusculoskeletal disorders of the low back, knee, and upper extremities. For example, workers who labored with their hands above shoulder level (i.e., acromium) have a greater incidence of injuries compared with those whose hands are generally kept below that level.[39]

Awkward postures involving hand, shoulder, and finger disability are becoming prominent, as are localized contact stresses from manual positions in which the arms are not supported or doing construction work with instruments the ergonomics of which are nonphysiologic.[32]

Vibration (mechanical oscillations) have become incriminated in causing or contributing to musculoskeletal soft tissue injuries. These vibrations may involve the whole body or only one extremity. Their pathomechanics remain unclear. Temperature extremes have also been incriminated but much remains to be confirmed as their pathomechanisms.[40]

Damage from repetitive motions and sustained efforts are becoming a major concern in workplace injury and disability. All the harmful aspects of repetitive efforts remain, as yet, unclear, but undoubtedly they relate to fatigue, extreme metabolic demands,[41,42] and psychologic aspects.

Feuerstein and Hickey[25] feel there must be a bridging of understanding between classic ergonomics and the workplace, as well as in the clinic in evaluation of the disability, its prevention, and modification, both in the workplace as a whole, and in the work of the person in the workplace. Rehabilitation demands this knowledge so that *return to work* is feasible and that the subsequent job demands are realistic. Thus even though function is not totally restored, there is an implication all the other aspects of disability have been ameliorated.

REFERENCES

1. Bureau of Labor Statistics: Occupational Injuries and Illnesses in the United States by Industry. Bulletin 2379, U.S. Department of Labor, U.S. Government Printing Office, Washington, 1989.
2. Melles, T, McIntosh, G, and Hall, H: Provider, Payer, and Patient Outcome Expectations in Back Pain Rehabilitation. J Occup Rehabil 5:57–69, 1995.
3. Feuerstein, M: Workers' compensation reform in New York state: A proposal to address medical ergonomic, and psychological factors associated with work disability. J Occup Rehabil 3:125–134, 1993.
4. California Department of Insurance, Office of Policy Research: Lowering workers' compensation insurance costs by reducing injuries and illnesses at work. Sacramento, 1993.
5. Human Resources Development Canada: Occupational injuries and their cost in Canada 1988–1992. HRDC, Ottawa, 1993.
6. Wegner, JA: Treatment standards for work-related injuries. J Occup Rehabil 3:135–143, 1993.
7. Chaffin, DB and Fine, LJ (eds): A National Strategy for Occupational Musculoskeletal Injuries—Implementation Issues and Research Need. U.S. Department of Health and Human Services, Center for Disease Control and Prevention, National Institute for Occupational Safety and Health, DHHS (NIOSH) Publication No. 93-101, Washington, DC, 1993.
8. Spitzer, WO, Le Blanc, FE, and Dupuis, M: Scientific approach to the management and activity-related spinal disorders. Spine 12:7S, 1987.
9. State of Minnesota, Department of Labor and Industry: Emergency rules relating to workers' compensation: Treatment parameters. Minnesota Status Section 176:83, subdivision 5, parts 5221.6010 to 5221.8900.
10. Feuerstein MA: A multidisciplinary approach to the prevention, evaluation, and management of work disability. J Occup Rehabil 1:5–12, 1991.
11. Habeck RV, Leahy MJ, Hunt MA, et al: Employer factors related to workers compensation claims and disability management. Rehab Council Bull 34:210–226, 1990.
12. Department of Labor, Occupational Safety and Health Administration: Ergonomic safety and health management: Proposed rule 29CFR, Part 1910. Federal Register: 34192-34200, 1992.
13. Armstrong TJ, Buckle P, Fine LJ, et al: A conceptional model of work-related neck and upper limb musculoskeletal disorders. Scan J Work Environ Health 19:73–84, 1993.
14. King PM: Back injury prevention programs: A critical review of the literature. J Occup Rehabil 3:145–158, 1993.
15. Bergquist, M and Larsson, U: Acute low back pain in industry: A controlled prospective study with special reference to therapy and confounding factors. Acta Orthop Scand Suppl A70:97–110, 1977.
16. Hurri, H: The Swedish back school in chronic low back pain. Part II: Factors predicting the outcome. Scand J Rehab Med 21:41–44, 1989.
17. Mattmiller, AW: The California back school. Physiotherapy 66:118–121, 1980.
18. Walker, JM: The difference between disability and impairment: A distinction worth making. J Occup Rehab 3:167–172, 1993.
19. American Medical Association Guides to the Evaluation of Permanent Impairment, ed 3. American Medical Association, Chicago, 1988, p 236.
20. McBride, ED: Disability Evaluation: Principles of treatment of Compensable Injuries, ed 4. JB Lippincott, Philadelphia, 1948.
21. American Medical Association Committee on the Rating of Physical and Mental Impairment: Guides to the Evaluation of Permanent Impairment, ed 1. American Medical Association, Chicago, 1984.
22. American Medical Association Council on Scientific Affairs: Guides to the Evaluation of Permanent Impairment, ed 2. American Medical Association, Chicago, 1984.

23. Galvin, D, Habeck, R, and Kirchner, K: Leadership forum on disability management. Washington Business Group on Health, October 1992.
24. Walker, J: Injured worker helplessness: Critical relationships and systems levels appropriate for intervention. J Occup Rehab 2:201–209, 1992.
25. Feuerstein, M and Hickey, PF: Ergonomic approaches in the clinical assessment of occupational musculoskeletal disorders. In Turk, DC and Melzack, R (eds): Handbook of Pain Assessment. Guildford Press, New York, 1992 pp 71–99.
26. Deyo, RA and Tsui-Wu, YJ: Descriptive epidemiology of low back pain and its related medical care in the United States. Spine 12:264–268, 1987.
27. Knapp, DA and Koch, H: The management of new pain in office-based ambulatory care. National Ambulatory Medical Care Survey. 1980 and 1981. National Center for Health Statistics. Advance data from Vital and Health Statistics, No. 97 (DHHS Pub. No. PHS 84-1250). Public Health Service, Hyattsville, 1984.
28. Chaffin, DB and Andersson, GBJ: Occupational Biomechanical Models, ed 2. Wiley Interscience, Philadelphia, 1991.
29. Putz-Anderson V (ed): (1988) Cumulative trauma disorders—A manual for musculoskeletal diseases of the upper limbs. Taylor and Francis, Philadelphia, 1988.
30. Mayer TG, Gatchel RJ, Mayer H, et al: A prospective two-year study of functional restoration in industrial low back injury. JAMA 258:1763–1767, 1987.
31. Cannon, IJ, Bernacki, EJ, and Walter, SD: Personal and occupational factors associated with carpal tunnel syndrome. J Occup Med 23:255–262, 1981.
32. Mitchell, RI and Carmen, GM: Results of multicenter trial using an intensive active exercise program for the treatment of acute soft tissue and back injuries. Spine 15:514–521, 1990.
33. Christensen, JM, Miller, DA, and Gill, RT: Human factors definitions revisited. Human Factors Society Bulletin 31:7–8, 1988.
34. Keyserling, WM, Armstrong, TJ, and Punnett, L: Ergonomic job analysis: A structured approach for identifying risk factors associated with overexertion injuries and disorders. Appl Occup Environ Hygiene 6:353–363, 1991.
35. Feuerstein, M, Sult, S, and Houle, M: Environmental stressors and chronic low back pain. Life events, family and work environment. Pain 22:295–307, 1985.
36. Magora, A: Investigation of the relationship between low back pain and occupation: III. Physical requirements: Sitting, standing and weight lifting. Indust Med Surg 4:5–9, 1972.
37. Cailliet, R: Low Back Pain Syndromes, ed 5. FA Davis, Philadelphia, 1995.
38. Cailliet, R: Pain: Mechanisms and Management. FA Davis, Philadelphia, 1993, p 102.
39. Byelle, A, Hagberg, M, and Michaelsson, G: Clinical and ergonomic factors in prolonged shoulder pain among industrial worker. Scand J Work Environ Hlth 5:205–210, 1979.
40. Grandjean, E: Fitting the task to the man: A textbook of occupational ergonomics. Philadelphia: Taylor and Francis, 1988.
41. U.S. Government Printing Office, U.S. Department of Labor, Dictionary of Occupational Titles (ed 4), Washington, DC, 1977.
42. Astrand, PO and Rodahl, K: Textbook of Work Physiology, ed 3. McGraw-Hill, New York, 1986.

CHAPTER 17

Neuromusculoskeletal Basis of Soft Tissue Pain and Impairment

Soft tissue pain, impairment, and disability has been discussed in this book as related to every specific organ system in the body. A generalization, however, is pertinent to associating all organ systems using a common denominator. The process by which the tissues within an organ system are traumatized, injured, or inflamed must be considered.

All soft tissues—muscles, ligaments, tendons, joint capsules, and even articular surfaces (cartilage)—depend on normal neurophysiologic function (Fig. 17–1). When impairment and dysfunction (Fig. 17–2) with resultant tissue structural damage are present, an indication that *neuromusculoskeletal* function was altered in a soft tissue injury may be assessed.[1]

Neuromuscular function imposed on anatomic structures of the moving part, that is, joints of the shoulder, elbow, and knee and the intervertebral disks of the cervical and lumbar spine (Fig. 17–3) must assume these structures to be normal, that is, that the articular cartilages secrete normal lubricant, that the capsules have adequate elasticity, and that the intervertebral disks have adequate hydration. Faulty *neuromuscular* activity causes equally faulty anatomic articular soft tissue motion with potential anatomic structural damage (Figs. 17–4 and 17–5) causing nociceptive (painful) impulses (Fig. 17–6) that further mitigate subsequent proper neuromuscular action.

The neurophysiology of normal motor control is well understood, albeit not yet completely documented. A motor neuron and all its target muscle fibers together are termed a **motor unit**. The largest motor units involve the

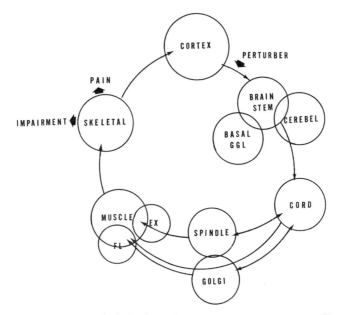

Figure 17–1. Neuromusculoskeletal mechanism. An activity is normally initiated within the cerebral cortex. Impulses pass through the midbrain and are coordinated by the cerebellum (cerebel) and the basal ganglia to the cord. The cord neurons activate the specific muscles performing the activity, which are coordinated by the spindle system and the Golgi apparatus. The muscles are divided into flexors (FL) and extensors (EX) with reflex reciprocal inhibition. The muscles activate the skeletal system to perform the required act. Perturbers can impair the sequence, which causes malfunction and impairment with resultant pain. These perturbers are numerous and include impatience, anxiety, anger, depression, fatigue, improper training, faulty ergonomics, and so on. The faulty skeletal activity that results causes mechanical dysfunction and skeletal (soft tissue) impairment with structural changes. Pain and disability result.

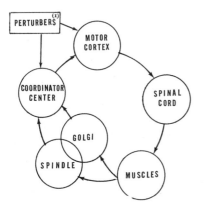

Figure 17–2. Perturber influence on neuromuscular mechanisms. The normal neuromuscular sequence of activity originating at the motor cortex transmitted to the muscle through the spinal cord, coordinated from feedback by the Golgi and spindle systems can be impaired by perturbers. Some of the perturbers are anxiety, fatigue, anger, distraction, and depression (see text).

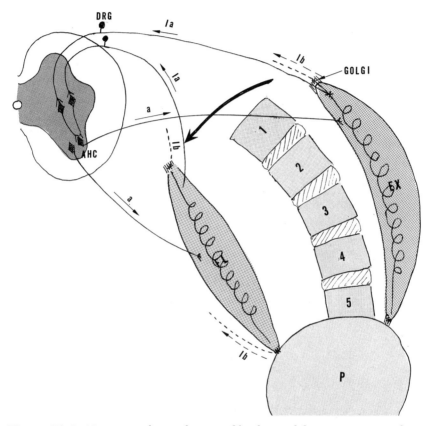

Figure 17–3. Neuromuscular mechanism of lumbosacral function. As a specific example of neuromusculoskeletal function as depicted in Figure 17–1, the lumbosacral
spine (pelvis [P], and 1–5 lumbar vertebrae) is depicted in flexion (*large curved arrow*). Flexion is activated by the abdominal flexors (FL) with the erector spinae extensors (EX) decelerating the action and reciprocally relaxing as the flexors are activated.
Action is coordinated by neural reflexes via the spindle system (*Ia*), the Golgi organs via
Ib, through a single synapse in the cord to the anterior horn cells (AHC) that activates
the extrafusal muscle fibers through *a* fibers. The dorsal root ganglia is intermediate to
the sensory (proprioceptive) impulses.

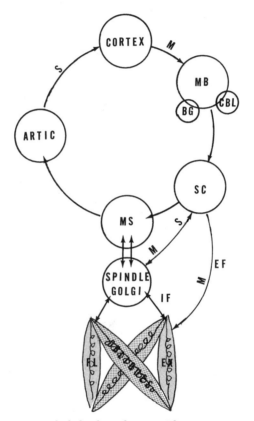

Figure 17–4. Neuromusculoskeletal mechanism: Flexion-extension and obliques. As most articular functions (ARTIC) subserved by muscular (MS) contractions cause flexion (FL) and extension (EX), there is also usually rotational forces subserved by the oblique muscles. The neurologic mechanism described in Fig. 17–1 is shown: the CORTEX initiates the plan and evokes motor (M) patterns, which are coordinated at the midbrain (MB) with the basal ganglia (BG) and cerebellum (CBL). These impulses are transmitted to the spinal cord (SC) where the muscles (MS) are innervated. The spindle system and the Golgi apparatus precisely coordinate the extrafusal muscle (EF) fibers via motor fibers. The intrafusal fiber (IF) are both motor (M) and sensory (S) to the spindle and Golgi systems. Appropriate strength, length, and speed of muscle contraction with reciprocal relaxation (agonist-antagonist) results.

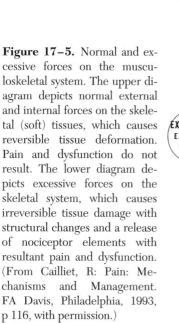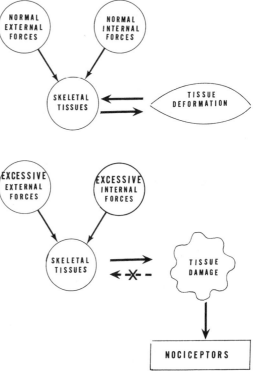

Figure 17–5. Normal and excessive forces on the musculoskeletal system. The upper diagram depicts normal external and internal forces on the skeletal (soft) tissues, which causes reversible tissue deformation. Pain and dysfunction do not result. The lower diagram depicts excessive forces on the skeletal system, which causes irreversible tissue damage with structural changes and a release of nociceptor elements with resultant pain and dysfunction. (From Cailliet, R: Pain: Mechanisms and Management. FA Davis, Philadelphia, 1993, p 116, with permission.)

greatest number of muscle fibers, thus drawing on the largest nerve cell bodies within the central nervous system (CNS).

There is thus a simple tenet—the *size principle*—[2] that determines the number of motor units recruited to achieve a specific activity. Mostly smaller and less excitable motor unit neurons are *turned on* with less stimulus by small adjustments in the number of muscle fibers activated.

These small motor units are made up of red muscle fibers with high density of mitochondria and high fatigue resistance because they are *on* a large proportion of the time. Large motor units that are *turned on* for brief, but forceful, activity are mostly white or pink muscle fibers capable of high velocity and force for short periods. Such muscle fatigues more easily. Recruitment between these units is usually well coordinated.

Normal function of the intended act is initiated at the cortical level (see Fig. 17–1), which determines the type and degree of stimulation of the needed motor units necessary to complete that act. Excessive force causes im-

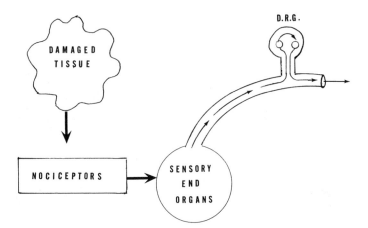

Figure 17–6. Sequence of tissue damage creating nociceptors. Tissue that has been damaged liberates chemical nociceptors, which stimulate the end organs of sensory nerve fibers, unmyelinated C and A alpha. The nerve fibers in turn release impulses in the dorsal root ganglion (DRG), which progress to the Rexed layers of the cord gray matter.

pairment because repeated activities cause fatigue. Pain and impairment results from the violated tissues.

Conscious sensations are termed **exteroceptors**, whereas the sensation affecting motor function are unconscious and termed **proprioceptors**. These latter fibers are located in the skin and in most soft tissues. Those in ligaments help stabilize joints Those fibers in muscles help coordinate neuromuscular action and so are stretch receptors (spindle system) and Golgi tendon organs. The spindle system (Fig. 17–7) has already been specifically discussed and illustrated in its relationship with the specific organ systems of the body elsewhere in this book.

Because spindle system organs are attached at both ends of the main muscle mass, they undergo the same relative length changes as the muscle. Golgi tendon organs are usually found in the tendons themselves or where the muscle attaches to the tendon. Functionally, Golgi organs are force transducers, which measure muscle tension.

Nerve axons connecting these organ systems to and from the spinal cord are termed **afferent** (to the cord) (Fig. 17–8) and **efferent** (from the cord). Afferents enter the cord through the dorsal root ganglion. Afferent fibers are termed **I** and **II** based on their axon diameter and high conduction velocity. Those from the spindle systems are Ia and from the Golgi organs Ib. Efferent nerve fibers that originate within the cord are myelinated and termed **alpha (A)**.

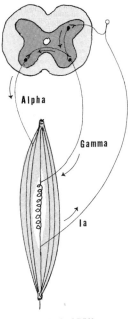

Figure 17–7. The spindle system. The spindle system (intrafusal fibers) elongate or shorten within extrafusal muscle fibers. It transmits proprioceptive information to the cord through Ia fibers that coordinate extrafusal muscle contraction through the alpha motor fibers. The spindle system is reset by impulses sent through the gamma fibers.

SPINDLE SYSTEM

STRETCH REFLEX

When an activated muscle is externally stretched, it contracts more completely than it had before it was stretched. It actually makes a greater effort to regain its original length. This is the *stretch reflex*. The length and tension are mediated (afferent) to the cord through the Ia and Ib fibers. These interact within the cord substance to the efferent (motor) nerve cell bodies through a single synapse; thus connection is very rapid.

Central interaction with the afferents of the agonist muscles allow the opposing (antagonist) muscles to relax reciprocally. Coordinated neuromusculoskeletal action ensues and automatically compensates for muscular fatigue.

Most, if not all, muscular actions are multidirectional. A rotatory component occurs in most joints, if such motion is violated, tissue damage results. Velocity and acceleration of normal activities have also been considered and are being studied to measure how pertinent they are in normal function.[3]

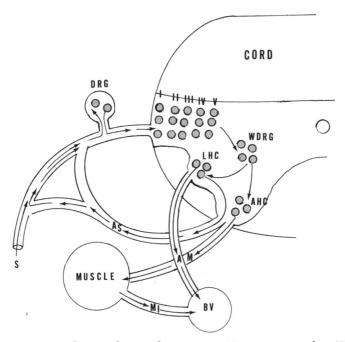

Figure 17–8. Neurologic pathways of nociception. Nociceptor impulses (S) arising from damaged tissues enter the Rexed layers I, II, III, IV, and V of the cord gray matter via afferent fibers of the dorsal root ganglion (DRG). Layers I and II are the substantia gelatinosum. Interneural fibers then transfer the impulses to the lateral spinal thalamic tracts (not shown) to the hypothalamus, limbic system, thalamus, and then to the cortex for interpretation. Nociceptive impulses transmit to the wide dynamic range ganglia (WDRG) where neurons transmit to the lateral horn cells (LHC) to initiate sympathetic autonomic response and to the anterior horn cells (AHC) to initiate motor response. The efferent fibers (A) from the lateral horn cells (LHC) innervate blood vessels (BV), sweat glands, and hair follicles (not shown). Afferent autonomic fibers transmit sensations (AS) to the WDRG. The skeletal muscles innervated by efferents (M) from the AHC cause protective segmental spasm. Persistent sustained contraction of the muscles initiate autonomic impulses to the blood vessels (MI) with resultant ischemia.

SUPRASPINAL MOTOR CENTERS

The spinal segment of neuromuscular system control is also moderated at a higher level (Fig. 17–9):[4] the brainstem, motor cortex, basal ganglia, and cerebellum. Each level processes and redirects incoming sensory information. The expected musculoskeletal function thus occurs with some expected physi-

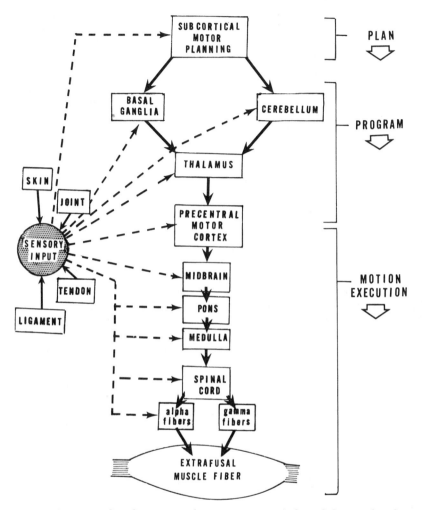

Figure 17–9. Spinal and supraspinal motor centers. (Adapted from Schmidt RF. Fundamentals of Neurophysiology. Springer-Verlag, New York, 1978.)

ologic fatigue but each end organ—joints, ligaments, capsules, and tendons—functions properly, efficiently, and painlessly.

Faulty function of this neuromuscular sequence ends in impairment of the end organs with attendant pain and dysfunction. Neuromuscular skeletal system impairment explains the mechanism by which soft tissue pain, impairment, and ultimately, disability occurs.[5] External forces (Fig. 17–10) are, of course, also a factor in causing soft tissue injury, but this finding is readily ascertained by taking an adequate history and seeking confirmation with radio-

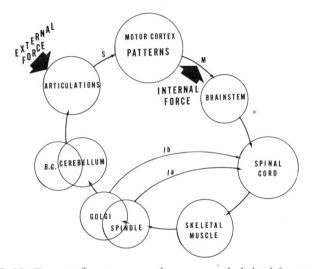

Figure 17–10. Forces influencing normal neuromusculoskeletal function. The neuromusculoskeletal patterns contained within the cortex and the brainstem (termed **neuromatrix**) are activated when a physical activity is contemplated. The motor action (M) activates the spinal cord efferents, which are monitored by the spindle system and the Golgi apparatus. The feedback mechanism to the cord is through the Ia and Ib fibers. The cerebellum and basal ganglia (BG) have already centrally coordinated the patterns. The final motor action results from musculotendonous action on the articular systems of the body with lever action. Sensory feedback (S) is from the joint capsules, tendons, and ligaments. Dysfunction occurs when there are abnormal or excessive external or internal forces imposed. Skeletal structures are deformed. (From Cailliet, R: Pain: Mechanisms and Management. FA Davis, Philadelphia, 1993, p 113, with permission.)

logic studies and bone scans. Internal forces are more difficult to measure, as regards mechanism of pain and cause of impairment.

Impaired *internal* neuromusculoskeletal function can thus occur at the cortical level with faulty expectations and inappropriate *job* action. Impairment of the intended action may also be altered by *perturbers*. Faulty ergonomics in the workplace also add distractions to the normal neuromusculoskeletal sequence.

Ultimately, it is the painful and impaired musculoskeletal component that brings the patient to the physician. Most tests are directed toward the damaged tissues, as is most treatment. Evaluation of the *neuro*musculoskeletal component ultimately divulges the factors that caused the condition and indicates appropriate treatment protocols to relieve symptoms, improve function, and prevent recurrences.

REFERENCES

1. McMahon, TA: Reflexes and motor control. In McMahon, TA: Muscles, Reflexes and Locomotion. Princeton University Press, Princeton, 1984, pp 139–167.
2. Henneman, E, Somjen, G, and Carpenter, D: Excitability and inhibitability of motorneurons of different sizes. J Neurobiol 28:599–620, 1965.
3. Marras, WS, Lavender, SA, Leurgans, SE, et al.: Biomechanical risk factors for occupationally reated low back disorders. Ergonomics 28:377–410, 1995.
4. Schmidt, RF: Motor Systems. In Schmidt, RF, (ed): Fundamentals of Neurophysiology, ed 2. Springer-Verlag, New York, 1978, pp 158–204.
5. Cailliet, R: Pain: Mechanisms and Management. FA Davis, Philadelphia, 1993.

Index

Page numbers followed by f indicates figures; page numbers followed by t indicates tables.

A-delta neurons, 22, 23, 149
Abdominal muscles, strength testing, 133–134,
    134f, 135f
Abduction
    forefoot, 449
    hip joint, 368, 371f
Abductor digiti quinti, 448
Abductor pollicis longus, 305, 306f, 319
Absolute stenosis of the lumbar spine (ASLC),
    159
Acetabulum, 362, 366f, 367
Acetylcholine, 40
Achilles tendon rupture, 464–465, 465f
Achondroplastic spinal stenosis, 159
Acquired spinal stenosis, 159
Acromioclavicular joint, 261, 289, 291, 292f,
    293
Acromium, 260–261, 271
Actin, 6, 65, 66
Active range of motion, cervical spine, 189,
    190f
Activities of daily living, 511–512
Acute pain
    compared to chronic pain, 34
    exercise and, 92
    foot, 443
    interrupting pathways of, 87
    psychologic aspects, 490
    treatment, 88
Adaptive supersensitivity, 51
Adduction
    forefoot, 449
    hip joint, 368
Adenosine triphosphate (ATP), 6, 74
Adenylate cyclase, 85
Adhesive capsulitis, 278, 278f, 279f
Adjustments, defined, 157
Adrenal gland, 41

Adrenergic blockade, 42
Adrenocorticotropic hormone (ACTH), 33, 93
Adson test, 244, 244f, 246, 247
Afferent nerves
    defined, 62, 522
    neuroanatomic physiology, 15, 26
    spindle cell: gamma system, 67, 69, 71
Agonist-antagonist action
    elbow, 307
    spindle cells, 62–63
    trunk/abdominal muscles, 118
    wrist and hand, 326
Agoraphobia, 492, 493–494
Alar ligament, 172, 176
Algodystrophy, 49, 471
Algogens, 16, 74, 76, 88, 149
Alpha-1 adrenoreceptors, hyperalgesia and,
    46–47, 47f
Alpha motor neurons, 67, 71, 522
Alpha receptors, 42
Alpha-training procedure, 490
Amine oxidase, 42
Amino acids, 28
Amygdala, defined, 84
Analgesics. *See also* Nerve blocks
    exercise and, 93
    pharmacologic sites of action, 36f
    physiologic basis, 28, 31, 84–86
Angle of anteversion, 362, 365f
Angle of inclination, 362, 364f
Anisotonic contraction, 7
Ankle injuries
    evaluation, 435–436
    mechanisms of, 433–435
    strains and sprains, 433–435
    stress fractures, 439
    subtalar joint, 439, 441
    treatment, acute injury, 436–437, 439

Ankle joint
   during gait, 455f
   functional anatomy, 428, 430f, 431f, 432f
   leg-ankle-foot RSD syndrome, 479–487
Annular fibers, intervertebral disk, 103, 107f,
      108f
Annulus fibrosus, 106f, 112, 195, 200f
Anterior cruciate ligament
   functional anatomy, 390, 396f
   injuries, 412, 413–415
Anterior foot, 428
Anterior horn cell (AHC), muscle spasm and,
      16, 19f
Anterior interosseous syndrome, 332, 333f
Anterior knee pain, 420–425
Anterior longitudinal ligament, 106, 109, 110,
      197
Anterior scalene syndrome, 246–248
Anterior stress test. See Drawer sign
Anterior talofibular ligament, 428
Antidepressants, 54, 75, 77–78, 86
Anxiety, 102, 492–495
AO joint. See Occipital-atlas joint
Apley test, 419, 421f
Apprehension test, 271, 277f
Arachidonic acid, 16, 71, 74
Arc slide, joint motion, 260f
Arcade of Struthers, 338
Arches, foot, 451, 453f
Arcuate ligament, 297, 298f
Arnold-Chiari syndrome, 174
Arthritis
   degenerative, 377–380, 382, 425f
   localized, 452
Arthroplasty, 380
Ascending sensory pathways, spinal cord, 21f
Ascending tracts, spinal cord, 20, 22f
Aspartic acid, 28
Ataxia, 179–180, 184
Athletics. See Repetitive strain injury
Atlantoaxial joint (C1–C2)
   clinical entities of, 194
   functional anatomy, 171–173, 184
   movement, 173f, 183, 184f, 191f
   occipital neuralgia, 174
Atlas (C1)
   clinical entities of, 194
   functional anatomy, 171
   ligaments, 172f
   movement, 172f
ATPase, muscle contraction and, 6
Audio analgesia, 490
Autonomic nervous system (ANS). See also
      Parasympathetic nervous system;
      Sympathetic nervous system
   compared to somatic, 37, 39f
   connection with somatic, 19–20, 62, 65f
   connective tissue, 2
   functional anatomy, 37–46, 38f

peripheral, transmission sequence, 39f
   spinal pain, role in, 113
Axis (C2), 172f, 194. See also Atlantoaxial joint
Axon reflex, 76
Axonal transport, 315, 316f, 327, 328f,
      473–474
Axonotmesis, 8

Babinski sign, 206
Back pain, 232. See also Low back pain; Lower
      cervical spinal complex; Upper cervical
      spinal complex
"Back schools," 510
Ballottement test, 410f
Baseball elbow, 300, 302
Beck Depression Inventory, 499
Benign aspect of pain, 490
Beta receptors, 42
Biofeedback, low back pain, 155
Black's molecular concept, pain perception, 33
Blind zone, cervical cord injury, 206–207, 207f
Blood flow
   lower extremity, 479, 482f
   therapeutic heat and, 90
Blood pressure, inactivity and, 11
Blood volume, inactivity and, 10
Body mechanics
   faulty, 120
   low back pain and, 92, 113–116, 114f, 115f,
      155
Bone mass, inactivity and, 11
Boutonniere deformity, 348, 349f
Braces
   application, standing/seated, 163f
   cervical, 210, 212f
   patellofemoral joint, 423f
   spinal stenosis, 161
   spondylolisthesis, 162
Brachial plexus
   anterior scalene syndrome, 246
   functional anatomy, 241f, 242f, 251f, 252f,
      253f
   injuries, 251–254
   thoracic outlet syndrome, 239, 240, 243
Brachial plexus compression (BP test), 255
Brachial plexus traction test (BPTT), 245f,
      245–246
Bradykinin, as nociceptor, 15, 74, 88, 149
Brain
   injury, with whiplash, 205
   pain perception and, 32–34
   ventricular system, 42, 42f
Brisement, 281, 288f
Bruxism, 219
"Bucket handle" meniscus tear, 417
Bunions, 452
Burning pain. See Causalgia
Bursitis, elbow, 302

Calcaneocuboid joint, 449
Calcium, 6, 65, 66
Callus formation, 453, 454
Cancer, pain of, 16
Canes/crutches, use of
    ankle injuries, 437, 439
    degenerative arthritis, hip, 378
    weight bearing, hip joint, 375, 375f
Capitular radial articulation, 295
Capsules. See Joint capsules
Carpal tunnel syndrome
    flexor tendon factors, 312–315, 321f
    functional anatomy, 310–315, 311f, 312f,
        313f, 314f
    pathophysiology, 78, 315–317, 321f,
        324–327
    similarity to tennis elbow, 307
    steroid injection technique, 323
    treatment, 317–329
Carpals, 354
Cartilage
    collagen type IX role in, 5f
    femoral head, of the, 369f
    menisci, 415
Casts
    ankle injuries, 437
    spondylolisthesis, 162
Catecholamines, 54, 75, 93
Caudal blocks, 96, 150, 485, 486f
Causalgia. See also Reflex sympathetic
        dystrophy
    defined, 470, 472
    post-sympathectomy, 46
    spinal cord tracts and, 16
Central pain, defined, 207
Central pain of spinal cord origin (CCPS),
    208–209
Cerebral cortex, role in pain perception,
    32–34
Cervical collars
    therapeutic concepts, 180, 210
    types, 210f, 211f
Cervical nystagmus, 179
Cervical rib, 247
Cervical rib syndrome, 239, 246
Cervical spine. See also Hyperextension-
        hyperflexion
    clinical entities, 194–197
    contralateral flexion test, 245
    cord lesions, 206–209
    examination, 187–189, 191–193
    functional anatomy, 185f
    lower complex, 185–187
    movement, 186f, 187f, 191f, 192f
    neurologic examination, 198–206, 202f, 203f
    pain, neurophysiologic concepts, 66
    pain, treatment protocols, 209–216
    upper complex, 171–185
    zygapophyseal joint pain, 196–197

Cervical traction, anterior scalene syndrome,
    247
Cervical vertigo, 179
Cervical zygapophyseal joint pain, 196–197,
    214–216
Cervicodorsal outlet syndrome, 239
Cervicogenic headache. See Headache
Chemical mediators, pain, 15, 74–75. See also
    Nociceptors
Chiropractics, concept of, 156–158, 157f. See
    also Manipulation
Cholecystokinin, as nociceptor, 18
Cholinergic terminals, parasympathetic
    nervous system, 40
Chondromalacia patella, 420–421
Chordotomy, 16, 24–25, 26
Chronic fatigue syndrome (CFS), 52–54
Chronic musculoskeletal pain syndrome
    (CPMS), 66
Chronic pain
    defined, 34
    exercise and, 92
    foot, 443
    mechanisms, 34–37
    psychologic concepts, 102, 490, 491, 492,
        497–501
    treatment, 88
Chronobiology, pain perception and, 34
Circadian rhythms, pain perception and, 34
Clavicocostal syndrome, 239
Clawed phalanges, 445, 453
Clinical instability, defined, 158
Clonidine, 46
Cluster headaches, 28
Coactivation, agonist-antagonist action,
    trunk/abdominal muscles, 118
Coccyx, 383
Cocontraction, 65, 325, 326
Cold, application of. See Cryotherapy
Collagen
    functional characteristics, 3–4, 5f, 6
    in tendons, 6, 339–340
    types, 4
    viscoelastic properties, temperature and, 4,
        343
Collagen fibers
    as component, connective tissue, 1, 2
    intervertebral disk, 103–104, 105f, 107f
    menisci, 415–416
    molecular structure, 4f, 5f
Collars. See Cervical collars
Collateral ligaments. See also Lateral collateral
        ligament; Medial collateral ligament
    functional anatomy, 388, 391f, 392, 395, 400
    injuries, 407, 415
Compartment syndrome, defined, 125
Compression. See Nerve compression;
        Neurovascular compression syndromes
Concentration deficit, with whiplash, 206

Concentric contraction, 6
Concentric force, interspinous muscles, 109, 117
Conditioned stimuli, 497
Congenital spinal stenosis, 159
Congenital spondylolisthesis, 161
Congruent joints, 261f, 362, 363f
Connective tissue. *See also* Collagen; Muscle;
    Tendons
  dense, 3
  elongation, modalities for, 91
  formation of, 2, 2f
  functional characteristics, 1, 3–4
  grouping, 2–3
  injury/repair, 4, 6
  therapeutic heat and, 91
Contractures, functional, 66, 67
Contralateral pathways, spinal cord, 25
Cord, spinal. *See* Chordotomy; Spinal cord
Corsets
  application, standing/seated, 163f
  low back pain, 153
  spinal stenosis, 161
  spondylolisthesis, 162
Corticoptropin-releasing hormone (CRH), 43
Corticosteroids. *See* Steroids
Corticotropin-releasing hormone (CRH)
    neurons, 32
Cortisol, exercise and, 93
Costoclavicular syndrome, 248–249
Cranial outflow, preganglionic fibers, 38
Creep, defined, 4, 342
Crepitation
  acromioclavicular joint, 291
  sternoclavicular joint, 293
  TMJ syndrome, 219
Cross (transverse ligament), 171–172, 173f
Crossed nerve stretch, 138
Cruciate ligaments
  functional anatomy, 171, 390, 392f, 393f,
    394f, 396f, 397f, 400
  injuries, 410–415
Crush syndrome, carpal tunnel syndrome,
    326–327, 329, 329f
Crutches. *See* Canes/crutches
Cryotherapy
  ankle injuries, 437
  cervical pain, 209, 213
  epicondylalgia (tennis elbow), 306
  knee injuries, 424
  low back pain, 149
  physiologic basis, 89
Cubital tunnel, 297, 298f
Cubital tunnel syndrome, 335, 337f, 337–339
Cumulative trauma disorders (CTD), 102, 324.
    See also Repetitive strain injury

D-CPP NMDA antagonists, 28
De Quervain's disease, 351, 352f

Deconditioning. *See* Immobilization/inactivity
Degenerative arthritis
  hip joint, 377–380, 378f, 382
  patellofemoral disease, 425f
Degenerative cuff disease, 271, 275f
Degenerative spinal stenosis, 159
Degenerative spondylolisthesis, 161
Demyelination, 8
Dens, 171–172, 183
Dense connective tissue, 3
Depression, mental
  chronic pain and, 102
  circadian rhythms, pain perception and, 34
  as perturbers, neuromuscular control, 115
  psychological testing, 498
  tricyclic antidepressants, physiologic basis, 54
Dermatomes
  cervical root levels, 184f
  hand and fingers, 193, 198f, 298, 299f
  levels, nerve root impingement, 140t, 142
  lower extremity, 143f, 481f
  upper extremity, 243f
Descending pain control system, 31
Descending tracts, spinal cord, 20, 22f
Developmental spinal stenosis, 159
Diabetic foot, 465–467
Diathermy, 90
Disability. *See also* Low back pain
  defined, 123, 511
  lower cervical segment, pain and, 195
  psychologic aspects, 501–503
  workers' compensation and, 507
Disability Management Program, 511
Discogenic mechanical pain, 122
Dislocations
  knee, 409
  pelvis, 384
  shoulder, 289, 289f, 290f
  wrist and hand pain, 354–357
Distal transverse metacarpal arch, 354
Dizziness. *See* Vertigo
Dorsal horn
  afferent sensory fibers entering, 20f, 26, 27,
    27f
  nociceptive transmission to, 77f
  reflex sympathetic dystrophy, 476, 476f
Dorsal motor nucleus, 38
Dorsal root ganglia (DRG)
  cubital tunnel syndrome, 339
  failed opioid modulation of pain, 48f
  muscle spasm and, 16, 19f, 20
  reflex sympathetic dystrophy, 476, 476f
Dorsal thalamic system, 24
Double-crush theory, carpal tunnel syndrome,
    326–327, 327f, 329
Down regulation, defined, 53
Drawer sign
  ankle joint, 435, 436, 436f
  · knee joint, 410, 411f, 412f

Drop foot, 123
Drop sign, rotator cuff tear, 271, 277f
Dural sheath, 109, 110, 111f
Dural sign, hamstring flexibility, SLR test, 131,
    137–138, 138f

Eccentric contraction, 6
Eccentric force, interspinous muscles, 109, 117
Edema
    epineural, 315, 317, 318
    with lower extremity RSD syndrome, 483
    soft tissue injury and, 16, 89
Edinger-Westphal, nucleus of, 38
Efferent nerves, 65, 522
Effusion, knee, 405, 407, 410f, 416, 418
Elastin fibers, 1, 2
Elbow joint
    baseball elbow, 300, 302
    epicondylalgia, 302, 305–307
    functional anatomy, 295, 296f, 297f
    nerve damage, 297–298, 300
    trauma, 295, 297
Electrolyte balance, inactivity and, 9–10
Electromyographic (EMG) testing
    carpal tunnel syndrome, 319
    pronator teres syndrome, 331
    thoracic outlet syndrome, 246
Electronystagmographic (ENG) testing, 185
Elongated pedicle spondylolisthesis, 162
Elongation
    modalities for, 91, 94
    plastic deformation, 91, 150
    tendons, 340–342
Emotions
    exercise and, 93
    low back pain, malingering and, 148
    pain perception and, 35–37, 43, 91
    as perturbers, neuromuscular control, 115
    tension exacerbates thoracic outlet
        syndrome, 240
Employers. See Workers' compensation
End-point, determination of, 189, 194
Endorphins (enkephalins)
    actions, neurophysiologic basis, 28
    exercise and, 93
    fibromyalgia and, 75–76
    pain perception and, 33, 37, 84
Entrapment syndromes
    interdigital nerve, 456, 458f
    pain of, neurophysiologic concepts, 66
    sciatic nerve, 162
Epicondylalgia (tennis elbow), 300, 302, 303f,
    304f, 305–307, 307f
Epidural blocks, 150, 152f, 485, 486f
Epinephrine
    action, alpha and beta receptors, 42
    secretion, postganglionic fibers, 40, 41–42
Epitenon, defined, 343

Epithelial tissue (skin)
    functions, 1
    in lower extremity RSD syndrome, 483, 484
    quality of pain in, 87
Ergonomics
    defined, 513
    low back pain and, 92, 116–117, 121, 153
    occupational musculoskeletal disorders and,
        510, 513–514
    shoulder complex, 281
    spondylolisthesis, 162
    TMJ syndrome and, 224
    wrist and hand pain, 356, 357
Exercise therapy. See also Strengthening
        exercises; Stretching exercises
    active vs. passive, 91
    after cryotherapy, 89
    ankle injuries, 435, 437, 439
    carpal tunnel syndrome, 321–322, 322f
    cervical pain, 213–214
    glenohumeral joint, 280
    hip joint, 380, 381f, 382f
    low back pain, 102, 150–151, 153, 154f, 155
    physiologic basis, 91–94
    shoulder complex, 282f–288f
    spondylolisthesis, 162
    TMJ syndrome and, 224, 229f, 230f
Extension. See also Hyperextension
    cervical spine, 171, 178, 186, 192f
    hip joint, 368
    knee, 388, 390, 394f, 395f, 399, 400
    lumbar spine, 135, 137f
    lumbosacral spine, 106
    wrist, 312
Extensor pollicis longus
    rupture, 349, 350f
    test, radial nerve, 305, 306f
Extensor tendinitis, 351
Extensor tendons, injury to
    anatomic zones, 345f
    mallet finger, 346, 347f, 348
    rupture, extensor pollicis longus, 349, 350f
    rupture, middle phalanx, 348–349, 349f,
        350f
    suturing, 344
Exteroceptors, defined, 61, 522
Extracellular water, 9
Extrafusal fibers, 62, 64, 340
Exudate, defined, 89
Eysenck personality test, 499

Facet arthrosis syndrome, 125
Facet(s). See also Zygapophyseal joints (facets)
    injury, diagnosis of, 196
    jammed, 156
    lower cervical segment, 185–186
    patella, 401, 403f
    upper thoracic pain and, 232

Facial expression, pain and, 495–496
Fajersztain test, 138
Fast-twitch fibers (type II)
  fibromyalgia syndromes, 78, 79, 79f
  muscle stiffness and, 71
  terminal in laminae, 20
Femoral nerve, 376, 398, 399
Femoral nerve stretch test, 140, 140f
Femorotibial joint, 388, 389f, 390f
Femur, 362, 367–368, 369, 369f. *See also*
  Knee joint
Fibro-osseous case, shoulder, 267, 269f
Fibroblasts, 4, 6
Fibromyalgia syndromes
  diagnostic criteria, 73–74
  low back pain and, 125
  management, 77–79
  occipital neuralgia and, 173
  pathophysiology, 74–77
  terminology, 73
Fibroplasia, 4, 6
Fibrositis, 72
Fingers
  dorsiflexion, 300, 301f
  flexion, 312
  fractures and dislocations, 355
  shoulder-hand-finger RSD syndrome, 471,
    478f
Finkelstein's test, 351
Five "D" syndrome, of pain, 491
5–hydroxytryptophan, 86
Flexion. *See also* Hyperextension-hyperflexion
  cervical spine, 171, 178, 186, 186f, 191f,
    192f
  fingers, wrist and hand, 312–315, 313f, 314f,
    324–326
  hip joint, 368
  knee joint, 388, 390, 394f, 395f, 399, 400
  lumbosacral spine, 106, 109, 113–115, 114f
Flexion contracture, hip, 378, 380
Flexor carpi ulnaris, 336f, 338–339, 353–354
Flexor digitorum profundus, 337f, 339
Flexor digitorum profundus tendons, 310, 312
Flexor digitorum superficialis, 312
Flexor pollicis longus tendon, 310, 312
Flexor tendinitis, 351, 353f, 353–354
Flexor tendon injury, 344–345, 346f
Foot. *See also* Ankle joint
  diabetic, 465–467
  functional anatomy, 428, 429f, 430f, 431f
  during gait, 455f
  leg-ankle-foot RSD syndrome, 479–487
Foot pain
  Achilles tendon rupture, 464–465, 465f
  chronic, 443, 445
  evaluation, 442
  hallux rigidus, 461–462, 462f
  hallux valgus, 459–461, 460f, 461f
  hammertoe, 462–464, 463f, 464f

heel, 446–448
  interdigital neuritis (Morton's neuroma),
    456, 458
  march fracture, 458–459, 459f
  Morton's syndrome, 454, 456, 456f
  normal foot, criteria for, 441–442
  strain, acute, 443, 444f, 446f
  transverse tarsal joints, 449, 451–464
Fractures
  ankle joint, 439
  foot, 458–459
  pelvis, 384, 385f, 386f, 387
  wrist and hand, 354–357, 356f
Froment sign, 338
Frozen shoulder, 279, 280
"Frozen shoulder-hand-finger syndrome," 478f
Full-blown syndrome, reflex sympathetic
  dystrophy, 49
Functional anatomy, defined, 102
Functional contracture (trigger point), 66,
  67
Functional syncytium, defined, 29
Fusiform motorneurons, 69–70

G protein, 85
GABA (gamma-aminobutyric acid), 494
Gait
  disorders, with cervical pathology, 179,
    184–185
  disorders, with low back pain, 123
  foot and ankle during, 443, 451, 452–453,
    455f
  foot pain, 442
  heel pain, 447
  hip joint motion, 369, 371, 373f, 374f
Gamma motor neurons. *See* Spindle cell
  (gamma system)
Gastrocnemius-soleus muscle, 142–143
Generalized myofascial syndrome, 72
Genu valgum and genu varum, 377f
Glenohumeral joint
  diagnostic procedures, 271, 277–279
  dislocation, 289, 289f
  functional anatomy, 259–261, 260f, 261f,
    262f, 265f, 268f, 269f
  history and examination, 270–271
  muscular action, 261
  pathogenic factors, 267
  treatment, 279–281
Glenoid fossa, 260, 262f, 266
Glutamic acid, 28
Gluteus maximus, 142–143
Golgi tendon organs, 62, 180f, 181f, 340, 395,
  522
Gray rami communicantes, 41
Greater occipital nerve, 177f, 179
Greater superior occipital nerve, 174, 175f
Guildford cervical brace, 212f

Guillain-Barré syndrome, 482
Guyon's canal, 333, 335f, 353

H⁺, as nociceptor, 15
Hallux rigidus, 461–462, 462f
Hallux valgus, 459–461, 460f, 461f
Hammertoe, 453, 462–464, 463f, 464f
Hamstring flexibility, low back pain and,
    130–131, 133f, 136
Hand. See Wrist and hand
Head of the femur. See Femur
Headache
    cervicogenic, 183, 184, 194, 197, 199–201,
        206
    migraine, 28
    occipital neuralgia and, 176, 178
    tension, 187
Health care system. See Workers'
    compensation
Heart rate, inactivity and, 11
Heat therapy
    cervical pain, 209, 213
    low back pain, 149
    physiologic basis, 89–91
Heel cord stretching exercises, 437, 438f
Heel pain, 446–448, 448f
Hemarthrosis, knee injury, 407, 416
Hemoglobin, inactivity and, 11
Hemorrhage, AO joint meniscus, 196, 197,
    201f
Hip joint
    degenerative arthritis, 377–380, 382
    functional anatomy, 362, 363f, 364f, 365f,
        366f, 366–368, 367f
    motions, 370f, 371, 371f, 372f, 375, 375f
    pain mechanisms of, 375–376
    pelvic trauma, 383–384, 387
Histamine, as nociceptor, 15, 16, 18, 76, 88,
    149
Histamine test, brachial plexus injuries, 254
Hoffmann sign, 206
Honeymoon paralysis, 331
Hormones, pain perception and, 33, 34f, 43
Horner's syndrome, 253, 254
Humeroulnar joint, 295
Humerus, 260, 261, 262f, 266
Hydrotherapy, 90
Hyperabduction syndrome, 239, 250, 250f
Hyperalgesia
    interdigital neuritis, 458
    low back pain, 149
    primary/secondary, 88, 149
    reflex sympathetic dystrophy, 46–51
Hyperexcitability, nervous system, 28
Hyperextension
    knee, 390
    lumbosacral spine, 126, 135, 137f

Hyperextension-hyperflexion, cervical spine
    (whiplash), 176, 179, 187, 194, 199f,
    200, 201–206
Hypertonus, fibromyalgia syndromes, 76
Hypochondriasis, psychological testing, 498
Hypothalamopituitary-adrenocortical system,
    32, 43
Hypothalamus, 28, 34
Hypothalmosympathoadrenocortical system,
    32
Hypothalmosympathoadrenomedullary system,
    43
Hypothyroidism, compared to fibromyalgia, 76
Hypoxia
    causes of, 65
    as nociceptor, 15, 74
Hysteria, psychological testing, 498

Iatrogenic disorders, 87, 159
Ice, application of. See Cryotherapy
Idiopathic spinal stenosis, 159
Idiopathic thoracic outlet syndrome, 243
Iliofemoral ligament, 367
Immobilization/inactivity
    acromioclavicular joint, 292f, 293
    cervical, 209–210
    disadvantages of, 6, 153, 343
    knee injuries, 409
    metabolic effects of, 9–11
    phalanges, interphalangeal joints, 355, 355f
Impairment, defined, 511
Impingement. See Nerve root impingement
Inactivity. See Immobilization/inactivity
Incongruent joints, 261f, 363f
Independent medical evaluation, 508
Inflammatory mediators, pain. See Nociceptors
Infraclavicular brachial plexus lesions,
    251–252
Inhibitory impulses, transmission of, 26, 27f
Injections. See Intra-articular injections; Local
    injections
Injury(ies). See also Nerve injury; Repetitive
    strain injury; Soft tissue injury
    cervical, 181, 183f, 187. See also
        Hyperextension- hyperflexion
    elbow, 295, 297
    shoulder complex joints, 270, 270f
Innominate bones, 383, 384
Interdigital neuritis (Morton's neuroma), 456,
    457f, 458
Interleukin-1 (IL-1), 74
Interspinous muscles, 109
Intervertebral disk
    as functional unit, lumbosacral spine,
        103–113, 104f
    lower cervical spine, 195
    walking, physiologic effects of, 155f

Intervertebral foramen, neural contents, 109,
110f
Intra-articular injections
cervical zygapophyseal joints, 214–216
glenohumeral joint, 280–281, 281f, 288f
hip joint, 378, 379f
Intracellular cyclic AMP (cAMP), 85
Intracellular water, 9
Intrafusal muscle fibers, 61f, 62, 63f
Intrapsychic, defined, 501
Intrathecal pressure, tests to increase, 143,
146–147
Intrinsic muscle stiffness, 67
Inversion stress test, ankle, 435, 436, 436f
Ipsilateral nucleus ventralis, 24, 25
Ischemia
elicits paresthesia, 16
with lower extremity RSD syndrome, 483,
484
results in pain, 74
serotonin and, 86
Ischiofemoral ligaments, 367
Isokinetic contraction, 6
cervical pain, 214
ROM testing, cervical spine, 191
Isometric contraction
cervical pain, 209, 213–214
ROM testing, cervical spine, 191
Isotonic contraction, 7
Isthmic spondylolisthesis, 161

Jackson's sign, 255
Jogger's foot, 443, 445f
Joint capsules
adhesive capsulitis, 278
capsular tears, 271, 277f
as component of soft tissue, 1
hip joint, 367, 367f, 368f
zygapophysial, 106

Kernig test, 147, 148f
Ketamine, 28
Knee injury
anterior knee pain, 420–425
clinical evaluation, 404–425, 411f
collateral ligaments, 407–410
cruciate ligaments, 410–415
rotational, 409
"stop and cut," 408f
Knee joint
aspiration, technique of, 424f
functional anatomy, 399–400
knee-ankle-foot RSD syndrome, 479
ligaments, 388–395, 389f, 391f, 393f, 396f,
397f
menisci, 397–398
muscles, 398–399

nerve supply, 398
posterior structure, medial aspect, 402f
Kocher manipulation, 289, 290f
Kyphosis, 113, 114, 247

L-tryptophan, 77
Labrum, 367
Lachman test, 412, 413f, 414f
Lactic acid, 71
Laminae I through IV, nociceptor terminals,
19–20, 20f
Lasegue test. See Straight leg raising (SLR)
(Lasegue test)
Laser heat therapy, 90
Lateral collateral ligament
ankle joint support, 428, 432f, 433f
functional anatomy, 388
injuries, 409–410, 434f
Lateral femoral cutaneous nerve, 376, 376f
Lateral flexion
cervical spine, 186, 192f
lumbosacral spine, 106, 126, 129
Lateral plantar nerve, 446, 448f
Learned stimuli, 497
Leg-ankle-foot RSD syndrome, 479–487
Leucine, 28
Leukotrienes, as nociceptors, 16, 18, 74
Lhermitte's sign, 255
Lifting
faulty technique, 115f
strength assessment, 118
tridimensional forces, trunk flexion, 117f,
117–118
Ligaments
ankle joint, 428, 432f, 433f, 433–435
as component of soft tissue, 1
elbow, 295
foot, 451, 455f
hip joint, 367, 367f
knee, 388–395, 389f, 390f, 391f, 393f, 396f,
397f
low back pain and, 124
pelvis, 384f
scapuloclavicular, 263
subtalar joint, 439, 441, 441f
upper cervical complex, 171–172, 172f,
173f, 174f, 176
wrist and hand, 310, 312, 314
zygapophyseal joints (facets), 106
zygapophysial joints (facets), 109
Limbic system, 34, 43, 84
Limited symptom panic attacks, 493
Limp. See Gait
Litigation, 502, 503, 510
Local injections
cervical pain, 209, 213
elbow joint, 300, 306
interdigital neuritis, 458

piriformis muscle, 164
plantar fascial, 450f
Locked joints
  C2 on C3, rotation and, 178f
  facets, 212
  knee, 418, 419
  manipulation, 156, 212
  manual therapy and, 94
  TMJ syndrome, 222f, 223
Locus coeruleus (LC), 24, 42–43
Longitudinal arch, 451, 454f
Longitudinal metacarpal arch, 354
Loose connective tissue, 2
Lordosis, low back pain and
  assessment with sitting, 123
  exercise therapy for, 151
  mechanisms of, 129f
  normal body mechanics, 113, 114
  tests for, 127–128, 130f
Low back disorders (LBD)
  causes, 101–102, 109
  classification, 118–119
Low back pain
  body mechanics, normal, 113–116
  exercise therapy, 91, 92
  facet pathology/examination, 125–126
  free dynamic measurement, 120
  functional anatomy, 103–113
  hamstring flexibility, 130–131, 133f
  heat therapy, 90
  history, 116–122
  intrathecal pressure, tests to increase, 143,
    146–147
  lateral and rotational flexibility, 129, 131f,
    132f
  lordosis, tests for, 127–128
  lumbar disk pain/examination, 126–127
  lumbar extension, 135, 137f
  lumbar flexion, 128–129, 130f, 131f
  malingering, 148–149
  manipulation, 94
  nerve root involvement, determination of,
    140–143
  neurologic examination, objective, 136–138,
    140
  neurophysiologic concepts, 66
  overview, 101–103
  pathophysiology, 78
  physical examination, 122–123, 127–133
  piriformis syndrome, 162, 164
  sciatic radiculitis, tests for, 147
  spinal stenosis, 158–161
  spondylolysis/spondylolisthesis, 161–162
  standard tests, 127–133
  strength testing, 118–119, 133–135
  tissue sites/examination, 124–126
  treatment, 149––158
Lower cervical spinal complex, 185–187, 189,
  195

Lower extremity
  dermatomes, 143f
  reflex sympathetic dystrophy, 470, 479–487
Lumbar extension, strength testing, 135, 136f,
  137f
Lumbar flexion, low back pain and, 128–129,
  130f, 131f
Lumbar motion monitor (LMM), 120, 120f,
  121
Lumbar pelvic rhythm, 115
Lumbosacral angle, abnormal, 127–128, 128f
Lumbosacral spine
  disk pain, 126–127
  functional anatomy, 103–113
  neural tissue, 109–113
  normal body mechanics, 113–116
  stenosis, 158–161
  zygapophyseal joints, 105–109
Luschka, recurrent nerve of, 110, 112

Maigne's technique, 213
Major reflex sympathetic dystrophy, 470–471,
  479
Malingering, 148–149, 490, 502
Mallet finger, 346, 347f, 348, 348f
Manipulation
  cervical, 212–213
  frozen shoulder, 280, 281
  knee joint, 419
  low back pain, 156–158
  mandible, 222f
  physiologic basis, 94–95
  tennis elbow, 307f
Manual therapy, pain relief, 94–95
March fracture, 458–459, 459f
McMurray test, 418–419, 421f
Mechanical pain, 122, 208
Medial collateral ligament
  ankle joint support, 428, 432f, 433f
  functional anatomy, 388, 391f, 392, 397
  injuries, 395, 407, 411f, 414–415, 435f
Median nerve
  compression, 311, 315, 327f
  functional anatomy, 193f, 194f, 310, 311f,
    318f, 325f
Medullary-pontine catecholamine neurons, 32
Memory deficit, with whiplash, 206
Meniscus(i)
  acromioclavicular joint, 291, 292f
  injuries, 415–419, 417f, 418f, 419f, 420f
  knee joint, 397–398, 398f, 399, 399f, 400,
    415–419
  lower cervical segment, 185, 186
  microscopic structure, 416f
  TMJ syndrome, 218
  zygapophyseal joints, 106, 196, 197
Meralgia paresthesia, 376f
Metabolic effects, injury and inactivity, 9–11

Metacarpals, 354, 354f
Metatarsal arch, 451
Metatarsal heads, 451, 452
Metatarsalgia, 451, 452–454
Methionine, 28
Microphages, 4
Middle foot, 428
Middle perforating bundle, 416
Middle plexus (trunk) lesions, 254
Migraine, 28
Milgram test, 143, 146, 146f
Minnesota Multiphasic Personality Inventory
    (MMPI), 492, 498, 498f
Minor reflex sympathetic dystrophy, 470–471,
    479
Mitochondrial monoamine oxidase (MAO), 54
Mobilization, 94–95. See also
    Immobilization/inactivity
Modulation, pain impulses, 27–32
Moist heat, application of, 90
Morphine, 85, 86
Morton's neuroma, 456, 457f, 458
Morton's syndrome, 454, 456
Motor control, 69–71, 179–181, 517, 521,
    524–526
Motor unit, defined, 517
Motor vehicle accidents (MVA), 471. See also
    Hyperextension- hyperflexion, cervical
    spine
Mucopolysaccharide gel, intervertebral disk,
    103, 104
Multi-ascending synaptic pathways (MAS), 22,
    22f, 24
Muscle fatigue
    fibromyalgia syndromes, 78–79
    low back pain and, 92
    soft tissue dysfunction and, 7
Muscle spasm
    algogens, irritating effects of, 74
    analgesic nerve blocks, 96
    exercise ad, 93
    manipulation, concepts of, 156
    neural patterns causing, 16, 18f, 19f, 151
    protective, 67, 69, 72
Muscle tension
    induces pain, 490–491, 491f
    neuroanatomic physiology, 66–67
Muscle(s). See also Range of motion; Strength
    testing; Strengthening exercises;
    Stretching exercises
    cervical pathology, as component of, 179
    as component of soft tissue, 1, 60
    contractions, types of, 6–7
    contractions induce pain, 491f
    dysfunctional, cause fatigue, 78–79
    elbow, 295, 303f
    functional anatomy, 6–9
    hardness, palpating areas of, 72
    head and neck, 176f

knee joint, 398–399
low back pain, 124
lumbosacral spine, 109
microscopic structure, 7f
neck, proprioception/motor control,
    179–181
neuromusculoskeletal function, 517–526
oxidative/glycolytic, 78
painful, become silent, 64, 67, 151
physical examination, low back pain and, 125
reflex-mediated stiffness, 67
relationship, specific nerve roots, peripheral
    nerves, 142t
shoulder complex, 261, 263, 266–267
stiffness, intrinsic, 67
stiffness, secondary, 71
wasting, 9
Musculotendinous mechanism, 63, 68f, 340,
    342f
Musculotendinous mechansim, 182f
Myelinated nerves, 15, 26, 27–28, 74, 327,
    329f
Myofascial pain, 66
Myofascial pain dysfunctional syndrome of the
    temporomandibular articulation,
    217–218
Myofascial pain syndrome (MPS), 73
Myofilaments, 6
Myogenic mechanical pain, 122
Myoneural junctions, tenderness, 143, 145f
Myosin, 65, 66
Myotome levels, nerve root impingement,
    140t, 142, 144f

N-methyl-D-aspartic acid (NMDA), 28
Naffziger test, 146f, 146–147
Naloxone, 37, 93
Narcotics, physiologic basis, 28
Neck. See Cervical spine
Nerve blocks
    cervical spine, 205–206
    diagnostic, 95
    facet pathology/examination, 126
    low back pain, 112, 150, 151f, 152f
    in lower extremity RSD syndrome, 485,
    486f, 487
    obturator, 378, 380f
    occipital neuralgia, 176
    physiologic basis, 95–96
Nerve compression. See also Neurovascular
    compression syndromes
    cubital tunnel syndrome, 335, 337–339
    pathophysiology, 315–317, 326–329
    pronator teres median, 329–332
    ulnar, 332–334
Nerve injury
    degeneration, tourniquet-induced, 10f
    degrees of, 9f

radial, 298, 300
soft tissue dysfunction and, 7–9
ulnar, 297–298
Nerve regeneration, 8, 11f
Nerve root impingement
dermatome/myotome levels, 141t
muscles, peripheral nerves, relationship of, 142t
neurologic determination of, 140, 142–143
Nerve(s)
cervical zygapophyseal joints, 185–186
as component of soft tissue, 1
conduction testing, carpal tunnel syndrome, 319
hip joint, 375–376
knee joint, 398
lower extremity, 480f
occipital neuralgia and, 174, 175f, 177f
reaction to cold, 89
severed, forming a neuroma, 45f
severed, forming *spouts*, 44–45
types that transmit pain, 15, 16
vertebral functional unit, 109–110, 110f, 111f, 112f, 112–113
Neuralgia
occipital, 173–174, 176, 178–179
postherpetic, spinal cord tracts and, 16
Neurasthenia, 72
Neurogenic claudication, spinal stenosis, 160
Neurogenic inflammation, 76
Neuromas, 45f, 425f, 474f
Neuromatrix, 32–33, 526f
Neuromusculoskeletal function
flexion/extension and obliques, 520f
lumbosacral function, 519f
normal, 517, 518f, 521–522, 526f
stretch reflex, 523
supraspinal motor centers, 524–526
"Neuron theory," 29
Neurons
function in ANS, 38, 40, 40f
neuromatrix, thalamus and cortex, 32
wide dynamic range, 476, 478
Neuropeptides, 28, 31, 76, 88, 149
Neuropraxia, 7–8
Neurosignature, defined, 32–33
Neurotransmission
physiology of, 29f, 29–31, 30f, 31f
reflex sympathetic dystrophy, 472–478
Neurotransmitters
defined, 29
as paraneurons, 33–34
Neurovascular compression syndromes
anterior scalene, 246–248
brachial plexus compression, 255, 256f
brachial plexus injuries, 251–254
costoclavicular, 248–249
hyperabduction, 250
lesions of the cord, 254–255

lesions of the trunk, 254
thoracic outlet, 239–246
Neurovascular reflex sympathetic dystrophy, 471
NMDA (N-methyl-D-aspartic acid), 28
"No man's land," suturing in, 344, 346f
Nociceptive impulses
neuromuscular function and, 517
soft tissue injury and, 16
transmission/inhibition, dorsal horn, 26, 27f, 27–29
Nociceptor sites
ankle, 435
defined, 16
glenohumeral joint, 266, 267
hip joint, 375
intervertebral disk, 105
nerve blocks and, 95
zygapophyseal joint ligaments, 106
Nociceptors
activate alpha-1 adrenoreceptors, 46, 47f
defined, 16
neuroanatomic physiology, 15, 19–20, 20f, 21f, 475, 476, 524f
norepinephrine, response to, 45
soft tissue injury and, 17f, 18–19
spindle cell system and, 64, 65
Nodes of Ranvier. *See* Ranvier, nodes of
Nomogenic disorder, 87
Nonsteroidal anti-inflammatory agents (NSAIDs)
cubital tunnel syndrome, 339
degenerative arthritis, hip, 378
epicondylalgia (tennis elbow), 306
knee injuries, 424
physiologic basis, 16
Norepinephrine
chronic fatigue syndrome and, 53, 54
intradermal, hyperalgesia in RSD, 46, 47–48
mood/anxiety disorders, 494
as neurochemical mediator, 28, 42, 43, 44–45, 476
urinary levels, in fibromyalgia syndromes, 75
Nuclear bags, 62
Nuclear chains, 62
Nucleus, intervertebral disk, 103, 104, 108f
Nucleus of Edinger-Westphal, 38
Nucleus of Perlia, 38
Nucleus pulposus, 105f
Nystagmus, 179, 180, 185

Obturator nerve, 398
Obturator nerve block, 378, 380f
Occipital-atlas joint (O-C1)
clinical entities of, 194
functional anatomy, 171, 184, 196, 197
ligaments, 172f

Occipital-atlas joint (O-C1)–*Continued*
    movement, 172f, 191f
    as nociceptor site, 184, 199–200
Occipital neuralgia, 173–174, 176, 178–179
Occupational musculoskeletal disorders, 507.
    See also Repetitive strain injury
Odd facet, patella, 402
Odontoid process (dens), 171–172, 183
Opiates, receptors in CNS, 84, 85
Opioids
    actions, neurophysiologic basis, 28
    exogenous, opium/morphine as, 85
    failed modulation of pain, 47–48, 48f
    peripheral mechanism, 85, 86
Orthotic devices. *See also* Braces; Cervical
    collars; Splints
    metatarsalgia, 454
    shoes, modified, 451f, 454, 458, 460, 462,
        462f, 464, 466f, 467f, 467–468, 468f
    TMJ syndrome, 223f
Osteopathy, 156
Osteoporosis, 377, 484
Overuse syndrome. *See* Repetitive strain injury

Pain. *See also* Chronic pain; Hyperalgesia; Low
        back pain; Psychologic aspects, pain
    chronic fatigue syndrome and, 52–54
    defined, 14–15, 101
    mediation, sympathetic nervous system,
        37–46
    modulation, concept of, 27–32
    neuroanatomic basis, 14–27
    neuronal pathways of, 475f
    perception, ANS role, 38f
    perception, cerebral cortex role, 32–34
    qualities, 87
    transmission, 29–31, 33–34, 35f, 35–37
    types, 23
    upper thoracic, 232
Pain, treatment modalities. *See also* Exercise
        therapy; Nerve blocks
    manual therapy, 94–95, 156–158
    pharmacologic sites of action, pattern
        interruption, 36f
    pharmacology, 84–87
    physical intervention, 87–91
Pain behavior, 495–496, 497
"Pain Estimate Chart," 500f
Painful arc, glenohumeral joint, 271, 276f, 277
Palmar creases, wrist and hand, 311f, 323f
Pancoast's tumor, 243
Panic disorders, 492–495
Parachlorophenylalanine (pCPA), 86
Paraffin, hot, 90
Paraneurons, 33–34
Paraplegia, 206, 482
Parasympathetic nervous system, 38, 40, 53
Paresis, 298, 482

Paresthesia
    carpal tunnel syndrome, 318, 319
    defined, 16
    mechanisms of, 320f
    thoracic outlet syndrome, 240
    ulnar nerve injuries, 298
    upper cervical spine injury, 206
    wrist and hand, 315
Passive range of motion, cervical spine, 189,
    190f
Patella
    facets of, 401, 403f
    physiologic motion, 422f
Patellofemoral joint, 388, 389f, 401–404,
    420–425, 423f
Pectoralis minor, 250
Pectoralis minor syndrome, 239
Pelvic tilt, 127
Pelvis
    functional anatomy, 366f, 383f, 383–384,
        384f
    injuries, 383–384, 385f, 386f, 387
Pendular exercise, frozen shoulder, 279, 280f
Periaqueductal gray (PAG) matter, 25, 77, 85
Peridural blocks, 96, 150
Peripheral nerves
    functional anatomy, 317f
    microscopic structure, 8f
    relationship, specific nerve roots, muscles,
        142t
Perlia, nucleus of, 38
Peroneal muscles, 433, 437
Peroneal nerve, 409
Personality disorders, 102
Perturbers, neuromusculoskeletal function
    and, 115, 116, 121, 155, 518f
Phalanges, motions with stance/walking, 445,
    447, 456, 462–463, 463f
Phalen test, 319
Phantom pain, 16
Pharmacologic treatment, pain, 84–87
Phobias, 492, 493
Phospholipids, as nociceptors, 16
Physical therapy, cervical neck pain, 215
Physical tone, collagen fibers, 4
Pinch strength, thumb, 333f, 334
Piriformis syndrome, 162, 163f, 164
Placebo therapy, 485, 490
Plantar fascia, 447, 449f
Plantar fascitis, 450f, 451f
Plantarflexion, ankle, 433, 464–465
Plastic deformation, 91, 150
Polypeptides, as nociceptors, 18, 33
Positron emission tomography (PET), 16
Post-traumatic osteoporosis, 471
Post-traumatic stress, 499
Posterior cruciate ligament, 390, 400
Posterior foot, 428
Posterior interosseous nerve, 300, 301f

Posterior longitudinal ligament, 106, 109, 110
Posterior talofibular ligament, 433
Posterior thigh muscles, 399, 400, 401f
Posterior tibialis, 445
Postganglionic fibers, ANS, 40, 41, 42
Posture
  anterior scalene syndrome, 246, 247
  cervical pain, 214, 215f, 216f, 217f
  degenerative cuff disease, 271, 274f
  fibromyalgia syndromes, 76
  low back pain, 92, 153
  lumbar lordosis, 127–128
  neck muscles, 179
  normal body mechanics, 113–116
  TMJ syndrome, 222f, 224, 224f, 225f, 226f,
    227f, 228f
Potassium (K+), as nociceptor, 15, 74
Preganglionic fibers, ANS, 37–38, 40–41, 41f
Primary fibromyalgia syndrome (PFS), 72–73
Primary hyperalgesia, 88, 149
Projection (transmission) fibers, 26
Pronation, foot, 445, 447f, 447–448, 449, 451
Pronator teres syndrome, 329–332, 330f
Proprioception
  ankle joint, 435, 437
  knee joint, 392, 415
  upper cervical spine, 179–181
Proprioceptors
  defined, 61, 522
  types, 62
Prostaglandin E, as nociceptor, 16, 74
Prostanoids, 85
Protective muscle spasm, 67, 69
Proximal metacarpal arch, 354
Pseudoclaudication, spinal stenosis, 160
Psychologic aspects, pain
  low back, 102, 121, 155, 489, 490
  malingering, tests for, 148–149
  pain behavior, 495–496
  panic and anxiety disorders, 492–495
  reflex sympathetic dystrophy, 476
  secondary gain concept, 501–503
  soft tissue pain, concepts of, 489–492
  testing, psychological, 497–501
  TMJ syndrome, 225
Pubic rami, 384, 386f
Pubofemoral ligament, 367
Pulsed electromagnetic fields, as heat therapy,
  90

Quadriceps, 399, 400, 402
Quadriceps angle (Q angle), 404, 405f, 406f
Quadriceps mechanism, 400f, 403f, 404f
Quadriplegia, 206, 482

Radial nerve
  functional anatomy, 197f, 300f, 301f, 305f
  injuries, 298, 300
  testing, 306f
Radial pulse, obliteration of, 244, 245
Radicular pain
  brachial plexus lesions, 255, 256f
  cervical, 207, 209
  defined, 136
Radiohumeral and radioulnar articulation, 295
Range of motion
  cervical spine, 189, 190f, 191–193
  hip joint, 368, 370f, 371f, 372f
  limitations, low back pain, 118, 129
Ranvier, nodes of, 8, 10f, 327, 328f
Raynaud's syndrome, 46, 76
Recovery (collagen), 4, 341
Recruitment, motor unit, patterns of, 78–79
Recurrent nerve of Luschka, 110, 111f, 112
Recurrent pain, 34, 87
Referred pain
  degenerative arthritis, hip joint, 378
  neurophysiology, 66, 71
  upper cervical spine injury, 205
  zygapophyseal joints, 201f
Reflex-mediated muscle stiffness, 67
Reflex sympathetic dystrophy (RSD)
  clinical manifestations, 472
  diagnosis, 48–49
  hyperalgesia in, 46–51
  leg-ankle-foot syndrome, 479–487
  lower extremity, 470, 471, 479–487
  major/minor, 470–471
  neural mechanisms of, 472–478
  spinal cord injuries and, 208
  terminology of, 471–472, 472–478
  types/classification, 49–51
  upper extremity, 470, 471, 478
Rehabilitation. See also Exercise therapy
  ankle injuries, 437, 439
  degenerative arthritis, hip, 382
Relative stenosis of the lumbar spine (RSLC),
  159
Repetitive strain injury. See also Carpal tunnel
    syndrome; Ergonomics
  ankle, 435, 439
  anterior scalene syndrome, 247
  cubital tunnel syndrome, 335, 337–339
  elbow joint, 300, 302, 305–307
  flexor carpi ulnaris tendinitis, 353
  hip joint, 377
  hyperabduction syndrome, 250
  low back, 101–102, 116–117
  medial collateral ligament, 395, 414
  pathophysiology, 71
  shoulder complex, 270–271, 271f, 272f,
    273f, 281
  tendinitis, 343
  ulnar nerve, 333
  wrist and hand, 355–357
Reserpine, 42, 86

Rest. *See* Immobilization/inactivity
Reticular fibers, 1, 2
Reticular network theory, 29
Reticular system, mid-brain, 24, 25f
Rheumatoid arthritis, 76
Rhomboid fossa, 42
Rim lesions, 195, 200f
Rotation
    cervical spine, 171, 178, 178f, 186, 187f, 192f
    hip joint, 363f, 368
    knee, 390, 394f, 395f, 396f, 397f, 399
    leg, with ankle supination, 441, 444f
    lumbosacral spine, 106, 109, 129
Rotator cuff injuries, 271, 274f, 275f
Rotator cuff muscles, 260, 264f, 267f, 269f
Rotatory instability test, 413, 414f
Ruffini nerve endings, 395
Rule of the moment arm, 314

Sacral outflow, preganglionic fibers, 38
Sacroiliac joints, 383, 384, 386f
Sacrum, 383, 387
Safety, workplace, 510
Sarcoplasmic reticulum, 65
Scalene anticus syndrome, 239, 242f
Scalene foramen, 246
Scalene muscles, 239, 241f, 246
Scalene syndrome, 244, 329
Scapula, 260, 261, 262f, 266f
Scapular elevation exercise, 247, 248f, 249f, 291
Scapuloclavicular ligaments, 263, 266f
Scar tissue, formation of, 4, 6
Sciatic nerve
    entrapment, 162
    functional anatomy, 375–376, 398
    stretch, 136–138
Sciatic radiculitis, tests for, 147
Sciatica, defined, 136
Scoliosis, functional, 123
Secondary gain, 501–503
Secondary hyperalgesia, 88, 149
Semmes-Weinstein test, 315, 319, 319f
Serotonin (5–hydroxytryptamine, 5–HT)
    mood/anxiety disorders, 494
    as neurochemical mediator, 16, 28, 29, 74, 75, 76, 77, 86
    occipital neuralgia and, 174
Sesmoid disease, 452
Shear
    cervical neck, 204–205
    knee joint, 390, 396f
    low back pain and, 118, 119
Shimizu reflex, 206–207, 207f
"Shin splints," 445f
Shoes. *See* Orthotic devices
Shoulder complex
    acromioclavicular joint, 289, 291, 293

dislocation, 289, 289f, 290f
    glenohumeral joint, 259–288
    joints of, listed, 259
    sternoclavicular joint, 293
Shoulder-hand-finger RSD syndrome, 471, 478f
Shrugging abduction, 271, 276f
signe de plateau, 247
"Silent" muscles, 64, 67, 151
Sit-up/sit-back abdominal strength testing, 133–134, 134f, 135f
Sitting, assessment, trunk movements, 123, 124f
Sjögren's syndrome, 76
Skin. *See* Epithelial tissue
Sleep disturbances
    circadian rhythms, pain perception and, 34
    fibromyalgia and, 73, 74, 75, 76, 77
Slow-twitch fibers (type I)
    crush syndrome, neural compression, 327, 329
    fibromyalgia syndromes, 78–79, 79f
    muscle stiffness and, 71
    terminal in laminae, 20
Soft tissue injury(ies). *See also* Reflex sympathetic dystrophy
    low back pain and, 124–126
    metabolic effects of, 9–11
    neuromusculoskeletal function and, 517–526
    neurophysiology, 16, 18–19, 72, 149, 521f, 522, 522f
    nociceptors, 15, 17f
    vasochemical sequelae of, 17f
Soft tissue(s)
    defined, 1
    functional characteristics, 1–9
    palpation, cervical spine examination, 188–189
Somatic nervous system, 2, 19–20
Somatoform disorders, 102
Somatokinin, as nociceptor, 18
Spasticity, pathophysiology, 70, 70f
Spinal canal contents, 159f
Spinal cord
    ascending tracts, 16, 20, 21f, 22f
    autonomic-somatic cord level interaction, 62, 65f
    cervical, lesions of, 206–209
    contralateral pathways, 25
    descending tracts, 20, 22f
    dysesthesia pain, 208
    neurovascular compression lesions of, 254–255
    pain transmission and, 16
Spinal manipulation. *See* Manipulation
Spinal stenosis, 158–161, 159f
Spindle cell (gamma system)
    autonomic-somatic cord level interaction, 62, 65f

cervical spine injury and, 179, 180, 180f, 181f, 182f
coordination, muscle length, contraction, tension, 66f
higher cortical control, 62, 64f
interneuronal role, pathophysiology of spasticity, 70, 70f
intrafusal muscle, 61f, 63f
motor neurons, 69–71
musculotendinous mechanism, 68f, 340, 342f
neuroanatomic physiology, 60–72, 523f
peripheral afferents, influence of, 69f
proprioceptive autonomic control, 67f
regulation of, 69–71
secondary feedback loop, 71
Spinoreticulothalamic tract (SRTT), 23, 23f
Spinothalamic tract (STT), 20, 22–23, 25, 26
Splay foot, 455f
Splints
ankle injuries, 437, 439
elbow pain, 300, 306
extensor tendon rupture, middle phalanx, 348–349
frozen shoulder, 281
pronator teres syndrome, 332
wrist and hand, 321, 322f
Spondylolisthesis, 161f, 161–162
Spondylolysis, 161–162
Sports. See Repetitive strain injury
Spouts, 44
Sprains, ankle, 434–435, 437
Sprouting, 50
Spurling's sign, 202f, 255
Stance phase, gait, 369, 371, 374f
Standing
foot pain and, 442
hip joint motions, 367, 371, 374f, 375
Steppage gait, 123
Sternoclavicular joint, 261, 293, 293f
Steroids
injections, carpal tunnel, 323
injections, cervical neck pain, 215
injections, cubital tunnel syndrome, 339
injections, glenohumeral joint, 281
Straight leg raising (SLR) (Lasegue test)
abdominal strength testing, 133
facet pathology/examination, 126
hamstring flexibility, 130
lumbar disk pain, 127
performance of, 136–138, 138f, 139f, 140
piriformis syndrome, 162
well leg, 138, 147
Strains
ankle, 434–435
foot, 443, 444f, 446f
Strength testing
evaluation of, 74–75
low back pain, 118–119, 133–135

Strengthening exercises
ankle injuries, 437
applications, 64–65
cervical pain, 213
knee joint, 419
low back pain, 153, 155
scalene muscles, 247, 248f, 249f
shoulder complex, 278, 280, 287f
TMJ syndrome and, 224, 230f
Stress, emotional
fibromyalgia and, 73
pain perception and, 31–32, 34, 43
Stress, mechanical. See also Ergonomics
collagen formation/function and, 4, 6
muscle stiffness and, 71
Stress and strain curve, tendons, 340–342
Stress fractures
ankle, 439
foot, 458–459
Stretch reflex, 62–64, 523
Stretching exercises
cervical pain, 209
low back pain, 150, 153
physiologic basis, 94–95
Stroke volume, inactivity and, 11
Structural pain, defined, 122
Subclavian artery
anterior scalene syndrome, 246
functional anatomy, 242f
thoracic outlet syndrome, 239, 240
Subluxation
atlantoaxial joint, 183, 184f
lower cervical spine, 186
manipulation, concepts of, 156
temporomandibular joint, 219
upper cervical spine, 194
Substance abuse, 102
Substance P, as nociceptor, 15, 18–19, 75, 76, 77, 85, 88, 149
Subtalar joint
functional anatomy, 439
injuries, 442f, 443f
Subtalar joint, 441
Sudeck's atrophy, 471
Supination
ankle, 433
foot, 444f, 449, 451
Supinator test, radial nerve, 305, 306f
Supraclavicular brachial plexus lesions, 251–252
Supraclavicular space, 239, 240f
Supraoptic nuclei (SON), 34
Supraspinal motor centers, 524–526, 525f
Sustentaculum tali, 441
Suturing tendons, 344, 345, 346f, 349
"Swayback." See Lordosis
Swing, in joint motion, defined, 260f
Swing phase, gait, 369, 374f, 451
Sympathalgia, 471
Sympathectomy, 45–46

Sympathetic nervous system
    chronic fatigue syndrome and, 53
    functional anatomy, 38, 40–43
Sympathetically independent pain (SIP), 471
Sympathetically maintained pain (SMP), 49,
        88, 471, 477f
Sympatheticotonia, 43
Sympathin, classes of, 42
Symphysis pubis, 384, 386f
Synapse, neuroanatomic physiology, 29f
Syncytium, defined, 29
Syndrome response, defined, 31
Synovitis, degenerative joint disease, 377,
        378f

Talocalcaneal joint, 439, 440f, 441, 441f, 443f
Talonavicular joint, 449
Talus, 428, 431f
Tardy ulnar palsy, 338
Tarsal arch, 451
Temperature
    collagen viscoelastic properties and, 4
    reflex sympathetic dystrophy and, 50–51
Temporomandibular pain and dysfunction
        syndrome (TMPDS)
    classification, 216–217
    diagnosis, 219, 223
    disorders, 218t
    fibromyalgia and, 73
    functional anatomy, 217–219, 218f, 219f,
        220f, 221f, 222f
    management, 223f, 223–225
    muscle disorders, 219t
    neurophysiologic concepts, 66
Tender points (TP), 73
Tendinitis
    extensor compartments, 351
    flexor compartments, 351, 353–354
    wrist and hand, 311, 339–343, 346–354
Tendon nodule, formation of, 351, 352f
Tendon(s)
    blood supply, 315f
    as component of soft tissue, 1
    components of, 6
    injuries, Achilles tendon rupture, 464–465
    injuries, anatomic zones of, 345f
    injuries, rupture, 340, 343–344
    low back pain, 125
    wrist and hand, 310–315, 326f, 339–354
Tennis elbow. *See* Epicondylalgia (tennis
        elbow)
Tenosynovitis, 311, 312, 315, 316
Tension headache, 187, 199
Thalamus, neural pathways, 23f, 23–25, 24f
Thermal agents. *See* Cryotherapy; Heat
        therapy
Thoracic outlet syndrome
    diagnosis, 244–246

etiologies, 245
functional anatomy, 239
paresthesia with, 206
symptoms and signs, 240, 243–244
Thoracic pain, upper, 232
Thoracolumbar outflow, preganglionic fibers,
        38
Thyroxine, 33
Tibia, 388, 390, 394f, 400, 428
Tilt board exercises, ankle, 435, 437, 437f,
        438f
Tinel sign, 319, 331, 338
Tonic motor units, 79
Topographic zones, 44
Total body weight, inactivity and, 9
Total hip replacement, 380, 382
Traction
    cervical, 211, 213f
    hip, 380, 381f
    low back pain, 155
    physiologic basis, 94–95
    TMJ syndrome and, 224–225, 231f
Traction injuries, brachial plexus, 252
Transcutaneous electrical nerve stimulation
        (TENS)
    low back pain, 155
    lower extremity RSD syndrome, 485
    physiologic basis, 27
Transmitter-receptor mismatch, 31, 31f
Transudate, defined, 89
Transverse acetabular ligament, 367
Transverse arches, 451, 453f
Transverse carpal ligament
    functional anatomy, 310, 312, 312f, 316
    release of, 324, 324f
Transverse (cross) ligament, 171–172, 173f,
        176
Transverse tarsal joints, 449, 452f
Trauma. *See* Injury(ies)
Traumatic angiospasm/venospasm, 471
Triceps paralysis, 254
Tricyclic antidepressants, 54, 75, 77–78
Tridimensional activities, spine, 117f,
        117–118, 119–120, 120f
Trigeminal nerve
    functional anatomy, 219f, 220f
    type of pain transmitted, 23
Trigeminal neuralgia, 26
Trigger fingers, 351, 353f
Trigger points, 66, 67, 71–72, 213
Tropocollagen trihelix fiber, 4f, 340, 340f,
        341f
Trunk, neurovascular compression lesions of,
        254
Tryptophan, 75, 77
Tyrosine-glycine-glycine-phenylalanine-
        leucine, 84
Tyrosine-glycine-glycine-phenylalanine-
        methionine, 84

Ulnar nerve
  compression, 332–334, 335, 337–339
  functional anatomy, 195f, 196f, 298f, 299f,
    334f, 336f
  injuries, 297–298
Ultrasound, therapeutic use, 90, 213
Unconditioned stimuli, 497
"Undesirable patients," 496
Unmyelinated C nerve fibers, 15, 20, 22, 27, 74
Up regulation, defined, 53
Upper cervical spinal complex
  clinical entities, 194
  examination, 181, 183–185
  functional anatomy, 171–173, 172f, 173f
  muscular component, cervical pathology,
    179
  neck muscle proprioception/motor control,
    179–181
  occipital neuralgia, 173–174, 176, 178–179
  range of motion testing, 189
Upper extremity
  dermatomes, 243f
  reflex sympathetic dystrophy, 470, 471,
    478
Upper plexus (trunk) lesions, 254
Upper thoracic pain, 232
Urinary tract, trauma to, 383, 387

VA system, 43
Valsalva maneuver, 147, 147f
Ventricular system, brain, 42, 42f
Ventrobasal thalamic system, 24
Vertebral artery, 174, 176f, 177f
Vertebral functional unit, 103–113, 112f
Vertigo, 179, 185, 206
Vibration tests, nerve compression, 315, 319
Viscoelastic properties
  actomyosin bounds of muscle, 67
  collagen, temperature and, 4, 91, 343
  osteoligamentous tissues, 109
  plastic deformation, 150
Volume transmission (VT), 30f, 30–31, 32
VT system, 43

Walking, for low back pain, 153, 154f, 155f
Wall-Melzak Gate Theory, 27f, 28
Water balance, inactivity and, 9–10
Weather changes
  fibromyalgia and, 73
  thoracic outlet syndrome and, 240
Weight bearing
  ankle injuries, 439
  hip joint, 371, 374f, 375f
  low back pain, 123
  pelvis, 383
Well leg straight-leg raising test, 138, 147
Whiplash. See Hyperextension-hyperflexion,
    cervical spine
White rami communicantes, 40, 41f
Wide dynamic range (WDR) neurons, 476, 478
"Winging" of the scapula, 252, 253
Wiring transmission (WT), 29f, 30f, 30–31, 32
Work. See Repetitive strain injury
Workers' compensation. See also Ergonomics
  disability and impairment, 511–512
  low back pain, claims for, 101, 149
  medical report, 512
  problems with the system, 507–508
  proposed remedies, 508–511
Wrist and hand. See also Carpal tunnel
    syndrome; Fingers
  anterior interosseous syndrome, 332
  cubital tunnel syndrome, 335–339
  dislocations, 354–357
  fractures, 354–357
  innervation, 300, 301f
  pronator teres median nerve compression,
    329–332
  shoulder-hand-finger RSD syndrome, 471,
    478f
  tendon problems, 339–354
  ulnar nerve compression, 332–334

Zygapophyseal joints (facets)
  cervical, 185–186, 196–197, 201f, 214–216
  functional anatomy, 105–109, 108f
  pathology/examination, 125–126